American Cancer Society
Atlas of
Clinical Oncology

Series Volumes

Blumgart, Jarnagin, Fong	*Hepatobiliary Cancer*
Cameron	*Pancreatic Cancer*
Carroll	*Prostate Cancer*
Char	*Cancer of the Eye and Orbit*
Clark, Duh, Jahan, Perrier	*Endocrine Tumors*
Eifel, Levenback	*Cervical, Vulvar and Vaginal Cancer*
Ginsberg	*Lung Cancer*
Grossbard	*Malignant Lymphomas*
Ozols	*Ovarian Cancer*
Pollock	*Soft Tissue Sarcomas*
Posner, Vokes, Weichselbaum	*Esophagus, Stomach and Small Bowel Cancer*
Prados	*Brain Cancer*
Raghavan	*Germ Cell Tumors*
Rice, Taylor	*Endometrial and Uterine Cancer*
Shah	*Head and Neck Cancer*
Shipley	*Urothelial Cancer*
Silverman	*Oral Cancer*
Sober, Haluska	*Skin Cancer*
Wiernik	*Adult Leukemias*
Willett	*Colon and Rectal Cancer*
Winchester, Winchester	*Breast Cancer*
Yasko	*Bone Cancer*

American Cancer Society
Atlas of
Clinical Oncology

Editors

GLENN D. STEELE JR, MD
University of Chicago

THEODORE L. PHILLIPS, MD
University of California

BRUCE A. CHABNER, MD
Harvard Medical School

Managing Editor

TED S. GANSLER, MD, MBA
Director of Health Content, American Cancer Society

American Cancer Society
Atlas of
Clinical Oncology
Breast Cancer

David J. Winchester, MD, FACS
Associate Attending, Department of Surgery
Evanston Northwestern Healthcare
Evanston, Illinois
Assistant Professor of Surgery
Northwestern University Medical School
Chicago, Illinois

David P. Winchester, MD, FACS
Chairman, Department of Surgery
Evanston Northwestern Healthcare
Evanston, Illinois
Professor of Surgery
Northwestern University Medical School
Chicago, Illinois

2000
B.C. Decker Inc.
Hamilton • London

B.C. Decker Inc.
4 Hughson Street South
P.O. Box 620, L.C.D. 1
Hamilton, Ontario L8N 3K7
Tel: 905-522-7017; 1-800-568-7281
Fax: 905-522-7839
E-mail: info@bcdecker.com
Website: http://www.bcdecker.com

ISBN 1–55009–112–3
Printed in Canada

Sales and Distribution

United States
B.C. Decker Inc.
P.O. Box 785
Lewiston, NY U.S.A. 14092-0785
Tel: 905-522-7017/1-800-568-7281
Fax: 905-522-7839
e-mail: info@bcdecker.com
website: http://www.bcdecker.com

Canada
B.C. Decker Inc.
4 Hughson Street South
P.O. Box 620, L.C.D. 1
Hamilton, Ontario L8N 3K7
Tel: 905-522-7017/1-800-568-7281
Fax: 905-522-7839
e-mail: info@bcdecker.com
website: http://www.bcdecker.com

Japan
Igaku-Shoin Ltd.
Foreign Publications Department
3-24-17 Hongo, Bunkyo-ku,
Tokyo 113-8719, Japan
Tel: 3 3817 5676
Fax: 3 3815 6776
e-mail: fd@igaku.shoin.co.jp

U.K., Europe, Scandinavia, Middle East
Blackwell Science Ltd.
Osney Mead
Oxford OX2 0EL
United Kingdom
Tel: 44-1865-206206
Fax: 44-1865-721205
e-mail: info@blackwell-science.com

Australia
Blackwell Science Asia Pty, Ltd.
54 University Street
Carlton, Victoria 3053
Australia
Tel: 03 9347 0300
Fax: 03 9349 3016
e-mail: info@blacksci.asia.com.au

South Korea
Seoul Medical Scientific Books Co.
C.P.O. Box 9794
Seoul 100-697
Seoul, Korea
Tel: 82-2925-5800
Fax: 82-2927-7283

South America
Ernesto Reichmann, Distribuidora
de Livros Ltda.
Rua Coronel Marques
335-Tatuape, 03440-000
Sao Paulo-SP-Brazil
Tel/Fax: 011-218-2122

Foreign Rights
John Scott & Co.
International Publishers' Agency
P.O. Box 878
Kimberton, PA 19442
Tel: 610-827-1640
Fax: 610-827-1671

Contributors

JOEL R. BERNSTEIN, MD
Department of Radiology
Evanston Northwestern Healthcare
Evanston, Illinois
Screening and Diagnostic Imaging

WILLIAM D. BLOOMER, MD
Department of Radiology
Evanston Northwestern Healthcare
Evanston, Illinois
Breast Cancer and Radiation Therapy

DAVID R. BRENIN, MD
Columbia-Presbyterian Medical Center
New York, New York
Unusual Breast Pathology

WENDY R. BREWSTER, MD
Department of Obstetrics and Gynecology
University of California
Irvine, California
*Estrogen Replacement Therapy for
Breast Cancer Survivors*

MASSIMO CRISTOFANILLI, MD
Department of Breast Medical Oncology
MD Anderson Cancer Center
Houston, Texas
*Breast Cancer Risk and Management:
Chemoprevention, Surgery, and Surveillance*

PHILIP J. DISAIA, MD
Department of Obstetrics and Gynecology
University of California
Irvine, California
*Estrogen Replacement Therapy for Breast Cancer
Survivors*

WILLIAM L. DONEGAN, MD
Department of Surgery, Sinai Samaritan
Medical Center
Milwaukee, Wisconsin
Carcinoma of the Breast in Men

GEOFFREY C. FENNER, MD
Evanston Northwestern Healthcare
Evanston, Illinois
Breast Reconstruction

RICHARD E. FINE, MD
The Breast Center
Marietta, Georgia
Image-Directed Breast Biopsy

ROBERT A. GOLDSCHMIDT, MD
Department of Pathology
Evanston Northwestern Healthcare
Evanston, Illinois
Histopathology of Malignant Breast Disease

HANINA HIBSHOOSH, MD
Columbia University, College of Physicians and
Surgeons
Columbia-Presbyterian Medical Center
New York, New York
Unusual Breast Pathology

GABRIEL N. HORTOBAGYI, MD
Department of Breast Medical Oncology
MD Anderson Cancer Center
Houston, Texas
*Breast Cancer Risk and Management:
Chemoprevention, Surgery, and Surveillance*

JAN M. JESKE, MD
Department of Radiology
Evanston Northwestern Healthcare
Evanston, Illinois
Screening and Diagnostic Imaging

JANARDAN D. KHANDEKAR, MD
Department of Medicine
Evanston Northwestern Healthcare
Evanston, Illinois
Surveillance of the Breast Cancer Patient

DAVID W. KINNE, MD
Columbia-Presbyterian Medical Center
New York, New York
Unusual Breast Pathology

MICHAEL A. LaCOMBE, MD
Department of Radiology
Evanston Northwestern Healthcare
Evanston, Illinois
Breast Cancer and Radiation Therapy

LAURIE H. LEE, PA-C
Division of General Surgery
Evanston Northwestern Healthcare
Evanston, Illinois
Surgical Management of Ductal Carcinoma In Situ

GERSHON Y. LOCKER, MD
Division of Hematology
Evanston Northwestern Healthcare
Evanston, Illinois
Adjuvant Systemic Therapy of Early Breast Cancer

HENRY T. LYNCH, MD
Creighton University
Omaha, Nebraska
*Genetics, Natural History, and DNA-Based
Genetic Counseling in Hereditary Breast Cancer*

JANE F. LYNCH, BSN
Creighton University
Omaha, Nebraska
*Genetics, Natural History, and DNA-Based
Genetic Counseling in Hereditary Breast Cancer*

DOUGLAS E. MERKEL, MD
Division of Hematology-Oncology
Evanston Northwestern Healthcare
Evanston, Illinois
Treatment of Metastatic Breast Cancer

DAN H. MOORE II, PhD
Geraldine Brush Cancer Research Institute
Pacific Medical Center
Department of Epidemiology and Biostatistics
University of California
San Francisco, California
Prognostic and Predictive Markers in Breast Cancer

THOMAS A. MUSTOE, MD
Division of Plastic Surgery, Northwestern University
Medical School
Chicago, Illinois
Breast Reconstruction

LISA NEWMAN, MD, FACS
Department of Surgical Oncology
University of Texas, MD Anderson Cancer Center
Houston, Texas
*Breast Cancer Risk and Management:
Chemoprevention, Surgery, and Surveillance*

PHILIP N. REDLICH, MD, PhD
Department of Surgery
Medical College of Wisconsin
Milwaukee, Wisconsin
Carcinoma of the Breast in Men

STEPHEN F. SENER, MD
Division of General Surgery
Evanston Northwestern Healthcare
Evanston, Illinois
Surgical Management of Ductal Carcinoma In Situ

S. EVA SINGLETARY, MD, FACS
MD Anderson Cancer Center
Houston, Texas
Locally Advanced Breast Cancer

MARGARET A. STULL, MD
Department of Radiology
University of Illinois
Chicago, Illinois
Screening and Diagnostic Imaging

ANN D. THOR, MD
Department of Pathology
Evanston Northwestern Healthcare
Evanston, Illinois
*Prognostic and Predictive Markers in Breast
Cancer*

DAVID J. WINCHESTER, MD, FACS
Department of Surgery
Evanston Northwestern Healthcare
Evanston, Illinois
Northwestern University Medical School
Chicago, Illinois
*Evaluation and Surgical Management of Stage I
and II Breast Cancer*

DAVID P. WINCHESTER, MD, FACS
Department of Surgery
Evanston Northwestern Healthcare
Evanston, Illinois
Northwestern University Medical School
Chicago, Illinois

Contents

Preface

The organization of this book reflects a logical, stepwise evaluation and treatment of the patient with breast cancer. It emphasizes the importance of early detection, but highlights a move toward risk identification and reduction. The understanding of the breast cancer patient has evolved from the radical mastectomy for all patients to a tailored approach employing aggressive applications of treatment modalities according to their respective risk reductions.

Despite shifting efforts to identify high-risk patients and address their risk with pre-emptive strategies, there remains a worldwide educational challenge to adopt early detection screening guidelines. Although there is continuing progress in implementing mortality reducing surveillance guidelines as reflected by the increased prevalence of preinvasive breast cancer, the full spectrum of disease remains a challenge to the medical community. The high prevalence of breast cancer continues to drive improvements in all areas of detection, diagnostic evaluation, disease characterization, multimodality therapy, quality of life issues, and, finally, in the treatment of patients whose disease has extended beyond our capabilities to detect or contain local or regional cancer.

One of the most important innovations in the understanding of breast cancer has been the identification of genetic mutations that have allowed the opportunity to intervene with proven surgical or chemopreventive strategies for high-risk patients. Diagnostic imaging technology continues to provide increased resolution and precision, resulting in an enhanced ability to preserve tissue. The surgical treatment of breast cancer is in the process of taking another significant step forward, with the development of sentinel lymph node biopsy. The definition of prognostic factors has helped to guide important adjuvant therapy decisions. Moving beyond the regimented doctrines of an overwhelming preoccupation of cancer treatment, immediate reconstruction with microvascular surgery and other techniques have provided an answer to some of the physical and psychological challenges of breast cancer. Recognition of other competing causes of mortality in the breast cancer survivor has led to a more comprehensive consideration of hormone replacement therapy to address quality of life issues and to reduce the risk of cardiovascular disease and osteoporosis. In the patient with metastatic disease, the introduction of novel forms of treatment, such as with Herceptin, has led to significant improvements in survival. In total, these innovations represent significant progress and provide important directions for future interventions.

One of the biggest challenges to the clinician has been the recognition of improved methods of diagnosis and treatment and utilization of these improvements despite ingrained practices. This pattern is well documented by the great variation observed nationally in the implementation of breast preserving surgery and the utilization of adjuvant treatment.

It is the goal of this book to identify significant improvements in each area of breast cancer diagnosis and treatment, and to help accelerate the dispersion of this knowledge to an ever-broadening spectrum of physicians and scientists who are dedicated to preventing and treating one of the most common afflictions of women.

We wish to thank our distinguished authors for their timely and expert contributions to this effort. We also wish to thank the American Cancer Society, particularly Ted Gansler, for a helpful review of this book.

DJW
DPW

To our parents, for their example and knowledge, and to Marilyn, Doris, Eric, Laura, Elena, and Colin, who have allowed us to spend their time working on this project.

David J. Winchester

David P. Winchester

Genetics, Natural History, and DNA-Based Genetic Counseling in Hereditary Breast Cancer

HENRY T. LYNCH, MD
JANE F. LYNCH, BSN

The extraordinary advances in molecular genetics during the past decade have established beyond doubt that there is a Mendelian inherited basis for a subset of virtually all forms of cancer.[1] Specifically, more than 30 hereditary cancer syndromes have been shown to harbor germ-line mutations. These culprit molecular genetic factors include oncogenes such as the *RET* proto-oncogene for the multiple endocrine neoplasia type 2 syndromes, the mismatch repair genes (*hMSH2*, *hMLH1*) in hereditary nonpolyposis colorectal cancer (HNPCC) of the Lynch I and Lynch II syndrome variants, and tumor suppressor genes. Examples of the latter include *APC*, which predisposes to familial adenomatous polyposis (FAP), and *BRCA1* and *BRCA2* mutations in hereditary breast cancer, the subject of this chapter.

In the United States in 1999, it was projected that 176,300 new cases of carcinoma of the breast would be diagnosed, and 43,700 would die from this disease.[2] The current authors estimate that approximately 10 percent (17,600) of these newly diagnosed patients will manifest a hereditary breast cancer (HBC) disorder, the most common of which will be the hereditary breast-ovarian cancer (HBOC) syndrome.[3] It is the purpose of this chapter to update what is known about HBC, including its genetic and phenotypic heterogeneity, natural history, genetic counseling issues, and cancer control implications.

GENETICS

The combination of carcinoma of the breast and ovary in families, now known as the HBOC syndrome, was first reported in the early 1970s.[4–6] The molecular genetic discoveries that confirmed beyond any doubt the hereditary basis for HBC and HBOC have progressed at an explosive rate, particularly over the past decade. This avalanche of knowledge was heralded by the gene linkage study of Hall and colleagues,[7] which identified a locus on chromosome 17q for families with site-specific breast cancer. Subsequently, Narod and colleagues[8] reported that this same locus was responsible for the HBOC syndrome. The culprit gene, now known as *BRCA1*, was then cloned.[9] More recently, a second breast cancer susceptibility locus on chromosome 13q, known as *BRCA2*, was identified by linkage analysis[10] and subsequently cloned.[11]

Approximately 45 percent of all hereditary breast cancer-prone families, including those characterized as HBOC, owe this condition to mutations of the *BRCA1* gene;[12] a slightly lower percentage is due to *BRCA2* mutations. Initial studies estimated that carriers of the *BRCA1* germ-line mutation harbor a lifetime risk for breast cancer of about 85 percent[12,13] and a risk for ovarian cancer that ranges between 40 and 66 percent.[12,13] Carriers of the *BRCA2* mutation, on the other hand, have a lifetime risk of breast cancer of about 85 percent, but their risk for ovarian cancer is somewhat lower (10 to 20 %).[12,13] Male *BRCA2* mutation carriers have an approximate 7 percent lifetime risk for breast cancer. Other cancers occurring in *BRCA2* mutation carriers include carcinoma of the pancreas, head and neck, and intraocular malignant melanoma. Males who are harbingers of germ-line mutations in *BRCA1/BRCA2* will have a two- to three-fold increased lifetime risk for prostate cancer.

These initial breast and ovarian cancer gene penetrance risks were based upon publications of highly extended pedigrees selected because of their profound familial cancer aggregations; they are thereby biased in the direction of cancer excess. In contrast, recent observations of breast and ovarian cancer occurrence in the Ashkenazi Jewish founder mutations (185delAG and 5382insC mutations on the *BRCA1* gene, and 6174delT on the *BRCA2* gene) indicate that the lifetime risk for breast cancer is only 56 percent, and that of ovarian cancer 16 percent.[14]

Claus and colleagues[15] examined the family history of carcinoma of the breast and ovary in a data set involving 4,730 patients with breast cancer and 4,688 controls who were enrolled in the Cancer and Steroid Hormone Study. Attention was given to the association between family history of carcinoma of the breast and/or ovary and breast cancer risk when controlling for the carrier status of *BRCA1* and *BRCA2* mutations. The question examined pertained to whether the family history of carcinoma of the breast remained a predictive risk factor once the carrier status for *BRCA1* and/or *BRCA2* was given consideration. Findings disclosed that among those women "...with a moderate family history of breast cancer, that is, predicted noncarriers of *BRCA1*

and/or *BRCA2* mutations, family history remains a factor in predicting breast cancer risk. In families with breast and ovarian cancers, the aggregation of these two cancers appears to be explained by *BRCA1/BRCA2* mutation-carrier probability." This study clearly enunciates the need for obtaining a well-orchestrated cancer family history for the assessment of breast/ovarian cancer risk.

Previously, the best prediction of a patient's lifetime breast cancer risk was 50 percent. This estimate was based upon the patient's position in the pedigree, namely, having one or more first-degree relatives with a syndrome cancer in the direct genetic lineage of an HBC or HBOC family. The identification of the mutations for *BRCA1*[9] and *BRCA2*[11] now enables physicians and genetic counselors to predict a patient's lifetime risk for carcinoma of the breast and ovary, in context with the penetrance of these genes.

Cancer Family History and Mutation Search

The search for a germ-line mutation should be performed only on families with substantial evidence of a hereditary cancer syndrome. Therefore, to establish a hereditary breast cancer syndrome diagnosis, a detailed collection of a patient's cancer family history, with as much pathologic corroboration as possible, is mandatory. The family history may potentially constitute the most cost-beneficial component of a patient's medical workup; its collection and evaluation in the typical clinical setting, however, remains notoriously neglected.[16,17] This problem was well documented by David and Steiner-Grossman[17] through a survey of 76 acute care, non-psychiatric hospitals in New York City. Only four of the 64 reporting hospitals indicated that family history information was reported in their medical records. Such serious omissions must be resolved in order to enhance cancer control. Otherwise, the opportunity to search for germ-line cancer prone mutations may be lost. This is a pity since, when a cancer-causing mutation is identified, this information can, in concert with genetic counseling, be used effectively to benefit the patient and family members.

ASSESSMENT OF BREAST CANCER-PRONE FAMILIES

Building the case for hereditary cancer is frequently based upon the cardinal clinical features of hereditary cancer (namely, early age of cancer onset, pattern of multiple primary cancers [such as breast and ovarian cancer], vertical transmission of cancer, and increased number of cancer occurrences) (Table 1–1). It is virtually axiomatic that the larger the breast cancer-prone family, the greater the number of expected carcinomas of the breast or ovary. One can be more confident of a likely hereditary etiology for breast cancer if there is evidence for earlier age of onset of cancer, especially when there is familial clustering of these cancers, particularly ovarian cancer, among primary and secondary relatives (see Table 1–1). In such a setting, there is an increased probability that a germ-line mutation (*BRCA1*, *BRCA2*) will be found. On the other hand, when dealing with families that are small, there may be a limited number of patients with cancer, a deficit of

females, or the few cancers that are occurring may be in the paternal lineage. The overall effect is that it becomes exceedingly difficult to predict whether such a small family should be a candidate for searching for a mutation in *BRCA1* or *BRCA2*.

HETEROGENEITY AND HEREDITARY BREAST CANCER

Virtually all forms of hereditary cancer show significant genetic and phenotypic heterogeneity. For example, breast cancer occurs in significant excess in disorders associated with extra-breast cancer sites, such as Li-Fraumeni syndrome (Figure 1–1), Bloom's syndrome, Cowden's disease, ataxia-telangiectasia, the breast-gastrointestinal tract cancer syndrome, extraordinarily early-onset breast cancer (Figure 1–2), and the HBOC syndrome (Figure 1–3). Undoubtedly, other tumor combinations and/or hereditary syndromes which will qualify as hereditary breast cancer are yet to be identified. Space does not allow a discussion of each of these breast cancer-associated disorders (for more detail see Lynch and colleagues[18]).

Clearly, it is no longer appropriate to characterize hereditary breast cancer as a generic term. Rather, one must be more precise and denote the particular breast cancer-associated

Table 1–1. ESTIMATED PROBABILITY OF *BRCA1* MUTATION BASED ON FAMILY HISTORY

Family History	Probability of *BRCA1* Mutation (%)
Single affected person	
Breast cancer at < 30 years of age	12
Breast cancer at < 40 years of age	6
Breast cancer at 40–49 years of age	3
Ovarian cancer at < 50 years of age	7
Sister pairs	
Both with breast cancer at < 40 years of age	37
Both with breast cancer at 40–49 years of age	20
Breast cancer at < 50 years of age, ovarian cancer at < 50 years of age	46
Both with ovarian cancer at < 50 years of age	61
Families	
Breast cancer only, three or more cases at < 50 years of age	40
Two or more breast cancers and one or more ovarian cancers	82
Two or more breast cancers and two or more ovarian cancers	91

Reprinted with permission of author (Barbara Weber, MD) and publisher from Weber B. Breast cancer susceptibility genes: current challenges and future promises. Ann Intern Med 1996;124:1088–90.

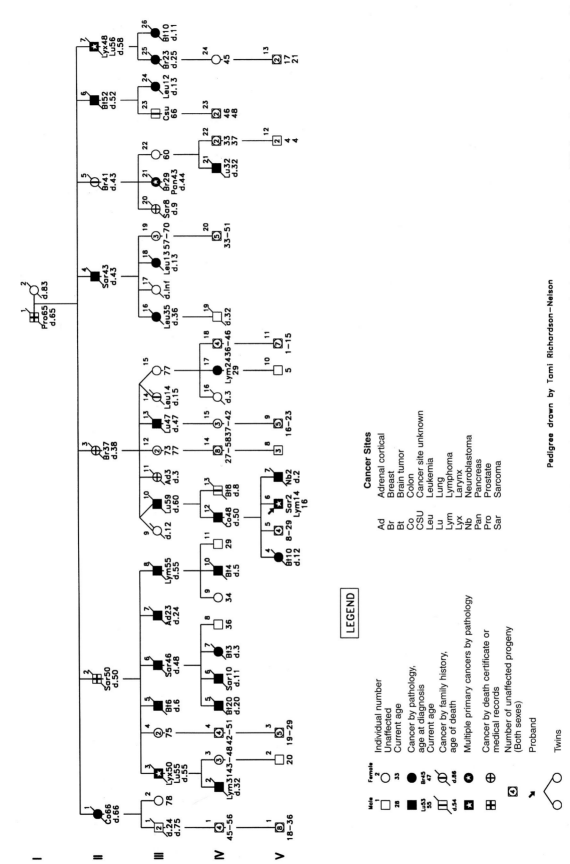

Figure 1–1. Updated pedigree of a family with sarcoma, breast cancer and brain tumors, lung and laryngeal cancer, and adrenocortical carcinoma (SBLA syndrome, also known as Li-Fraumeni syndrome). Reprinted with permission from Lynch et al. Genetic and pathologic findings in a kindred with hereditary sarcoma, breast cancer, brain tumors, leukemia, larygeal, and adrenal cortical carcinoma. Cancer 1978; 41:2055–64.

syndrome relating to a particular patient/family. Such syndrome identification is important not only for molecular genetic assessment but, moreover, for targeted surveillance and management purposes.

GENOTYPE-PHENOTYPE DIFFERENCES

More than 200 different *BRCA1* germ-line mutations have been identified in HBOC families. Certain types of these mutations may give rise to differing patterns of cancer occurrence. For example, Gayther and colleagues[19] suggest that the position of the *BRCA1* mutation has a significant influence on the ratio of breast to ovarian cancer in HBOC kindreds. Specifically, they reported that mutations in the 3' third of the gene are associated with a lower proportion of ovarian cancer. However, these findings must be reviewed cautiously. Serova and colleagues[20] were unable to confirm these findings. However, the findings of the latter did suggest that the risk of ovarian cancer is greater in families with mutations associated with reduced RNA levels. In the case of *BRCA2*, Gayther and colleagues[21] found that "... truncating mutations in families with the highest risk of ovarian cancer relative to breast cancer are clustered in a region of approximately 3.3 kb in exon 11 (*p* = .0004)." Further research in this area may establish links between specific mutations and specific cancer risk that will be extremely useful for genetic counseling. Until confirmation of these genotype-phenotype findings is more firmly established, however, the current authors prefer to withhold this information in the genetic counseling setting.

Most of the hereditary cases will harbor a *BRCA1* or *BRCA2* germ-line mutation. However, one should expect (albeit rarely) to encounter families where both *BRCA1* and *BRCA2* mutations are segregating, considering the high prevalence of carcinoma of the breast and ovary in the general population, coupled with the fact that approximately 5 to 10 percent of the total breast

cancer burden will be hereditary. Interestingly, Ramus and colleagues[22] reported a patient from a Hungarian family who manifested both breast and ovarian cancer and was found to have truncating mutations in *both* the *BRCA1* and *BRCA2* genes. This patient "... carried the 185delAG mutation in *BRCA1* as well as the 6174delT mutation in *BRCA2*. Both of these mutations are common in Ashkenazi Jewish breast cancer patients."[23–25] Recently, Liede and colleagues[26] identified an Ashkenazi Jewish kindred with three mutations, namely *BRCA1* 185delAG, *BRCA1* 5382insC, and *BRCA2* 6174delT. Each founder mutation has been shown to have a frequency of approximately 1 percent in the Ashkenazi population.[27–29]

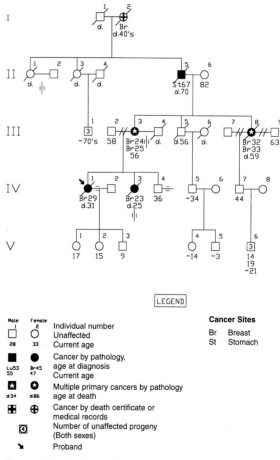

Figure 1–2. Pedigree of a family showing extremely early age of onset of hereditary breast cancer. Reprinted with permission from Lynch et al. Extremely early onset hereditary breast cancer (HBC): surveillance/management implications. Nebr Med J 1988; 73:97–100.

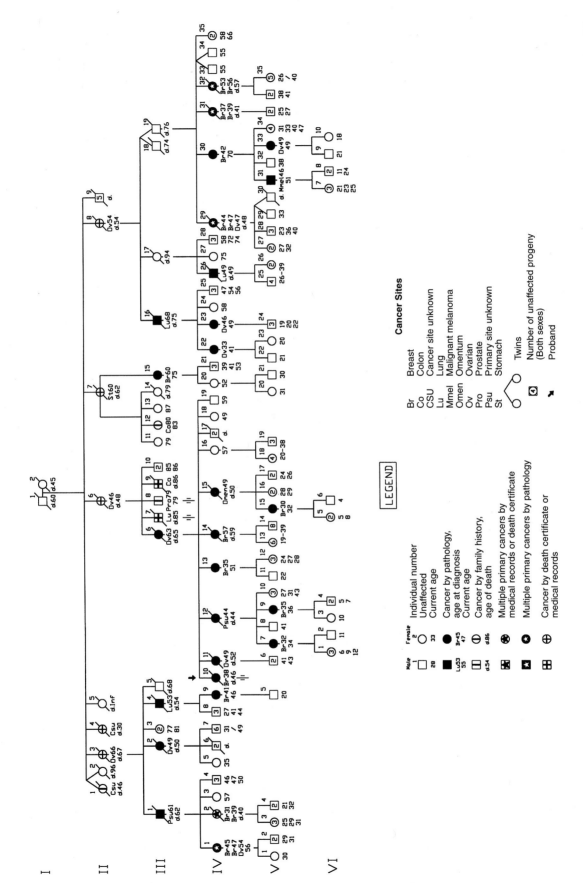

Figure 1–3. Updated pedigree of a large hereditary breast-ovarian cancer family. Adapted with permission from Lynch et al. Management of familial breast cancer, parts I and II. Arch Surg 1978;113:1060–71.

PATHOLOGY OF HEREDITARY BREAST/OVARIAN CANCER IN CONCERT WITH *BRCA1* OR *BRCA2* MUTATIONS

Pathology studies have shown differences between *BRCA1*- and *BRCA2*-related breast cancers when compared with sporadic controls. Specifically, Marcus and colleagues[30–32] have shown that *BRCA1* HBC has a highly distinctive pathology phenotype, consisting of an increased number of aneuploid cancers, more medullary carcinomas, and high proliferation rates as measured by DNA flow cytometry and mitotic grade, and lesser ductal carcinoma in situ (DCIS) than in nonfamilial cases. In alluding to high S-phase fraction in HBC and attributing it to the *BRCA1*-linked subset, it was suggested that the mutation resulted in enhanced cellular proliferation.[33] This prediction was borne out by the demonstration of the antiproliferative effect of *BRCA1* mRNA protein in vitro and in vivo[34–36] after the gene was cloned. The current authors have proposed a model for the *BRCA1* pathophenotype that considers the tumors to be in an advanced state of genetic evolution.[30]

In contrast, "other" HBCs (cases from HBC families with no *BRCA1* mutations, no 17q linkage, and a paucity of ovarian cancer affecteds, or with *BRCA2* mutations or 13q linkage) appear to lack the systematic high grade, aneuploidy, and high proliferation of *BRCA1* HBCs, and they are not deficient in in situ carcinoma.[30,31] This "other" group also has more invasive lobular, tubular, tubulolobular, and cribiform special type carcinomas, which we have designated as "tubular-lobular group" (TLG). Indeed, the excess of TLG and "no special type" (NST) invasive carcinomas with TLG "features" (10 to 50% tumor composition) parallels a trend for more lobular neoplasia (lobular carcinoma in situ and atypical lobular hyperplasia) in "other" HBC. These features are present in the subset of mutation-confirmed *BRCA2* HBC cases in the "other" HBC group,[32] which suggests that TLG carcinomas and lobu-

lar neoplasia are signatures of the *BRCA2* HBC phenotype.[32] In contrast, *BRCA1* HBC cases manifest a *deficit* of TLG carcinomas and lobular neoplasia.[32] Armes and colleagues[37] confirm an excess of TLG carcinoma (in their cases, pleomorphic lobular carcinomas) in *BRCA2* HBC in a population-based study of *BRCA2* cases that were not specifically recruited from large HBOC families.

The pathophenotype of *BRCA2* HBC may be more heterogeneous than *BRCA1* HBC when the amount of high-grade carcinoma in the syndrome is considered. There have been reports of *BRCA2* families with predominantly high-grade carcinomas.[38,39] However, we have not seen high-grade predominance in the four *BRCA2* families we have studied nor as the average phenotype of the "other" HBC group in which most Creighton *BRCA2* families would reside.[32] Similarly, the Breast Cancer Linkage Consortium has not observed unusually high grades in its *BRCA2* family series.[40] The higher grades reported from Iceland[39] and, to a lesser extent, from the Linkage Consortium,[40,41] may well be associated with a site on the *BRCA2* gene, in these cases the 999del5 mutation.[37]

Lakhani and colleagues[41] confirmed many of the original observations of Marcus and colleagues.[32,33,42] Specifically, they showed that "Cancers associated with *BRCA1* mutations exhibited higher mitotic counts ($p = .001$), a greater proportion of the tumor with a continuous pushing margin ($p < .0001$), and more lymphocytic infiltration ($p = .002$) than sporadic (ie, control) cancers. Cancers associated with *BRCA2* mutations exhibited a higher score for tubule formation (fewer tubules) ($p = .0002$), a higher proportion of the tumor perimeter with a continuous pushing margin ($p < .0001$), and a lower mitotic count ($p = .003$) than control cancers." These authors concluded that this histopathology information may improve the classification of breast cancers in those showing a positive family history for this disease. Specifically, employing multifactorial analysis results from their previous estimates, they found that 7.5 percent of individuals with breast cancer in Britain who had been diagnosed at between the ages of 20 and 29 years harbor a *BRCA1* mutation.[43] Further, "Assuming that the odds ratios from our analysis are independent of age, only about 2 percent of case subjects in this age group in whom the mitotic count is below 5 per 10 hpf, without continuous pushing margins, and in whom there is no lymphocytic infiltrate would be expected to carry a *BRCA1* mutation. By contrast, about 45 percent of case subjects in the 20- to 29-year-old group with 20 to 39 mitoses per 10 hpf, continuous pushing margins occupying more than 75 percent of the tumor perimeter, and a prominent lymphocytic infiltrate would be expected to be *BRCA1* carriers. The corresponding proportions based on mitotic count would be 4 and 16 percent."

RADIATION EFFECTS AND *BRCA1* AND *BRCA2* MUTATIONS

Questions have been raised relevant to potential carcinogenic risk of radiation exposure for women who harbor the *BRCA1* or *BRCA2* mutations. Scully and colleagues[44] raised the possibility that there may be an interaction between *BRCA1* and *BRCA2* gene products with respect to proteins involved in the repair of radiation-induced DNA errors. However, this issue remains controversial due to lack of confirmation of this risk in the past by other investigators.[45] Nevertheless, recent evidence has indicated that both *BRCA1* and *BRCA2* are associated with defective repair of radiation-induced DNA damage.[44,46]

In a study by Chabner and colleagues[45] of 201 patients, 29 of whom had positive family histories of breast cancer (a mother or sister previously diagnosed before the age of 50 years, or ovarian cancer at any age) and who had undergone breast-conserving surgery and radiation therapy for early-stage breast cancer, there was no evidence associated with a higher rate of "...local recurrence, distant failure, or second (nonbreast) cancers in young women with a family history (FH) suggestive of inherited breast cancer susceptibility compared with young women without an FH." As expected, the patients with a positive FH showed an increased risk of contralateral breast cancer. This matter of contralateral breast cancer must be given careful consideration when counseling women with positive family histories who are considering the option of breast conserving surgery and radiation therapy versus modified radical mastectomy. Given these findings, Chabner and colleagues[45] conclude that "... young women can be offered conservative surgery and radiation therapy as a reasonable option at breast cancer diagnosis." However, the investigators appropriately call attention to the limitations in their study: a relatively short follow-up time, small size of their cohort, and the absence of specific genetic findings on their patients, including an absence of *BRCA1* or *BRCA2* mutation findings.

OVARIAN CARCINOMA

Any discussion of the genetics of carcinoma of the breast must include ovarian cancer. This disease will affect approximately 1 percent of women in the United States during their lifetime, where it accounts for about 14,500 deaths annually[2] with a five-year survival rate of < 30 percent. The biological mechanism of transforming benign cells to carcinoma remains elusive, although it likely involves a multistep process requiring an accumulation of genetic lesions involving different gene classes. As mentioned, the etiologic association of ovarian cancer with breast cancer was first reported in the early 1970s in a series of breast cancer-prone pedigrees;[4–6,8] both *BRCA1* and *BRCA2* mutations were subsequently found to predispose to ovarian cancer. In *BRCA1*, the lifetime risk for ovarian cancer is in the range of approximately 50 percent, while in *BRCA2* the lifetime ovarian cancer risk is about 20 percent. Ovarian carcinoma is also an integral lesion in Lynch syndrome II.[47] Lynch and colleagues[48] have provided an extensive review of the genetics of ovarian cancer.

GENETIC COUNSELING

We believe that genetic counseling should be mandatory for patients who are at high risk for breast cancer and are contemplating DNA testing in the search for specific germ-line mutations. Counseling should take place *prior* to collection of DNA and at the time of *disclosure* of results. The ideal individual for initial gene testing in a family where a hereditary form of breast cancer is considered likely would be one who has had a syndrome cancer, particularly if diagnosed at an early age, and who is in the direct line of descent of syndrome cancer expression. The clinician's task during the genetic counseling process is to help the patient answer crucial questions which may arise during the genetic testing process. Importantly, patients need to decide whether to be tested for the presence of a germ-line mutation in *BRCA1* or *BRCA2*, once the facts are understood. They should be aware of the potential for fear, anxiety, apprehension, intrafamily strife, as well as insurance/ employment discrimination. Finally, they need to know the best type of medical management for them, based upon the test result.

Because there are a limited number of certified genetic counselors who have sufficient knowledge of oncology to effectively counsel cancer-prone families, the American Society of Clinical Oncology (ASCO) has recommended that, whenever possible, physicians should perform genetic counseling.[49] In its published position[49] on genetic testing for cancer susceptibility, ASCO recognizes that the clinical oncologist's role should be to document the family history of cancer, provide counseling with respect to a patient's inordinate lifetime cancer risk, and provide options for prevention and early detection to those families for whom genetic testing may aid in the genetic counseling process. Informed consent by the patient is considered to be an inte-

gral part of the process of genetic predisposition testing, on either a clinical or research basis. Predisposition testing should be performed on patients for whom there is a strong family history of cancer that is consonant with a likely hereditary etiology, where the results can be adequately interpreted, and where there is a potential to aid in the medical management of the patient and/or family members.

The American Society of Clinical Oncology also recognizes the need to strengthen regulatory authority over laboratories that provide cancer predisposition tests that will ultimately be used in making informed clinical decisions. In the interest of protecting patients and their families, ASCO endorses the adoption of legislation to prohibit discrimination by insurance companies or employers based on an individual's susceptibility to cancer. Finally, ASCO and the American Cancer Society prudently endorses the need for all individuals at hereditary risk for cancer to have, in concert with medical care, appropriate genetic counseling which should be covered by public and private third-party payers.

Figure 1–4 is an algorithm depicting the process used by the Creighton cancer genetic research team to ascertain, test, and counsel HBC/HBOC-prone families. Detailed information about the natural history of HBC/HBOC was provided and the pros and cons of DNA testing were discussed with more than 2,000 members of 29 large families with *BRCA1* mutations and 8 families with *BRCA2* mutations (Table 1–2).[50] The current authors found that the perceived risk for cancer was associated with the individual's position in the pedigree. There was a significant tendency to *overestimate* risk rather than *underestimate* it ($p < .001$) by a chi-square test from Fleiss and colleagues[51] (Table 1–3).

Fifty-seven family members who had provided blood samples several years ago declined the opportunity to receive the results of their DNA testing. Thirty of the 57 responded to an anonymous questionnaire by giving one or more reasons for declining. Their responses varied, but fear of insurance discrimination was cited by 37 percent of this group, and fear of a positive result was cited by 20 percent.

Of those choosing to learn their mutation status, the majority identified their children as a primary reason for being tested (Table 1–4).

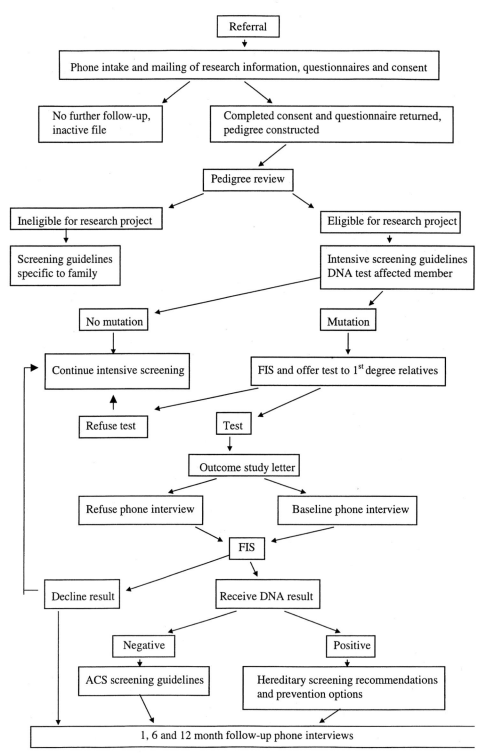

Figure 1–4. Algorithm for education and assessment of *BRCA1* and *BRCA2* families. Reprinted with permission from Lynch et al. Cancer. In press.

Table 1–2. DEMOGRAPHIC CHARACTERISTICS OF STUDY SUBJECTS IN 29 *BRCA1* FAMILIES AND 8 *BRCA2* FAMILIES

	BRCA1	BRCA2
Total number counseled and given gene status	339	85
Mutation positive	137 (40)	42 (49)
Mutation negative	198 (58)	43 (51)
Ambiguous	4 (1)	0
Male	89 (26)	20 (24)
Female	250 (74)	65 (76)
Age Group		
< 25	11 (4)	4 (6)
25-50	89 (36)	26 (40)
> 50	150 (60)	35 (54)
Cancer status		
Breast and/or ovarian cancer affected	59 (24)	16 (25)

Reproduced with permission of author and publisher from Lynch et al. An update on DNA-based *BRCA1/BRCA2* genetic counseling in hereditary breast cancer. Cancer Genet Cytogenet 1999;109:91–8.

Although most of these individuals freely chose to be tested, occasionally they reported pressure within the family either for or against their being tested.

Overall, 167 of 403 queried family members (41%) cited health management (especially surveillance for early detection and prophylactic surgery) as a reason for seeking genetic testing, making it the second most common reason reported. In the subgroup where mutation status information would have the greatest impact on recommendations for surveillance (women under the age of 40), 72 of 118 queried, or 61 percent, cited this reason (other subgroup data are not shown).

Patients' self reports indicated that currently the majority were having breast cancer screening tests at the recommended frequency (Table 1–5). Nevertheless, the majority said that they would consider increasing surveillance if the mutation test showed they were mutation carriers. Only a slim majority (13 of 25 overall) would consider decreasing surveillance if the test showed they were not mutation carriers. Sixty-two percent (59 of 95) of all women over the age of 25 years said they would consider prophylactic mastectomy if the test showed they were mutation carriers. Patient self reports indicated that a minority of these women are having CA-125 and

transvaginal ovarian ultrasound as often as recommended (Table 1–6). Most said they would consider increasing surveillance and/or having prophylactic oophorectomy if the test showed them to be mutation carriers. Note that all data on post-test management reflect what patients say they will consider in the decision-making process, not necessarily what they plan to do.

The emotional responses to disclosure of germ-line mutation results cannot always be anticipated. Our data show that the majority of patients who are negative express relief. However, some may experience disbelief or survivor guilt. Those who are told they do have the germ-line mutation express a variety of reac-

Table 1–3. ESTIMATE OF PERCEIVED RISK OF HARBORING A *BRCA1/BRCA2* MUTATION

Pedigree Risk*	Perceived Risk of Mutation Carriage (n (%))		
	< 50%	50%	> 50%
< 25%	27 (38.0%)	27 (38.0%)	17 (23.9%)
50%	44 (17.7%)	74 (29.8%)	130 (52.4%)
Affected/obligate gene carrier	3 (3.8%)	5 (6.3%)	71 (89.9%)

*These individuals tended to overestimate their risk more often than to underestimate it ($p < .001$) (chi square test[51]).
Reproduced with permission of author and publisher from Lynch et al. An update on DNA-based *BRCA1/BRCA2* genetic counseling in hereditary breast cancer. Cancer Genet Cytogenet 1999;109:91–8.

Table 1–4. REASONS FOR SEEKING RISK ASSESSMENT IN COUNSELED MEMBERS OF 29 BRCA1 FAMILIES AND 8 BRCA2 FAMILIES

	Counseled BRCA1 Individuals (n = 319)	Counseled BRCA2 Individuals (n = 84)
Top three reasons for seeking risk assessment		
Children	170 (53)	47 (56)
Surveillance/ prophylaxis	125 (39)	42 (50)
Curiosity	94 (29)	24 (29)

Reproduced with permission of author and publisher from Lynch et al. An update on DNA-based BRCA1/BRCA2 genetic counseling in hereditary breast cancer. Cancer Genet Cytogenet 1999;109:91-8.

tions, including acceptance because the results are not a surprise to them, relief of anxiety with the removal of uncertainty about their genetic risk status, a positive attitude in terms of prevention, feelings of sadness, or even anger. The genetic counselor must be responsive to all of these emotions.

At a baseline interview in a study by Lerman and colleagues,[52] breast-ovarian cancer-related stress symptoms were predictive of the onset of depressive symptoms in family members who were invited but declined testing. "Among persons who reported high baseline levels of stress, depression rates in decliners increased from 26 percent at baseline to 47 percent at one-month follow-up; depression rates in noncarriers decreased and in carriers showed no change (odds ratio [OR] for decliners versus noncarriers = 8.0; 95% confidence interval [CI] 1.9 to 3.5; $p = .0004$). These significant differences in depression rates were still evident at the six-month follow-up evaluation ($p = .04$)." It was concluded that in BRCA1/BRCA2-linked families, individuals showing high levels of cancer-related stress who ultimately declined genetic testing appeared to be at increased risk for depression. It was reasoned that they could derive benefit through education and counseling even though they might ultimately decline to be tested; these are the individuals who require monitoring for the potential occurrence of adverse psychological effects.

An important genetic counseling question is, Do patients who received information about their genetic risk status, including the presence of a BRCA1/BRCA2 germ-line mutation, heed surveillance and management recommendations? These recommendations include the need for increased frequency of mammography, breast self-examination, and physician breast examination. Recommendations for ovarian screening

Table 1–5. SURVEILLANCE PRACTICES AND ATTITUDES TOWARD PROPHYLACTIC MASTECTOMIES PRIOR TO GENETIC TEST RESULT DISCLOSURE*

		BRCA1	BRCA2
Bilateral mastectomies prior to the counseling session			
Breast cancer-affected		39/250 (16)	8/65 (12)
Breast cancer-free (Prophylactic)		23/250 (9)	3/65 (5)
Current surveillance practices‡			
Mammography	Ever	145/153 (95)	42/46 (91)
	As recommended	92/118 (78)	25/36 (69)
Physician BE	Ever	105/107 (98)	39/40 (97)
	As recommended	84/90 (93)	37/38 (97)
Self BE	Ever	102/116 (88)	38/42 (90)
	As recommended	54/88 (61)	27/37 (73)
If carrier, will consider prophylactic mastectomy†		51/77 (66)	8/18 (44)
If carrier, will consider increasing surveillance‡		62/65 (95)	24/25 (96)
If noncarrier, will consider decreasing surveillance‡		9/20 (45)	4/5 (80)

*In counseled female members of 29 BRCA1 families and counseled female members in 8 BRCA2 families (number/number queried† (percent)).
†The number queried varies from item to item since not all questions were asked and/or responded to within the genetic counseling setting.
‡Excluding women aged < 25 or with bilateral mastectomies.
BE= breast examination.
Reproduced with permission of author and publisher from Lynch et al. Cancer Genet Cytogenet 1999;109:91–8.

Table 1–6. SURVEILLANCE PRACTICES AND ATTITUDES TOWARD PROPHYLACTIC OOPHORECTOMIES PRIOR TO GENETIC TEST RESULT DISCLOSURE*

		BRCA1	*BRCA2*
Bilateral oophorectomies prior to the counseling session			
Ovarian cancer-affected		7/250 (3)	0/65 (0)
Ovarian cancer-free		83/250 (33)	5/65 (8)
Current surveillance practices‡			
CA-125	Ever	26/65 (40)	4/19 (21)
	As recommended	10/49 (20)	2/17 (12)
Ultrasound	Ever	32/71 (45)	11/25 (44)
	As recommended	11/51 (22)	2/16 (12)
Pelvic	Ever	86/96 (90)	50/51 (98)
	As recommended	64/79 (81)	45/46 (98)
If carrier, will consider prophylactic oophorectomy‡		72/81 (89)	10/20 (50)
If carrier, will consider increasing surveillance‡		50/53 (94)	25/26 (96)
If noncarrier, will consider decreasing surveillance‡		8/15 (53)	5/6 (83)

*In counseled female members of 29 *BRCA1* families and counseled female members in 8 *BRCA2* families (number/number queried† (percent)).
†The number queried varies from item to item since not all questions were asked and/or responded to within the genetic counseling setting.
‡Excluding women aged < 25 or with bilateral oophorectomies.
Reproduced with permission of author and publisher from Lynch et al. An update on DNA-based *BRCA1/BRCA2* genetic counseling in hereditary breast cancer. Cancer Genet Cytogenet 1999;109:91–8.

included transvaginal ovarian ultrasound, Doppler color bloodflow imagery, and CA-125. However, the patients were thoroughly educated about the *limitations* of ovarian cancer screening. The option of prophylactic mastectomy and/or prophylactic oophorectomy was also discussed during genetic counseling sessions.[50]

Preliminary data show that psychological assessment 6 months following *BRCA1/BRCA2* testing among unaffected individuals (both male and female) from HBOC families did not reflect adverse psychological effects.[53] However, with respect to screening, we did find that rates of adherence to mammography recommendations among mutation carriers was not increased. It was also noted that carriers of deleterious genes who said they would consider prophylactic surgery nevertheless showed low rates of actually adopting such options. However, these observations are based upon short-term experience; longer-term data will be required to determine how often women may opt for prophylactic surgery.[53]

PROPHYLACTIC MASTECTOMY

In a landmark study, Hartmann and colleagues[54] pursued the efficacy of prophylactic mastec-

tomy on a retrospective cohort study of all women with a breast cancer-positive family history who underwent bilateral prophylactic mastectomy at the Mayo Clinic between 1960 and 1993. These women were divided into high-risk versus moderate-risk groups based on their family history. Those at high risk showed pedigrees consistent with a single-gene, autosomal dominant predisposition to carcinoma of the breast, whereas those at moderate risk showed positive family histories that did not meet these high-risk criteria. To predict the number of breast cancers expected in these two groups had prophylactic mastectomies not been performed, the researchers used a nested-sister control study for the high-risk group and the Gail Model for the moderate-risk group. Their findings were based upon 693 women with a family history of breast cancer (214 high-risk and 425 moderate-risk) who had bilateral prophylactic mastectomies. Their median follow-up was 14.4 years, while the median age at prophylactic mastectomy was 43 (mean 42.4) years. The Gail Model prediction for breast cancer occurrence expected in the moderate-risk group was 37.4. However, only four breast cancers occurred following prophylactic mastectomy in this group (89.5% reduction, $p < .001$).

Breast cancer occurrences in the 214 high-risk probands were compared to their sisters who had not undergone prophylactic mastectomy. These 214 probands had a total of 403 sisters. Of keen interest was the finding that there have been 156 breast cancers in the sisters; 115 occurred before the sister proband's mastectomy, 38 after the sister proband's prophylactic mastectomy, and 3 with date unknown. In comparison, 3 of the 214 probands had developed breast cancer. This represents a > 90 percent reduction in the incidence of breast cancer with current follow-up. Breast cancer mortality was also reduced significantly in both the high and moderate-risk groups.

The investigators concluded that prophylactic mastectomy resulted in a significant reduction in the incidence of and mortality from breast cancer among these women with positive family histories of breast cancer. This information will be useful for genetic counseling.[54]

Schrag and colleagues[55] discuss the decision analysis involved in prophylactic mastectomy and oophorectomy and life expectancy outcome among patients with BRCA1 and BRCA2 germ-line mutations. They found that, on average, a 30-year-old woman harboring such a mutation would gain from 2.9 to 5.3 years of life expectancy from prophylactic mastectomy and from 0.3 to 1.7 years from prophylactic oophorectomy. These findings were dependent upon their cumulative risk of cancer. Gains in life expectancy also would decline with age at the time of prophylactic surgery. They would be minimal for a 60-year-old woman. Importantly, in women aged 30, an oophorectomy may be delayed for 10 years with minimal loss of life expectancy. This would allow women to complete their families. These investigators concluded that "On the basis of a range of estimates of the incidence of cancer, prognosis, and efficacy of prophylactic surgery, our model suggests that prophylactic mastectomy provides substantial gains in life expectancy and prophylactic oophorec-tomy more limited gains for young women with BRCA1 or BRCA2 mutations."

CONSERVATIVE VERSUS CONVENTIONAL SURGERY IN HEREDITARY BREAST CANCER

Should a patient with HBOC, particularly one who is harboring a BRCA1 or BRCA2 germ-line mutation, be managed differently from a patient with the more common sporadic form of this disease? We have taken the position that, because of the early age of breast cancer onset and excess lifetime risk for bilaterality, coupled with the potential deficiency of repair of radiation-induced DNA damage,[44] the patient should be given the option of total mastectomy as opposed to conservative ("lumpectomy") management, and seriously consider contralateral prophylactic mastectomy, assuming that the ipsilateral breast cancer is likely to have adequate control.

POTENTIAL FOR TARGETED BRCA1/BRCA2 MUTATION THERAPY

In addition to identifying cancer risk status through mutations such as BRCA1 and BRCA2, this knowledge has the potential to provide individualized highly-targeted molecular genetic therapies based upon mutation discoveries.[56] Specifically, once the functions of cancer susceptibility genes have been identified, knowledge as to how such gene-determined biochemical functions can be employed for targeted radiation and chemotherapy should emerge.

Abbott and colleagues[57] examined the protein product of the BRCA2 gene in terms of its having an important role in mediating repair of double-strand breaks in DNA. They identified a human pancreatic carcinoma cell line which lacked one copy of the BRCA2 gene and contained a mutation (617delT) in the remaining copy.[58] They performed in vitro and in vivo experiments in this cell line as well as with other carefully matched cell lines. They then examined double-strand break repair with attention given to sensitivity to drugs and radiation effect that induce double-strand breaks. Their findings disclose that "... *BRCA2*-defective cells are unable to repair the double-strand DNA breaks induced by ionizing radiation. These cells were also markedly sensitive to mitoxantrone, amsacrine, and etoposide... (two-sided $p = .002$) and to ionizing radiation (two-sided $p = .001$). Introduction of antisense *BRCA2* deoxyribonucleotides into cells possessing normal *BRCA2* function led to increased sensitivity to mitoxantrone (two-sided $p = .008$). Tumors formed by injection of *BRCA2*-defective cells into nude mice were highly sensitive (> 90% tumor size reduction, two-sided $p = .002$) to both ionizing radiation and mitoxantrone when compared with tumors exhibiting normal *BRCA2* function." Abbott and colleagues concluded that these *BRCA2*-defective cancer cells were highly sensitive to agents that contribute to double-strand breaks in DNA.

SURVEILLANCE AND MANAGEMENT FOR HEREDITARY BREAST CANCER

When the diagnosis of a hereditary breast cancer-prone syndrome has been established, the surveillance and management strategies are then melded to the natural history of the particular HBC syndrome. We recommend that patients receive intensive education regarding the natural history, genetic risk, and availability of DNA testing such as *BRCA1*, *BRCA2*, or *p53*, depending upon the hereditary breast cancer syndrome of concern. We initiate such education between the ages of 15 and 18 years but do not perform any DNA testing until the patient is > 18 years of age and has given informed consent.

When patients are 18 years old, the authors provide instruction in breast self examination (BSE) with physician assessment of their performance. Although the effectiveness of BSE has been controversial, the authors are convinced that it can be effective if the woman is

taught how to perform this procedure and demonstrates proficiency in doing so on return medical visits. When patients reach the age of 20 years, we begin semiannual breast examination by the physician and at age 25 initiate annual mammography.

With respect to ovarian cancer, we discuss transvaginal ovarian ultrasound, Doppler color bloodflow imaging, and CA-125, with their limitations, and initiate this at age 30 and perform it annually. The option of prophylactic bilateral oophorectomy is also discussed. If the patient is interested in this option and has completed her child bearing, the oophorectomy can be performed between the ages of 35 and 45 years.

CONCLUSION

It is necessary to keep an open mind about the pros and cons of DNA testing and genetic counseling and its translation into medical practice by the basic scientist, medical and molecular geneticist, physician, genetic counselor, and ethicist. For example, how does one interpret some of the ethical positions of today suggesting that genetic testing be limited to a research setting or even curtailed until specific benefit of such DNA testing can be more fully established?

Prodigious advances in science and technology (ie, better surveillance, more effective surgical management including data supporting prophylactic surgery, and improved molecular genetic technology with lower cost for germ-line mutation discovery) may resolve some of the concerns about molecular genetic testing that cause certain physicians, basic scientists, and ethicists to believe it should be limited. How does one educate these colleagues about newly emerging benefits of molecular genetic testing which could prove to be lifesaving?

Molecular genetic advances are occurring at such a rapid pace that it is exceedingly difficult to keep physicians fully informed of this progress. For example, it is predicted that the entire human genome will be identified by the year 2003.

The lay press strives to keep the public fully informed about the impact new gene discoveries may have on patients and their close relatives. Unfortunately, certain members of the media have overinterpreted the benefit of germ-line testing and have not fully dealt with some of its drawbacks. In turn, some molecular genetic laboratories have made testing appear to be the panacea for cancer control. Some may offer molecular testing without sufficient evidence that the family of concern merits testing. Genetic counseling may not be provided to those being tested. In spite of these misgivings, we believe that hereditary breast cancer patients, when properly counseled and DNA tested, will benefit immensely during this exciting era of molecular genetics.

Patients must be encouraged to meticulously examine their family histories of cancer. Should they be found to harbor a germ-line cancer predisposing mutation, this knowledge may be used to encourage screening and detect cancer at an early stage so that a cure might be possible and/or cancer prevented through the option of prophylactic surgery.

REFERENCES

1. Vogelstein B, Kinzler KW. The genetic basis of human cancer. New York: McGraw-Hill; 1998.
2. Landis SH, Murray T, Bolden S, Wingo PA. Cancer statistics, 1999. CA Cancer J Clin 1999;49:8–31.
3. Lynch HT, Lemon SJ, Durham C, et al. A descriptive study of BRCA1 testing and reactions to disclosure of test results. Cancer 1997;79:2219–28.
4. Lynch HT, Krush AJ. Carcinoma of the breast and ovary in three families. Surg Gynecol Obstet 1971;133:644–8.
5. Lynch HT, Krush AJ, Lemon HM, et al. Tumor variation in families with breast cancer. JAMA 1972;222:1631–5.
6. Lynch HT, Guirgis HA, Albert S, et al. Familial association of carcinoma of the breast and ovary. Surg Gynecol Obstet 1974;138:717–24.
7. Hall JM, Lee MK, Newman B, et al. Linkage of early-onset breast cancer to chromosome 17q21. Science 1990;250:1684–9.
8. Narod SA, Feunteun J, Lynch HT, et al. Familial breast-ovarian cancer locus on chromosome 17q12–q23. Lancet 1991;388:82–3.
9. Miki Y, Swensen J, Shattuck-Eidens D, et al. A strong candidate for the breast and ovarian cancer susceptibility gene BRCA1. Science 1994;266:66–71.
10. Wooster R, Neuhausen SL, Mangion J, et al. Localization of a breast cancer susceptibility gene, BRCA2, to chromosome 13q12–13. Science 1994;265:2088–90.
11. Wooster R, Bignell G, Lancaster J, et al. Identification of the breast cancer susceptibility gene BRCA2. Nature 1995;378:789–92.
12. Easton DF, Bishop DT, Ford D, Crockford GP, The Breast Cancer Linkage Consortium. Genetic linkage analysis in familial breast and ovarian cancer: results from 214 families. Am J Hum Genet 1993;52:678–701.
13. Easton DF, Ford D, Bishop DT, The Breast Cancer Linkage Consortium. Breast and ovarian cancer incidence in BRCA1 mutation carriers. Am J Hum Genet 1995;56:265–71.
14. Struewing JP, Hartge P, Wacholder S, et al. The risk of cancer associated with specific mutations of BRCA1 and BRCA2 among Ashkenazi Jews. N Engl J Med 1997;336:1401–8.
15. Claus EB, Schildkraut J, Iversen ES Jr, Berry D, Parmigiani G. Effect of BRCA1 and BRCA2 on the association between breast cancer risk and family history. J Natl Cancer Inst 1998;90:1824–9.
16. Lynch HT, Follett KL, Lynch PM, et al. Family history in an oncology clinic. Implications for cancer genetics. JAMA. 1979;242:1268–72.
17. David KL, Steiner-Grossman P. The potential use of tumor registry data in the recognition and prevention of hereditary and familial cancer. NY State J Med 1991;91:150–2.
18. Lynch HT, Lemon SJ, Marcus JN, et al. Breast cancer genetics: heterogeneity, molecular genetics, syndrome diagnosis, and genetic counseling. In: Bland KI, Copeland EMI, editors. The breast: comprehensive management of benign and malignant diseases. 2 ed. Philadelphia (PA): W. B. Saunders Company; 1998. p. 370–94.
19. Gayther SA, Warren W, Mazoyer S, et al. Germline mutations of the BRCA1 gene in breast and ovarian cancer families provide evidence for a genotype-phenotype correlation. Nat Genet 1995;11: 428–33.
20. Serova O, Montagna M, Torchard D, et al. A high incidence of BRCA1 mutations in 20 breast-ovarian cancer families. Am J Hum Genet 1996;58:42–51.

21. Gayther SA, Mangion J, Russell P, et al. Variation of risks of breast and ovarian cancer associated with different germline mutations of the *BRCA2* gene. Nat Genet 1997;15:103–5.

22. Ramus SJ, Friedman LS, Gayther SA, Ponder BAJ. A breast/ovarian cancer patient with germline mutations in both *BRCA1* and *BRCA2*. Nat Genet 1997;15:14–15.

23. Tonin P, Moslehi R, Green R, et al. Linkage analysis of 26 Canadian breast and breast-ovarian cancer families. Hum Genet 1995;95:545–50.

24. Neuhausen S, Gilewski T, Norton L, et al. Recurrent *BRCA2* 617delT mutations in Ashkenazi Jewish women affected by breast cancer. Nat Genet 1996;13:126–8.

25. Couch FJ, Farid LM, DeShano ML, et al. *BRCA2* germline mutations in male breast cancer cases and breast cancer families. Nat Genet 1996;13: 123–5.

26. Liede A, Metcalfe K, Offit K, et al. A family with three germline mutations in *BRCA1* and *BRCA2*. Clin Genet 1998;54:215–8.

27. Struewing JP, Abeliovich D, Peretz T, et al. The carrier frequency of the *BRCA1* 185delAG mutation is approximately 1 percent in Ashkenazi Jewish individuals. Nat Genet 1995;11:198–200.

28. Roa BB, Boyd AA, Volcik K, Richards CS. Ashkenazi Jewish population frequencies for common mutations in *BRCA1* and *BRCA2*. Nat Genet 1996;14:185–7.

29. Oddoux C, Struewing JP, Clayton CM, et al. The carrier frequency of the *BRCA2* 6174delT mutation among Ashkenazi Jewish individuals is approximately 1%. Nat Genet 1996;14:188–90.

30. Marcus JN, Watson P, Page DL, et al. Hereditary breast cancer: pathobiology, prognosis, and *BRCA1* and *BRCA2* gene linkage. Cancer 1996; 77:697–709.

31. Marcus JN, Page DL, Watson P, et al. *BRCA1* and *BRCA2* hereditary breast carcinoma phenotypes. Cancer 1997;80 Suppl:543–56.

32. Marcus JN, Watson P, Page DL, et al. *BRCA2* hereditary breast cancer phenotype. Breast Cancer Res Treat 1997;44:275–7.

33. Marcus JN, Watson P, Page DL, Lynch HT. The pathology and heredity of breast cancer in younger women. J Natl Cancer Inst Monogr 1994;16:23–34.

34. Thompson ME, Jensen RA, Obermiler PS, et al. Decreased expression of *BRCA1* accelerates growth and is often present during sporadic breast cancer progression. Nat Genet 1995;9: 444–50.

35. Rao VN, Shao N, Ahmad M, Reddy ESP. Antisense RNA to the putative tumor suppressor gene *BRCA1* transforms mouse fibroblasts. Oncogene 1996;12:523–8.

36. Holt JT, Thompson ME, Szabo CI, et al. Growth retardation and tumour inhibition by *BRCA1*. Nat Genet 1996;12:298–302.

37. Armes JE, Egan AJM, Southey MC, et al. The histologic phenotypes of breast carcinoma occurring before age 40 years in women with and without *BRCA1* or *BRCA2* germline mutations: a population-based study. Cancer 1998;83: 2335–45.

38. Collins N, McManus R, Wooster R, et al. Consistent loss of the wild type allele in breast cancers from a family linked to the *BRCA2* gene on chromosome 12q12–13. Oncogene 1995;10:1673–5.

39. Sigurdsson H, Agnarsson BA, Jonasson JG, et al. Worse survival among breast cancer patients in families carrying the *BRCA2* susceptibility gene. [abstract] Breast Cancer Res Treat 1996; 37:33.

40. Breast Cancer Linkage Consortium. Pathology of familial breast cancer: differences between breast cancers in carriers of *BRCA1* or *BRCA2* mutations and sporadic cases. Lancet 1997; 349:1505–10.

41. Lakhani SR, Jacquemier J, Sloane JP, et al. Multifactorial analysis of differences between sporadic breast cancers and cancers involving *BRCA1* and *BRCA2* mutations. J Natl Cancer Inst 1998;90:1138–45.

42. Eng C, Li FP, Abramson DH. Mortality from second tumors among long-term survivors of retinoblastoma. J Natl Cancer Inst 1993;85: 1121–6.

43. Ford D, Easton DF, Peto J. Estimates of the gene frequency of *BRCA1* and its contribution to breast and ovarian cancer incidence. Am J Hum Genet 1995;57:1457–62.

44. Scully R, Chen J, Plug A, et al. Association of *BRCA1* with Rad51 in mitotic and meiotic cells. Cell 1997;88:265–75.

45. Chabner E, Nixon A, Gelman R, et al. Family history and treatment outcome in young women after breast-conserving surgery and radiation therapy for early-stage breast cancer. J Clin Oncol 1998;16:2045–51.

46. Lim DS, Hasty P. A mutation in mouse Rad51 results in early embryonic lethal that is suppressed by a mutation in p53. Mol Cell Biol 1996;16:7133–43.

47. Watson P, Lynch HT. Extracolonic cancer in hereditary nonpolyposis colorectal cancer. Cancer 1993;71:677–85.

48. Lynch HT, Casey MJ, Lynch J, et al. Genetics and ovarian carcinoma. Semin Oncol 1998;25:265–81.

49. American Society of Clinical Oncology. Statement of the American Society of Clinical Oncology: genetic testing for cancer susceptibility. J Clin Oncol 1996;14:1730–6.

50. Lynch HT, Watson P, Tinley S, et al. An update on DNA-based *BRCA1/BRCA2* genetic counseling in hereditary breast cancer. Cancer Genet Cytogenet 1999;109:91–8.

51. Fleiss JL. Statistical methods for rates and proportions. 2nd ed. New York: John Wiley & Sons; 1981.

52. Lerman C, Hughes C, Lemon SJ, et al. What you don't know can hurt you: adverse psychologic effects in members of *BRCA1*–linked and *BRCA2*-linked families who decline genetic testing. J Clin Oncol 1998;16:1650–4.

53. Lerman C, Narod S, Schulman K, et al. BRCA1 testing in families with hereditary breast-ovarian cancer: a prospective study of patient decision-making and outcomes. JAMA 1996;275:1885–92.

54. Hartmann LC, Schaid DJ, Woods JE, et al. Efficacy of bilateral prophylactic mastectomy in women with a family history of breast cancer. N Engl J Med 1999;340:77–84.

55. Schrag D, Kuntz KM, Garber JE, Weeks JC. Decision analysis—effects of prophylactic mastectomy and oophorectomy on life expectancy among women with BRCA1 or BRCA2 mutations. N Engl J Med 1997;336:1465–71.

56. Livingston DM. Genetics is coming to oncology. JAMA 1997;277:1476–7.

57. Abbott DW, Freeman ML, Holt JT. Double-strand break repair deficiency and radiation sensitivity in BRCA2 mutant cancer cells. J Natl Cancer Inst 1998;90:978–85.

58. Goggins M, Schutte M, Lu J, et al. Germline BRCA2 gene mutations in patients with apparently sporadic pancreatic carcinomas. Cancer Res 1996; 56:5360–4.

2

Breast Cancer Risk and Management: Chemoprevention, Surgery, and Surveillance

MASSIMO CRISTOFANILLI, MD
LISA NEWMAN, MD, FACS
GABRIEL N. HORTOBAGYI, MD

In the past decade, the systematic use of mammography as part of diagnostic screening programs and the extensive use of stereotactic fine-needle biopsy techniques have greatly improved our ability to detect pre-invasive as well as microinvasive breast carcinomas. The consequent earlier detection of breast lesions is considered the most important factor explaining the recent decline in overall mortality from breast cancer observed in the United States.[1] This progress has translated into many efforts to gain insight into the biologic mechanisms responsible for cancer development and progression and to identify potential areas of intervention for prevention studies.[2]

About 20 percent of women diagnosed with proliferative breast disease display atypical hyperplasia, a condition associated with increased risk of breast cancer and probably a precursor to the disease.[3] The recognition of the importance of these benign breast lesions as risk factors and the identification of genetic alterations (*BRCA1, BRCA2, p53*) associated with genetic predisposition to breast cancer have spurred investigation in the areas of prophylactic surgery and chemoprevention in the management of women at high risk of breast cancer and directed attention to specific interventions and to the design of comprehensive surveillance programs.[4–6]

The development of effective chemoprevention strategies requires a systematic approach focusing on multiple investigational aspects of the problem including (1) a clear description of the specific risk factors that may be used in selecting cohorts of women at increased risk and as end points for chemoprevention studies; (2) the identification and preclinical evaluation of cancer chemoprevention agents and subsequent development of definitive, large-scale clinical trials; and (3) the identification and characterization of specific molecular biomarkers that may be quantitatively assessed and used as surrogate end-point biomarkers (SEBs) in future trials.

BREAST CANCER RISK ASSESSMENT

Chemoprevention is traditionally defined as the inhibition or reversal of carcinogenesis, before overt malignancy, by intervention with chemical agents. Most breast cancer chemopreventive studies are conducted within cohorts of women considered at high risk of the disease.[7] In the context of chemoprevention investigations, the most important cancer risk factors are considered to be those that can be measured quantitatively in the subject at risk. These factors are called risk biomarkers, and they can be used to identify cohorts for chemoprevention trials.[8]

Generally, the risk biomarkers are grouped in the following categories: (1) genetic predisposition, (2) carcinogen exposure, (3) carcinogen effect/exposure, (4) previous cancers, and (5) intermediate biomarkers. In some cases, risk biomarkers that are measurable and may undergo selective modulation by chemopreventive agents can be used as SEBs in clinical chemoprevention studies.[9] Today, there is not a single ideal risk biomarker or SEB for breast cancer, and the selection of high-risk subjects for breast cancer chemoprevention studies is generally done on the basis of the presence of proliferative atypical breast disease or epidemiologic and genetic factors known to increase a woman's risk of developing breast cancer.[10,11]

The quantification of the risk of developing cancer is usually estimated from epidemiologic models, which consider a variety of risk factors and project a cumulative risk for the development of disease over a finite period of time. Among the various models proposed, the model developed by Gail and colleagues is probably the most widely accepted.[12] Proposed in the original form in 1989 and subsequently modified, this model was designed to calculate the absolute breast cancer risk in women on the basis of the data from the Breast Cancer Detection Demonstration Project (BCDDP) that recruited 280,000 women in 28 centers in the United States in the mid-1970s. It represented an attempt to define the contribution of accumulated breast cancer risk from a number of risk factors combined in a multivariate logistic regression model. The variables identified included age of the patient, number of first-degree relatives with breast cancer,

Table 2–1. RISK FACTORS CONSIDERED FOR THE CALCULATION OF ABSOLUTE BREAST CANCER RISK

Risk Factor		Associated Relative Risk	Expansion Variables
Age at menarche (y)			
≥ 14		1.000	
12 to 13		1.099	A
< 12		1.207	
No. of breast biopsies			
Age < 50 y			
0 (0)		1.000	
1 (1)		1.698	
≥ 2 (2)		2.882	
Age ≥ 50 y			B
0 (0)		1.000	
1 (1)		1.273	
≥ 2 (2)		1.620	
Age at first-term live birth (y)	No. of first-degree relatives with breast cancer		
< 20	0 (0)	1.000	
	1 (1)	2.607	
	≥ 2 (2)	6.798	
20 to 24	0 (0)	1.244	
	1 (1)	2.681	
	≥ 2 (2)	5.775	
25 to 29 or nulliparous	0 (0)	1.548	C
	1 (1)	2.756	
	≥ 2 (2)	4.907	
≥ 30	0 (0)	1.927	
	1 (1)	2.834	
	≥ 2 (2)	4.169	

Absolute risk = A × B × C × 1.82 *
A × B × C × 0.93[†]

*Presence of atypical hyperplasia in biopsies.
[†]No atypical hyperplasia.
Adapted from Gail MH, Brinton LA, Byar DP, et al. Projecting individualized possibilities of developing breast cancer for white females who are being examined annually. J Natl Cancer Inst 1989;81:1879–86.

nulliparity or age at first live birth, number of breast biopsies, presence or absence of atypical hyperplasia, and age at menarche (Table 2–1). The individualized absolute risk can be estimated by combining the relative risk based on the woman's age and individual risk factors and then combining this information with an estimate of the baseline hazard rate for a woman with no risk factors.[12,13] In particular, women with a strong family history of breast cancer (2 first-degree relatives affected, or 1 first-degree and 2 second-degree relatives affected) or of breast and ovarian cancers (3 affected relatives with breast cancer and 1 relative with ovarian cancer) have a 25 percent or greater lifetime risk of developing breast cancer. A computer program called RISK has been subsequently developed and allows physicians to calculate a woman's absolute risk to develop breast cancer with 95 percent confidence interval bounds.[14]

Familial and Genetic Factors

Identification of cohorts at genetic risk for cancer is an appealing concept because it may offer the opportunity to explore the steps in breast carcinogenesis, from the inheritance of a predisposing mutation through the development of preinvasive lesions or overt malignancy. However, germline genetic changes are rare and reported in only a small proportion of women who will eventually develop breast cancer.[15]

Breast cancer attributed to a family history of the disease has been reported to account for 6 to 19 percent of all cases of breast cancer. Hereditary breast cancers, which constitute a proportion of these cases, are characterized by early onset, a high incidence of bilateral disease, association with other malignancies, and autosomal dominant inheritance. Genetic-linkage studies of families with multiple members with breast cancer have allowed major improvements in our understanding of the genetic alterations associated with hereditary predisposition. Such studies led to the discovery of germline mutations in the *BRCA1* and *BRCA2* genes.[16]

The *BRCA1* gene, a breast cancer susceptibility gene localized to chromosome 17q, was described for the first time in 1990. It is a tumor-suppressor gene postulated to be important in regulating the growth of breast epithelial cells and in the process of deoxyribonucleic acid (DNA) damage repair.[17] The breast cancer susceptibility gene *BRCA1* accounts for 45 percent of hereditary cases of breast cancer and 80 to 90 percent of hereditary cases of combined breast and ovarian cancers. The *BRCA1* mutations are found in approximately 7 to 12 percent of women with breast cancer of early onset. Mutations have been described as spreading evenly across the entire gene. The most commonly described mutation is a specific alteration causing a deletion of adenine and guanine (185delAG). This mutation is present in 1 percent of the Ashkenazi Jewish population and contributes to a risk of breast cancer as high as 21 percent among Jewish women. Women who carry a *BRCA1* mutation were initially estimated to have an 87 percent lifetime risk of breast cancer and a 44 percent lifetime risk of ovarian cancer.[18] Subsequent studies suggest risks of 56 percent and 16 percent, respectively.

More recent data from population-based studies suggest that *BRCA1* mutations account for only 10 to 20 percent of inherited breast cancer, and *BRCA2* mutations are responsible for half this fraction. The discrepancy between estimates from early studies is probably related to the fact that initial data were derived from linkage analysis that probably tends to overestimate the true incidence of *BRCA1* and *BRCA2* mutations in hereditary breast cancer.[19–21]

The breast cancer susceptibility gene *BRCA2*, localized to chromosome 13q, was described in 1994. Linkage studies suggest that 35 percent of high-risk families may have *BRCA2* mutations.[22] Male breast cancer, a rare condition that represents less than 1 percent of all cancer and 0.1 percent of cancer-related deaths in men, has been found to be associated with mutations in the *BRCA2* gene.[23]

Familial clustering of breast cancer has also been described in families diagnosed with Cowden syndrome and Li-Fraumeni syndrome, and more recently, ataxia-telangiectasia.[24,25] Cowden syndrome involves multiple hamartomatous lesions, especially of the skin, and mucous membranes, and carcinoma of the breast and thyroid. Li-Fraumeni syndrome, associated with a high incidence of *p53* mutations, consists of a familial aggregation of breast carcinomas, soft tissue sarcomas, brain tumors, osteosarcomas, leukemias, and adrenocortical carcinomas.

Hereditary breast cancer syndromes are clinically relevant because they raise the possibility of effective identification, through genetic testing, of patients at high risk and optimal quantification of the risk. In view of the high risk of developing an invasive breast cancer during their lifetime and in consideration of the imperfect nature of early detection, patients with hereditary breast cancer syndromes constitute an ideal target for chemoprevention studies.

Environmental Radiation Exposure

Epidemiologic observations suggest that exposure of breast tissue to ionizing radiation is associated with an increased risk of breast cancer. In particular, an increased risk of breast carcinoma has been clearly documented in young women that have survived atomic bombs, in patients who have undergone repeated fluoroscopies (eg, in patients with tuberculosis), and in patients treated with radiation for postpartum mastitis, thymic enlargement, and Hodgkin's disease.[26–37]

Treatment-associated second neoplasms have emerged as a major complication in patients cured of Hodgkin's disease. Sporadic cases of breast carcinoma after mantle irradiation for Hodgkin's disease were reported beginning in 1978, by which time clinical data on a large cohort of women treated and cured for their disease in the 1960s had become available.[25]

Subsequent reports directed attention to the carcinogenic risk associated with radiation exposure and the latency time between exposure and clinical manifestations of breast cancer. A latency period of at least 10 years is usually required in the majority of the patients; a shorter latency period (5 to 10 years) has been reported occasionally.[31]

These observational studies suggest that the carcinogenic process is related to two factors: the dose of radiation delivered and the person's age at the time of exposure. In general, young women (less than 30 years of age) represent a cohort with a higher relative risk compared with the risk for other age groups. The clustering of breast carcinoma in women irradiated for Hodgkin's disease at an early age is probably related to the increased sensitivity of the incompletely differentiated breast epithelium to the carcinogenic action of radiation.[33]

The high risk of breast carcinoma in young women with Hodgkin's disease treated with irradiation mandates regular follow-up with breast examination and yearly mammography starting within 8 years of completion of the radiation treatment.[37]

The hypothetical risk of breast cancer derived from prolonged screening needs to be mentioned. Using a risk estimate provided by the Biological Effects of Ionizing Radiation (BEIR) V Report of the National Academy of Sciences and a mean breast glandular dose of 4 mGy from bilateral mammography, with two views per breast, one can estimate that annual mammography of 100,000 women for 10 consecutive years beginning at age 40 years will result in, at most, 8 breast cancer deaths during their lifetime. On the other hand, researchers have shown a 24 percent mortality reduction from biennial screening of women in this age group; this will result in one life lost. An assumed mortality reduction of 36 percent from annual screening would result in 36.5 lives saved per life lost and 91.3 years of life saved per year of life lost. Thus, the theoretic radiation risk from screening mammography is extremely small compared with the established benefit from this life-saving procedure and should not unduly distract women under age 40 years who are considering screening.[38]

Intermediate Biomarkers

A key element in the control and prevention of invasive breast cancer is the recognition of early, preclinical changes with or without associated characteristic molecular abnormalities that may identify a woman as being at high risk for development of the disease.[39] These alterations, called intermediate biomarkers, may be used as SEBs and provide a more cost-effective and rapid means of testing chemopreventive interventions. To date, the most specific intermediate biomarkers for invasive breast cancer development are precancerous and preinvasive lesions, such as histologic changes of atypical hyperplasia, lobular carcinoma in situ (LCIS), and ductal carcinoma in situ (DCIS). Observations about the value of molecular alterations, for example, *c-erb*B-2 overexpression and *p53* accumulation, as markers of disease progression and increased risk in patients with benign breast conditions are contradictory.[40]

Intermediate biomarkers are essentially precancerous lesions identified as being directly on the control pathway to cancer. Their presence puts carriers at high risk for invasive disease. A hypothetical model of intraepithelial breast neoplasms postulates progression from focal aberrant ductal or lobular proliferation (hyperplasia) to cellular pleomorphism, disorganized growth, and abnormal growth (dysplasia), and, finally, focally invasive cancer.[41]

The histologic abnormalities, described by Page and colleagues[3] and collectively known as proliferative breast disease (PBD), are associated with increased risk of breast cancer; the lesions and associated risks of cancer development vary from moderate hyperplasia (two-fold risk), to atypical ductal hyperplasia (four-fold risk), to carcinoma in situ (CIS) (11-fold risk).[3,4,42]

The presence of these lesions in the contralateral breast of patients with a history of breast cancer has been associated with up to a 0.8 percent chance per year of developing a new primary tumor. In this context, these lesions appear to be the ideal target for chemo-prevention studies, the main advantage being the possibility of a more objective assessment of the effectiveness of interventions through repeated core biopsies.

In recent years, the availability of sensitive assays of DNA damage and genetic instability have prompted novel investigations and may help define subsets of women who are at high risk of developing breast cancer. Among the various molecular markers investigated, *p53* overexpression, dysplasia, and aneuploidy have been found to be associated with increased risk of invasive breast carcinoma.[43,44] Rohan and colleagues conducted a case-control study within a cohort of 4,888 Canadian women in the National Breast Screening Study (NBSS) who were diagnosed with benign breast disease. Case subjects were the women in whom breast cancer subsequently developed. The *c-erb*B-2 protein overexpression and *p53* accumulation were determined by immunohistochemical techniques. Accumulation of *p53* was associated with an increased risk of breast cancer (adjusted odds ratio 2.5), while *c-erb*B-2 protein overexpression was not.[44] Even with multiple methodologic problems, this investigation provides an interesting model for the clinical use of biomarkers in benign breast disease.

The design of prospective trials that includes the evaluation of *p53* status along with other markers studied in randomly obtained fine-needle aspirates may provide a unique opportunity to identify specific, measurable, intermediate biomarkers that may be used in short-term trials to verify the efficacy of chemopreventive agents.

ESTROGENS AND BREAST CANCER RISK

Endogenous Hormones

The controversy surrounding exogenous hormone use and breast cancer risk is predicated on the concept that breast carcinogenesis is a hormone-dependent process. The ability to control breast cancer with hormonal manipulation has been recognized since 1986, when Beatson reported on oophorectomy as a successful treatment for this disease.[45] Since that time several other epidemiologic, experimental and clinical lines of evidence have developed that also support this concept.[46]

It is well established that menstrual factors resulting in exposure of the breast to increased numbers of ovulatory estrogen cycles over a lifetime, such as early menarche (< 13 years), late menopause (> 50 years), and nulliparity can increase the risk of breast cancer.[46,47] Conversely, bilateral oophorectomy at a young age and interruptions of the menstrual cycle in the form of multiple pregnancies may confer a protective effect.[48]

The impact of pregnancy on the risk of breast cancer is strongest in the case of the first pregnancy occurring at a young age (before 20 years). The rate of proliferation of the ductal epithelium is normally high after puberty. The hormonal influences associated with pregnancy induce a process of terminal ductal and lobular stem cell differentiation, theoretically rendering the breast more resistant to carcinogenesis.[47,48] Henderson and colleagues hypothesized that completion of a full-term pregnancy is crucial for this protective effect because the rapid increase in free estradiol during the first trimester of pregnancy is "equivalent to several ovulatory cycles over a relatively short period of time." They hypothesized that failure to over-ride this estrogenic surge with the subsequent hormonal changes of advanced pregnancy (as occurs with first-trimester abortions) can result in increased risk of breast cancer.[49]

It is also well established that estrogen and progesterone exert proliferative effects on human breast tissue[49,50] and that estrogen can promote mammary tumorigenesis in animal models as well as in in vitro tissue cultures.[47–51]

Postmenopausal obesity has been associated with increased breast cancer risk, and this relationship appears to be mediated by age-related variations in estrogen metabolism. In the post-menopausal woman, androstenedione, synthesized in the adrenal gland, is the principal estrogen precursor following the decline of ovarian function. Increased conversion of androstenedione to estrone by fat cells that results in elevated levels of this predominant postmenopausal estrogen is reputed to be the underlying explanation for the increased risk of breast cancer seen in obese postmenopausal women.[47–52] In contrast, in premenopausal obese women, derangement of the estrogen-progesterone balance and subsequent menstrual disturbances result in a decreased risk of breast cancer.[50,53]

Male breast cancer is also likely to be related to factors resulting in abnormalities of estrogen metabolism, such as liver disease or genetic defects such as Klinefelter's syndrome.[53–55]

Exogenous Hormones

Oral Contraceptives

Oral contraceptives (OCs) have been marketed extensively over the past 30 to 40 years; worldwide users are estimated to be over 200 million women, and in the United States, it is projected that approximately 80 percent of all women will have used OCs by the age of 40 years.[48] Studies evaluating a possible association between OCs and breast cancer risk have been hampered by changes in the composition of OCs over time and by individual patient variation in the duration of use.[56–64]

Early evidence that OCs could significantly increase the risk of breast cancer was reported by Pike and colleagues in 1983.[56] In their case-control study of 314 breast cancer patients < 37 years of age and 314 matched controls, the use of OCs with a relatively high progesterone content for more than 6 years and starting use of OCs before age 25 years were associated with a relative risk of 4.9 for breast cancer development. Since that time, many studies have been conducted in the United States attempting to quantify the level of risk of breast cancer conferred by the use of OCs. The results of the largest studies are summarized in Table 2–2. Most studies[56–61,63] have been case-control studies, in which the rates of use of OCs among groups of breast cancer patients were compared with the rates of use of OCs among matched groups of noncancer patients. The results are relatively inconsistent, with some studies demonstrating an increased risk of breast cancer associated with use of OCs, whereas others demonstrate a protective effect associated with the use of OCs. It should be noted that in most studies, the relative risk estimate is close to unity, indicating that any effect of OCs is modest in magnitude. However, the high incidence of breast cancer in the United States suggests that even small increases in relative risk could translate into more cases of breast cancer.

One of the most widely quoted case-control studies on OCs and breast cancer is the Cancer and Steroid Hormone (CASH) Study by the Centers for Disease Control.[57] This project, first reported in 1983, evaluated 689 patients diagnosed with breast cancer between the ages of 20 and 54 years who were identified through the Surveillance, Epidemiology, and End Results (SEER) program. These patients were matched with 1,077 controls, and on initial analysis, the risk of breast cancer was lower for women that had been users of OCs than for women who never used OCs (relative risk, 0.9). Results of the CASH study were re-evaluated and reported in 1991 by Wingo and colleagues.[64] In this report, a particular focus was placed on the issue of OCs having variable, age-related associations with breast cancer risk. This analysis revealed a trend toward increased risk for users of OCs younger than 35 years (relative risk, 1.4), and a slight decrease in risk for users of OCs from 45 to 54 years of age (relative risk, 0.9).

The Nurses' Health Study[61] provides data regarding the relative risk of breast cancer among users of OCs followed up in a prospective fashion. In a cohort of more than 100,000 nurses with more than 1 million person-years of follow-up, no significant increase in breast cancer risk

Table 2–2. SUMMARY OF RANDOMIZED STUDIES EVALUATING THE RISK ASSOCIATED WITH THE USE OF ORAL CONTRACEPTIVES (OCs)

Study	Number of Patients	Age (y)	Years Use	Relative Risk
Pike[56]	314P	< 37	≥ 6	4.9
	314C			
CASH[57]	689P	< 55	> 4	1.1
	1,077C			
Stadel[58]	2,088P	< 45	> 4	1.1
	2,065C			
Miller[59]	521P	< 45	3–4	0.8
	521C		> 7	1.4
Jick[60]	127P	< 43	> 5	0.7
	174C		≥ 10	1.4
Romieu[61]	>118K	< 65	< 1	1.2
	Cohort		3	0.9

P = patients; C = controls; CASH = Cancer and Steriod Hormone Study, Centers for Disease Control.

was associated with the use of OCs. This relative risk was not affected appreciably by the duration of use, history of fibrocystic breast disease, or family history of breast cancer. These results were validated in an updated review of the Nurses' Health Study reported in 1997, with over 1.6 million person-years of follow-up.[62]

In 1996, a meta-analysis of 54 epidemiologic studies of OCs and breast cancer was published in *Lancet*.[65] This review compiled data on more than 53,000 breast cancer patients and more than 100,000 controls from 25 countries. Current users of OCs had a small but statistically significant increase in the risk of breast cancer (relative risk, 1.24; $p < .00001$), and this risk did not persist after 10 years following discontinuation of the OCs. The tumors detected in users of OCs were also found to be of earlier stage than those that were detected in women that did not use OCs. Two theoretical mechanisms could explain these findings. One explanation is related to the concept of estrogen acting as a promoter rather than as a cause of the neoplastic process. Under this circumstance, it would be expected that more tumors would be detected during and following use of OCs because the estrogen content would merely be expediting the clinical appearance of a pre-existing but previously occult tumor. The second explanation is that women who are users of OCs are necessarily receiving follow-up care, which presumably includes surveillance for breast cancer.

Hormone Replacement Therapy

The controversy surrounding hormone replacement therapy (HRT) and breast cancer is complicated not only by the prevalence of breast cancer but also by the fact that we live in an aging society. The health risks associated with the postmenopausal estrogen-deficient state, namely, cardiovascular disease and osteoporosis, are being faced by increasing numbers of women still in the prime years of their life.

Approximately one quarter of the American population is currently over the age of 55 years, and cardiovascular disease is the leading cause of death among postmenopausal women. Cardiovascular disease accounts for nearly three times as many deaths as cancer among women over the age of 65 years.[66] Osteoporosis afflicts approximately 25 million Americans, and it is estimated that half of all women will experience an osteoporotic fracture by the age of 75 years. In particular, hip fractures are a major problem; they are associated with a 34 percent mortality rate within 6 months, and the corresponding health-care costs are several billion dollars annually.[67]

Menopause also causes several other symptoms that have a significant adverse impact on the quality of life. Vasomotor symptoms are experienced by 80 percent of menopausal women; urinary incontinence, vaginal dryness, sleep disturbances, depression, anxiety, and memory losses are being reported increasingly and have all been related to changes in estrogen.[66,68–70]

Estrogen replacement therapy (ERT) in postmenopausal women has been proved to reverse several risk factors for cardiovascular disease, such as low high-density lipoprotein (HDL) cholesterol levels,[71] and ERT has been associated with a 40 to 60 percent reduction in complications of cardiovascular disease, such as

myocardial infarction and sudden death.[66,72–76] Estrogen replacement therapy also reduces rates of bone resorption by as much as 60 percent, thereby lowering rates of osteoporosis and osteoporotic fractures.[66,75,76] Unfortunately, ERT exerts a dose-dependent and duration-of-use–dependent proliferative effect on the uterine lining, and several studies have demonstrated an increased rate of endometrial cancer associated with ERT.[66,74,77–79] Results from the Postmenopausal Estrogen/Progestin Interventions (PEPI) trial, however, demonstrated that the addition of cyclic micronized progesterone to ERT negated the risk of endometrial hyperplasia (as measured by baseline and annual endometrial aspiration biopsy), without adversely affecting the favorable impact of ERT on the cholesterol profile.[71]

The effect of ERT on the risk of breast cancer remains an unresolved question. To date, no prospective, randomized study has been completed, and many of the patterns and inconsistencies demonstrated in the available data are similar to those seen in the published series of OC use and breast cancer. The results of several studies of HRT and breast cancer conducted in the United States and abroad are given in Table 2–3. The relative risk estimates[80–85] vary considerably. A protective effect was seen in the study by Gambrell and colleagues,[81] in which a relative risk of 0.3 was

Table 2–3. HORMONE REPLACEMENT THERAPY: BREAST CANCER RISK IN THE GENERAL POPULATION

Study	Year	Number of Women	Mean Number of Years Follow-Up	Relative Risk
Hoover[80]	1976	1,891	12	1.3
Gambrell[81]	1983	5,563	7	0.4
Hunt[82]	1987	4,544	6	1.59
Bergkvist[83]	1989	23,244	5.7	1.1
Mills[84]	1989	20,341	6	1.7
Colditz[85]	1995	23,965	16	1.321

associated with HRT (combined estrogen and progestin) among more than 5,500 women followed up at the Wilford Hall United States Air Force Medical Center. In this study, the relative risk estimate was calculated by comparing the observed breast cancer incidence with the incidence expected on the basis of the SEER program. Mills and colleagues[84] followed up a cohort of more than 20,000 Seventh Day Adventist women and found a relative risk of 1.7 associated with any history of HRT use; this relative risk increased to 2.5 for current HRT users, and to 2.8 for HRT users with a history of benign breast disease. In 1995, Colditz and colleagues[85] reported on findings from the Nurses' Health Study. A significant increase in the relative risk of breast cancer associated with current HRT use (relative risk, 1.32) was demonstrated.

Updated results of the Nurses' Health Study were published in 1997.[86] At the time of the updated report, more than 120,000 registered nurses had been followed up with biannual questionnaires since 1976, and more than 3,600 deaths had been documented. Several important findings were reported. Use of HRT was associated with significant decreases in mortality compared with nonuse (relative risk of death, 0.63). This benefit of HRT was strongest for women who had pre-existing risk factors for atherosclerotic heart disease (eg, current tobacco use, parental history of premature myocardial infarction, diabetes, or hypertension). For women considered to be at low risk for cardiac disease, there was a lesser benefit from HRT (relative risk of death, 0.89). After 10 years of HRT, however, mortality rates began to rise, predominantly from an increasing rate of breast cancer–related deaths.

In conclusion, the use of ERT and OCs appears to be associated with an increased risk of breast cancer, particularly in younger women.[87] In the presence of atherosclerotic disease and osteoporosis, the use of ERT seems to reduce the incidence of severe complications (eg, myocardial infarction and bone fractures) and appears to be associated with improved survival. Recommendation for routine use should be restricted to a select group of women, and the decision on treatment should be based on a detailed evaluation of the risk/benefit ratio.

BREAST CANCER CHEMOPREVENTIVE AGENTS

The importance of estrogens as breast cancer promoters has been sustained by direct and indirect observations since the 1960s. An important source of indirect evidence is provided by the relevant clinical observations derived from clinical trials of the adjuvant use of tamoxifen. Several large randomized studies have demonstrated that adjuvant therapy with the nonsteroidal antiestrogen tamoxifen citrate is associated with reduction in the risk of developing a second contralateral primary breast cancer by 30 to 50 percent.[88–90]

Table 2–4. SUMMARY OF ONGOING RANDOMIZED CHEMOPREVENTIVE TRIALS

Study	Agent	Number of Patients	Patient Population
BCPT-P1 (USA)[94]	TAM vs. placebo	13,388	High-risk, pre-/postmenopausal
Royal Marsden (UK)[93]	TAM vs. placebo	2,012	High-risk pre-/postmenopausal
National Tumor Institute (ITALY)[96]	TAM vs. placebo	5,408	Post-hysterectomy No risk of breast cancer, pre-/postmenopausal
MD Anderson Cancer Center (USA)[115]	TAM +/-4-HPR (pre-operative)	Ongoing	Ductal carcinoma in situ
National Tumor Institute (ITALY) 94[112]	4-HPR	2,972	History of breast cancer
STAR (USA)[94]	TAM vs. Raloxifene	Ongoing	High-risk, pre-/postmenopausal

BCPT = Breast Cancer Prevention Trial; NSABP = National Surgical Adjuvant Breast and Bowel Project; TAM = tamoxifen; 4-HPR = fenretinide (N-[4-hydroxyphenyl] retinamide, 4-HPR); STAR = Study of Tamoxifen and Raloxifene.

These observations confirm the central role for estrogens in the promotion of breast cancer and suggest an opportunity for developing a preventive strategy based on using selective antiestrogens to modulate estrogenic activity.

Preclinical data and clinical observations derived from clinical chemoprevention trials conducted in other malignancies indicated a potential activity of retinoids as chemopreventive agents. The major ongoing chemoprevention trials are listed on Table 2–4.

Tamoxifen

Tamoxifen is a nonsteroidal triphenylethylene derivative, which is generally classified as an antiestrogen with partial estrogen-agonist activity in some tissues. In fact, results from chemopreventive and adjuvant trials suggest that treatment with tamoxifen is associated with an increase in bone mineral density and decreased serum cholesterol, particularly in postmenopausal women.[91,92]

More importantly, the use of adjuvant tamoxifen following primary surgery for estrogen-sensitive early breast cancer has been associated with prolonged disease-free survival and reduction in the risk of death by 20 to 30 percent. One of the major arguments in favor of the use of tamoxifen as a chemopreventive agent is derived from the observation of a significant reduction in the incidence of primary tumors in the contralateral breast in women treated with adjuvant tamoxifen.[88,89,93,94]

The National Surgical Adjuvant Breast and Bowel Project (NSABP) and other European studies showed a reduction between 40 and 50 percent in the incidence of primary tumors in the contralateral breast among women taking tamoxifen as adjuvant therapy.[88,91,92] Among the European trials, the Stockholm trial, designed to evaluate the efficacy and toxicity of adjuvant tamoxifen (40 mg daily) for 2 years in postmenopausal patients (23 percent older than 50 years) with unilateral breast cancer, deserves particular mention.[90] This trial demonstrated a significant decrease in the incidence of contralateral breast cancer but also a six-fold increase in the incidence of endometrial cancer and an unexpected excess of gastrointestinal malignancies.

Of particular interest is the overview analysis of the major randomized trials of adjuvant tamoxifen among nearly 30,000 women with early breast cancer.[95] A recent update of this analysis demonstrated a reduction in the incidence of contralateral breast cancer incidence of 47 percent with 5 years of treatment. The proportional reduction in contralateral breast cancer appeared to be unrelated to the estrogen receptor (ER) status of the original tumor. The treatment appeared to be associated with a significant increase in the incidence of endometrial cancer and a slight, not significant increase in colorectal cancer (larger with only 1 year of tamoxifen).

In 1986, a pilot study was started in the United Kingdom to test the feasibility and toxicity associated with long-term tamoxifen treatment in women at high risk of breast cancer.[93] Between October 1986 and June 1993, a total of 2,012 women were accrued and randomly assigned to tamoxifen (20 mg/day) or placebo for up to 8 years. A total of 265 women were on HRT at entry and 131 were randomized to tamoxifen treatment. With a median follow-up of 36 months and with a compliance of 77 percent of the women assigned to the treatment arm, no obvious effect on bone mineral density was observed and only marginal effects on clotting factors. Tamoxifen was associated with a significant reduction in the serum cholesterol level. More importantly, there was an increased incidence of uterine fibromata and benign ovarian cysts; however, no increase in endometrial cancer incidence was reported.

On the basis of these encouraging data, in 1992, a large, multicenter, randomized, double-blind trial funded by the National Cancer Institute (NCI) was begun to test whether tamoxifen could prevent breast cancer in high-risk women.[94] The population at risk was defined, taking into account the following risk factors, as indicated by the Gail model: age, age at menarche and at first live birth, number of first-degree relatives affected, and, finally, the number of previous breast biopsies and the presence or absence of atypical hyperplasia.

The Breast Cancer Prevention Trial (BCPT-P1) enrolled 13,388 women older than 35 years between April 1992 and September 1997. The research, coordinated by the NSABP, involved more than 300 centers across the United States and Canada. The study was closed and preliminary results released 14 months earlier than planned.[94] In the median average follow-up time of 54.6 months, 89 cases of invasive breast cancer occurred in the group of women assigned to tamoxifen treatment (6,681 women) compared with 175 cases in the group assigned to placebo (6,707 women), corresponding to a 49 percent risk reduction. There was also a 50 percent reduction in the incidence of noninvasive breast cancer. Tamoxifen reduced the occurrence of ER-positive tumors by 69 percent, but no efficacy was seen in the prevention of ER-negative tumors. The risk reduction was not age dependent; the risk reduction in women aged 49 years or younger was 44 percent, and it was 55 percent in women older than 60 years. The NCI and the Endpoint Review, Safety Monitoring, and Advisory Committee agreed that the participants and their physicians should be told which treatment has been assigned because of the clear evidence that tamoxifen reduced breast cancer risk.

The Breast Cancer Prevention Trial was also designed to evaluate the possible benefit of tamoxifen in reducing cardiac events and osteoporosis-related complications. There was no difference between the tamoxifen group and the placebo group in the number of heart attacks, whereas there was a 19 percent reduction in the incidence of fractures of the hip, wrist, and spine (111 cases in the tamoxifen group versus 137 cases in the placebo group). Treatment with tamoxifen was associated with an increased incidence of endometrial cancer (33 cases versus 14 cases in the placebo group), in particular in women aged 50 years or older. A slight increase in the incidence of deep vein thrombosis and pulmonary embolism in the tamoxifen group was also reported; all these events were more frequently observed in women older than 50 years of age. Because of these reported complications, the decision about whether to use tamoxifen as a chemopreventive agent must be carefully weighed for every patient on the basis of an accurate evaluation of the patient's age group, personal breast cancer risks, and comorbid conditions.

Similar trials of tamoxifen for chemoprevention have been conducted in Italy and the United Kingdom.[96] The Italian study has completed accrual of 5,408 women who have had hysterectomy and have no factors associated with increased risk of breast cancer. Preliminary analysis at a median follow-up of 46 months did not show any difference in breast cancer incidence in the tamoxifen group compared with the placebo-control group.[96] Differences in the study populations, age distributions, history of HRT, and family history may account for the inability of studies to confirm the effectiveness of tamoxifen for chemoprevention.

Selective Estrogen Receptor Modulators

In the past decade, the reports of significant side effects associated with the prolonged use of tamoxifen have stimulated research directed toward the development of other selective estrogen receptor modulators (SERMs). Among the various products investigated, raloxifene has demonstrated antitumor activity and a favorable toxicity profile and is being further investigated.[97–99]

Preclinical data have shown that raloxifene, an antiestrogen with no estrogen-agonist effect on the uterus, inhibits mammary carcinogenesis in a rat model of breast cancer in a manner similar to tamoxifen when raloxifene is used in combination with *9-cis* retinoic acid.[97] Clinical trials have been started in an attempt to establish the role of raloxifene in preventing osteoporosis in postmenopausal women, and preliminary results from two randomized clinical trials have recently become available. The Multiple Outcomes of Raloxifene Evaluation (MORE) trial was specifically designed to evaluate the possibility of reducing the risk of fractures in postmenopausal women receiving raloxifene; a markedly reduced risk of newly diagnosed breast cancer was demonstrated with raloxifene compared with placebo (0.21% versus 0.82%).[100] Jordan and colleagues recently reported the results of a multicenter, double-blind randomized trial conducted in about 12,000 women. Treatment with raloxifene was associated with a 58 percent reduction in the risk of developing primary breast cancer.[101] These results have stimulated the design of a second major breast cancer prevention trial, the Study of Tamoxifen and Raloxifene (STAR) that will compare the toxicity, risks, and benefits of raloxifene with those of tamoxifen. Women enrolled in the study will be randomly assigned to receive either 20 mg of tamoxifen or 60 mg of raloxifene for 5 years, with follow-up planned for an additional 2 years.

A number of other SERMs have emerged (eg, toremifene, trioxifene, droloxifene, TAT-59) for clinical use.[102–105] The majority of these drugs are presently in phase I to II clinical trials and have already demonstrated their clinical activity in the management of breast cancer. They represent possible candidates for future chemoprevention studies.

Retinoids

Retinoids are a family of natural and synthetic compounds structurally related to vitamin A. They are a group of molecules capable of influencing many biologic functions, such as proliferation, differentiation, and induction of apoptosis.[106–109] Retinoids function via two types of nuclear receptors, the retinoid alpha-receptors (RARs) and the retinoid X receptors (RXRs), each of which is encoded by three genes.[93]

Preclinical data have demonstrated that carcinogen-induced mammary carcinomas are sensitive to the antiproliferative effects of retinoids. Enhanced sensitivity has been shown by estrogen receptor–positive cell lines, whereas estrogen receptor–negative cell lines have shown minimal sensitivity to these compounds.[110,111] The mechanisms of the antiproliferative effect are still being investigated. At least, in some cell lines, apoptosis, instead of differentiation, seems to be the prevalent mechanism of growth inhibition.[111]

A synthetic retinoid, fenretinide (N-[4-hydroxyphenyl] retinamide, 4-HPR), has demonstrated the capacity to inhibit the growth of breast cancer cell lines and chemically induced mammary tumors in rats, without the toxicity associated with other retinoids. This compound was the first retinoid to be tested in clinical trials and has been proved to be well tolerated at a daily dose of 200 mg with a 3-day monthly drug holiday.[112,113]

An Italian prospective randomized trial designed to evaluate the role of fenretinide in reducing the incidence of contralateral breast cancer began in March 1987. In July 1993, accrual of 2,972 women, age 30 to 70 years, with history of T1-2, N0 breast cancer was completed.[112] Preliminary data suggested that fenretinide can reduce the incidence of ovarian carcinomas.[113] Though safer than other retinoids in experimental models, fenretinide produced visual (dark adaptation) and ophthalmologic complaints (ocular dryness, lacrimation, conjunctivitis, photophobia) in 20 percent and 8 percent of women, respectively, at 5 years.[114] Such effects are thought to be caused by the reduction of plasma retinal levels, which occurs after administration of the retinoid.

In animal models, 9-*cis*-retinoic acid in combination with antiestrogens (tamoxifen or raloxifene) resulted in effective chemoprevention of a rat model of breast cancer induced by the carcinogen nitrosomethylurea.[97,111]

The University of Texas M. D. Anderson Cancer Center is presently investigating the role of tamoxifen and fenretinide in reducing the risk of invasive breast cancer in patients diagnosed with DCIS.[115] This phase II trial is accruing women presenting with small breast lesions and mammographic calcifications suspicious for malignancy. After histologic confirmation through core biopsies, participants are randomly assigned to receive tamoxifen, fenretinide, or a combination of both. The treatment is planned for 3 weeks before definitive surgery. An important objective of this trial is to perform a detailed quantitative assessment of biomarkers to be used as surrogate end points. The proposed SEBs include estrogen and progesterone receptors, nuclear retinoid receptors, transforming growth factor (TGF)-β, *HER-2/neu*, proliferation (Ki-67 immunostaining), angiogenesis (factor VIII) markers, and chromosomal aberrations. This trial is expected to provide insight into the biologic mechanisms of antiestrogens and retinoids, or the combination of both, in reducing the progression of DCIS to invasive cancer.

Dietary Interventions

Epidemiologic observations of large international differences in the incidence of breast cancer have provided a basis for formulating hypotheses on a possible relation between diet and the development of cancer. The age-adjusted incidence of breast cancer varies from 22 per 100,000 in Japan to 68 per 100,000 in the Netherlands.[116] The ratio of breast cancer mortality between the United States and Japan is 3:1 for premenopausal women and 8:1 for postmenopausal women.[117] These important differences may possibly be related to fat intake and total calories in the diet. Clinical data collected from case-control studies have demonstrated a positive correlation between diets high in fat and meat and breast cancer.[118–122] Experimental studies have shown that omega-6 polyunsaturated fatty acids (PUFAs) contained in high-fat diets promote both mammary tumorigenesis and cell proliferation in chemically induced mammary tumors, whereas omega-3 PUFAs, contained in fish oil, can inhibit these effects.[119,120]

Heterocyclic amines, a group of mutagenic compounds identified in cooked foods, seem to be related to the increased risk of breast cancer associated with high intake of well-done meat. Recently, a case-control study among 41,836 women demonstrated that women who consumed well-done meats, including hamburger, beef steak, and bacon, had higher adjusted odds ratios for breast cancer (up to 4.62), if they consumed all three different meats well done.[121]

These data have provided the rationale for diet interventions, consisting of a low-fat diet and fish-oil supplements, that have been found to be able to produce increases in total omega-3 PUFAs in adipose tissue and in the ratio of omega-3/omega-6 PUFAs in patients with breast cancer.[120] The Canadian Diet and Breast Cancer Prevention Study Group has conducted a multicenter randomized trial involving women with breast densities detected on mammography and showed that after 2 years of a low-fat diet, with less than 15 percent of calories from fat, there was a significant reduction in the number of radiographic abnormalities.[122] Adjuvant dietary recommendations of 15 percent of calories from fat for women with postmenopausal breast cancer are currently being evaluated in the Women's Intervention Nutrition Study and in the Women's Healthy Eating and Living Study.[123]

The role of alcohol consumption and smoking are also being extensively investigated as possible risk factors for breast cancer. While the majority of the studies has documented that high alcohol intake is associated with a significant increased incidence of breast cancer, no definitive pathogenetic role for active or passive smoking has been demonstrated.[124,125]

The use of natural products contained in essential oils and soy-based products, for example, the monoterpenes limonene and perillyl alcohol and the isoflavonoid genistein, all showed preclinical evidence of tumor regression.[126–129] The effects of limonene and limonene-related monoterpenes, perillyl alcohol and perillic acid, on cell growth, cell cycle progression, and expression of cyclin D1 has been investigated in T-4D, MCF-7, MDA-MB-231 breast cancer cell lines. The results revealed that limonene-related monoterpenes caused a dose-dependent inhibition of cell proliferation. Of the three monoterpenes tested, perillyl alcohol was the most potent and limonene was the least potent inhibitor of cell growth. Growth inhibition induced by perillyl alcohol and perillic acid was associated with a fall in the proportion of cells in the S phase, accumulation of cells in the G1 phase, and a decrease in cyclin D1 mRNA levels.[128] The potential preventive role of genistein, a component of soy, has been evaluated in rats. Pharmacologic doses of genistein given to immature rats enhance mammary gland differentiation, resulting in a significantly less proliferate gland that is not as suspectible to mammary cancer.[129] These components are presently being tested in several clinical chemopreventive studies.

SURGICAL PROPHYLAXIS AND MODULATION OF RISK

Prophylactic Mastectomy

It seems intuitive that mastectomy would be an effective means of preventing breast cancer, especially in this era of immediate reconstruction techniques that produce cosmetically acceptable results. However, animal models as well as clinical data from trials in humans have confirmed that this is not always the case. Studies have demonstrated that even total mastectomy (defined as removal of the entire breast, including the nipple-areolar complex, but sparing the axillary contents) is frequently incomplete; microscopic amounts of breast tissue may be left in the skin flaps, attached to the pectoralis fascia and extending into the axilla. Temple and colleagues[130] evaluated 10 prophylactic mastectomy specimens from 5 patients considered to be at high risk for developing breast cancer. In this study, random frozen sec-

tion analyses (approximately 700 per breast) of the margins identified 3 cases of breast tissue extending into the pectoralis fascia, 1 case of pectoralis muscle involvement, 2 cases of inferior skin flap involvement, and 1 case of axillary tissue involvement. It would be expected that prophylactic subcutaneous mastectomy (defined as removal of all gross breast tissue, usually via an inframammary incision, but sparing the nipple-areolar complex) would result in additional breast tissue left on the skin flaps of the nipple-areolar complex.

The clinical significance of retained breast tissue in the setting of prophylactic mastectomy for humans is not yet defined. In the rodent model of mammary tumors and prophylactic mastectomy, it is clear that the extent of breast tissue removed does not clearly correlate with the extent of protection against breast cancer. Wong and colleagues[131] performed varying degrees of partial versus total mastectomy versus sham surgery in a series of rats, either before or after administration of the carcinogen DMBA; at 8 months of age, there were no significant differences in the number of carcinogen-induced tumors between any of the groups. Using a mouse model with a high incidence of spontaneous mammary tumor development (and therefore theoretically more similar to the human experience of spontaneous breast cancer incidence) Nelson and colleagues[132] similarly found no difference in the number of tumors that developed in mice that underwent either sham surgery, 50 percent mastectomy, or total mastectomy.

Data on prophylactic bilateral mastectomy in humans are limited. The often-cited studies by Pennisi and Capozzi[133] and Woods and Meland[134] in the plastic surgery literature each reported on at least 1,500 women who underwent subcutaneous mastectomies, and in both studies, the subsequent incidence of breast carcinoma was less than 1 percent. However, both these studies have been criticized for their limited applicability to truly high-risk women, since many of the prophylactic procedures were performed in women who would be considered at the present time to be at only low or intermediate risk for breast cancer. Detailed follow-up information is also lacking in these large series.

It remains to be determined if a prophylactic mastectomy is clearly indicated in women at high risk of developing breast cancer. Women with *BRCA1* mutations, who may have a cumulative breast cancer risk of 40 to 85 percent, would be the obvious candidates.

Schrag and colleagues[135] developed a statistical decision model to calculate the benefit that *BRCA1* or *BRCA2* mutation carriers might derive from prophylactic mastectomy. Using a risk-reduction estimate of 85 percent associated with prophylactic mastectomy, this study determined that a 30-year-old *BRCA1* mutation carrier would gain 2.9 to 5.3 years of life expectancy following preventive surgery. Lynch and colleagues[136] reported on the results of a series of women who had undergone extensive genetic counseling and subsequently tested positive for *BRCA1* gene mutations. Only 35 percent of these patients said they would consider undergoing prophylactic mastectomy. This finding underscores the complexity of identifying high-risk women who will benefit psychologically as well as clinically from preventive surgery.

In addition, there are many case reports documenting the failure of prophylactic total mastectomy to protect against breast cancer.[137–141]

However, very intriguing data were recently reported by Hartmann and colleagues from the Mayo Clinic.[142] A retrospective analysis was performed on 639 women with moderate or high risk for breast cancer (by family history) that had undergone bilateral prophylactic subcutaneous mastectomy between 1960 and 1993. The breast cancer incidence in these women was compared with the number of expected cases based on the Gail model and with the number of cases that occurred among female siblings who had not undergone prophylactic surgery; these estimations revealed an approximately 90 percent reduction in breast cancer

risk associated with prophylactic mastectomy.

Another patient population that might be considered to be suitable for prophylactic mastectomy is women with a history of unilateral breast cancer, in whom the risk of subsequent contralateral breast cancer is approximately 0.5 to 0.7 percent per year.[143] However, it has been argued that the risk of death from the primary cancer is still greater than the risk of developing a second primary cancer for the majority of breast cancer patients, making the survival benefit of prophylactic surgery questionable.[144] On the other hand, the rationale has also been offered that optimal immediate reconstruction cosmesis can be attained with bilateral transverse rectus abdominis myocutaneous (TRAM) flaps. To address this issue Kroll and colleagues[145] studied 88 patients with unilateral breast cancer who had undergone bilateral mastectomies with immediate breast reconstruction. Previously unsuspected invasive breast cancer was found in 3.4 percent of the contralateral mastectomy specimens.

The Society of Surgical Oncology has delineated categories of patients for whom prophylactic mastectomy may reasonably be considered on the basis of clinical features (and not including genetic testing results).[144] For women with no history of breast cancer, the indications include atypical hyperplasia, family history of premenopausal bilateral breast cancer, and dense, nodular breasts associated with atypical hyperplasia. For women with a known unilateral breast cancer, the indications for considering contralateral prophylactic mastectomy include diffuse microcalcifications, LCIS, a large, difficult-to-evaluate breast, history of LCIS, and family history of early-onset breast cancer.

Prophylactic Oophorectomy and/or Hysterectomy

Several studies have documented lower breast cancer incidence among women who underwent oophorectomy at a young age. The effect of hysterectomy on breast cancer risk is less clear, but it has been postulated that hysterectomy may have some secondary effects by affecting ovarian blood flow and ovulation. Schairer and colleagues evaluated 15,844 women undergoing surgery in the Uppsala health care region of Sweden and found a 50 percent reduction in breast cancer risk in those women who underwent bilateral oophorectomy prior to age 50 years, compared with the risk of the background population.[146] Hysterectomy alone had no consistent association with change in breast cancer risk. In a case-control series from Italy, women who underwent premenopausal oophorectomy with hysterectomy or hysterectomy alone had reduced relative risk of developing breast cancer (0.8 and 0.7, respectively).[147] However, given the importance of the ovarian function in maintaining cardiovascular and bone health, there are presently no indications for recommending these procedures as prophylaxis against breast cancer in any subset of patients.

CONCLUSIONS

The recently reported encouraging results with the use of tamoxifen and the ongoing clinical trials introducing SERMs (raloxifene), retinoids, and other approaches suggest an increasing awareness in physicians of the field of chemoprevention and its potentially enormous socioeconomic implications. Breast cancer chemoprevention is a field in constant evolution and has the potential to significantly affect the lives of thousands of women by reducing their risk of breast cancer.

In the last decade, the increasing information available on the differential contribution of genetic, dietary, and environmental factors has greatly improved our ability to determine the absolute breast cancer risk for every woman and properly select high-risk groups for interventional studies. Interestingly, the concomitant evaluation of histopathologic factors and multiple biomarkers has offered the opportunity to increase our understanding of the important biologic modifications associated with tumor progression. In the future, prospective clinical trials of chemoprevention strategies should be limited to high-risk populations identified on the basis of a combination of epidemiologic, histopathologic, and genetic data and should make use of SEBs to evaluate the efficacy of drug interventions. This approach will contribute greatly to reducing the patient population under study, eventually reducing the costs related to these investigations and helping to clarify the biology of each drug's mechanism of action.

The initial results of the BCPT-P1 have demonstrated, for the first time, the possibility of reducing the risk of breast cancer in a high-risk group of women, with a marginal toxicity. The ongoing STAR preventive trial is designed to determine if raloxifene has a chemopreventive efficacy comparable with tamoxifen with less associated toxicity. In the meantime, a longer follow-up of the BCPT-P1 trial will clarify if the treatment with tamoxifen represents a true preventive intervention or a treatment for preclinical conditions with consequent delaying of the onset of invasive breast cancer.

The potential role of dietary intervention in modifying the risk of breast cancer is probably presently underestimated; the ongoing clinical trials may contribute essential information to their potential clinical applicability.

In conclusion, more attention should be directed to the biologic relationships among hormone modulation, diet, and the risk of breast cancer to develop an "ideal lifestyle model" to propose for the high-risk groups. In this context, the role of prophylactic surgery, with the psychologic consequences related to the change in body image, even if associated with improved outcome in high-risk women, will come to be considered as a secondary, rather than a primary, option for breast cancer risk management.

REFERENCES

1. Chu KC, Tarone RE, Kessler LG, et al. Recent trends in U.S. breast cancer incidence, survival,

and mortality rates. J Natl Cancer Inst 1996; 88:1571–9.

2. Vogel VG. Subjects and recruitment strategies for a short-term phase II chemoprevention trial of breast cancer using surrogate endpoint biomarkers. J Cell Biochem 1993;17G:257–8.

3. Page DL, Dupont WD, Rogers LW. Atypical hyperplastic lesions of the female breast. A long-term follow-up study. Cancer 1985;55:2698–708.

4. Dupont WD, Page DL. Relative risk of breast cancer varies with time since diagnosis of atypical hyperplasia. Hum Pathol 1989;20:723–5.

5. Hill AD, Doyle JM, McDermott EW. Hereditary breast cancer. Br J Surg 1997;84:1334–9.

6. Tseng SL, Yu IC, Yue CT, et al. Allelic loss at *BRCA1, BRCA2*, and adjacent loci in relation to *TP53* abnormality in breast cancer. Genes Chromosomes Cancer 1997;20:377–82.

7. Sporn MB, Newton DL. Chemoprevention of cancer and retinoids. Fed Proc 1979;38:2528–34.

8. Kelloff GJ, Boone CW, Steele VE. Progress in cancer chemoprevention: perspectives on agent selection and short-term clinical intervention trials. Cancer Res 1994;54:2015S–24S.

9. Kelloff GJ, Boone CW, Crowell JA, et al. Surrogate endpoint biomarkers for phase II cancer chemoprevention trials. J Cell Biochem Suppl 1994;19:1–9.

10. Grizzle WE, Myers RB, Arnold MM, Srivastava S. Evaluation of biomarkers in breast and prostate cancer. J Cell Biochem Suppl 1994;19:259–66.

11. Fabian CJ, Kamel S, Zalles C, Kimler BF. Identification of a chemoprevention cohort from a population of women at high risk for breast cancer. J Cell Biochem 1996;25S:112–22.

12. Gail MH, Brinton LA, Byar DP, et al. Projecting individualized probabilities of developing breast cancer for white females who are being examined annually. J Natl Cancer Inst 1989;81:1879–86.

13. Benichou J, Gail MH, Mulvihill JJ. Graphs to estimate an individualized risk of breast cancer. J Clin Oncol 1996;14(1):103–10.

14. Smith J. New computer program assesses a woman's risk for developing breast cancer. J Natl Cancer Inst 1998;90(18):1332.

15. Lynch HT, Krush AJ. The cancer family syndrome and cancer control. Surg Gynecol Obstet 1971;132:247–50.

16. Marcus JN, Watson P, Page DL, et al. Hereditary breast cancer: pathobiology, prognosis, and *BRCA1* and *BRCA2* gene linkage. Cancer 1996;77:697–709.

17. Ford D, Easton DF, Petro J. Estimates of the gene frequency of BRCA1 and its contribution to breast and ovarian cancer incidence. Am J Hum Genet 1995;57:1457–62.

18. Struewing JP, Hartge P, Wacholder S, et al. The risk of cancer associated with specific mutations of BRCA1 and BRCA2 among Ashkenazi Jews. N Engl J Med 1997;336:1401–8.

19. Shattuck-Eidens D, Oliphant A, McClure M, et al. BRCA1 sequence analysis in women at high risk for susceptibility mutations. JAMA 1997;278:1242–50.

20. Couch FJ, DeShano M, Blackwood MA, et al. BRCA1 mutations in women attending clinics that evaluate the risk of breast cancer. N Engl J Med 1997;336:1409–15.

21. Iglehart JD, Miron A, Rimer BK, et al. Overestimation of hereditary breast cancer risk. Ann Surg 1998;228(3):375–84.

22. Krainer M, Silva-Arrieta S, FitzGerald MG, et al. Differential contributions of *BRCA1* and *BRCA2* to early onset breast cancer. N Engl J Med 1997;336:1416–21.

23. Prechtel D, Werenskiold AK, Prechtel K, et al. Frequent loss of heterozygosity at chromosome 13q12-13 with BRCA2 markers in sporadic male breast cancer. Diagn Mol Pathol 1998;7(1):57–62.

24. Malkin D, Li FP, Strong LC, et al. Germ line *p53* mutations in a familial syndrome of breast cancer, sarcomas, and other neoplasms. Science 1990;250:1233–8.

25. Swift M, Morrell D, Massey RB, Chase DL. Incidence of cancer in 161 families affected by ataxia-telangiectasia. N Engl J Med 1991;325:1831–6.

26. Tokunaga M, Land CE, Yammoto T, et al. Incidence of female breast cancer among atomic bomb survivors, Hiroshima and Nagasaki, 1950–1980. Radiat Res 1987;112:243–72.

27. Mackenzie I. Breast cancer following multiple fluoroscopies. Br J Cancer 1965;19:1–8.

28. Miller AB, Howe GR, Sherman GJ, et al. Mortality from breast cancer after irradiation during fluoroscopic examinations in patients being treated for tuberculosis. N Engl J Med 1989;321:1285–9.

29. Shore RE, Hildreth N, Woodard E, et al. Breast cancer among women given x-ray therapy for acute postpartum mastitis. J Natl Cancer Inst 1986;77:689–96.

30. Hildreth NG, Shore RE, Dvoretsky PM. The risk of breast cancer after irradiation of the thymus in infancy. N Engl J Med 1989;321:1281–4.

31. Goss PE, Sierra S. Current perspectives on radiation-inducted breast cancer. J Clin Oncol 1998; 16(1):338–47.

32. van Leeuwen FE, Klockman WJ, Hagenbeek A, et al. Second cancer risk following Hodgkin's disease: a 20-year follow-up study. J Clin Oncol 1994;12:312–25.

33. Kaldor JM, Day NE, Brand P, et al. Second malignancies following testicular cancer, ovarian cancer and Hodgkin's disease: an international collaborative study among cancer registries. Int J Cancer 1987;39:571–85.

34. Tucker MA, Coleman CN, Cox RS, et al. Risk of second cancers after treatment for Hodgkin's disease. N Engl J Med 1988;318:76–81.

35. Hancock SL, Tucker MA, Hoppe RT. Breast cancer after treatment of Hodgkin's disease. J Natl Cancer Inst 1993;85:25–31.

36. Sankila R, Garwicz S, Olsen JH, et al. Risk of subsequent malignant neoplasm among 1641 Hodgkin's disease patients diagnosed in childhood and adolescence: a population-based cohort study in the five Nordic countries. J Clin Oncol 1996;14:1442–6.

37. Aisenberg AC, Finkelstein DM, Doppke KP, et al. High risk of breast carcinoma after irradiation of young women with Hodgkin's disease. Cancer 1997;79(6):1203–10.

38. Feig SA, Hendrick RE. Radiation risk from screening mammography of women aged 40-49 years [Monogr]. J Natl Cancer Inst 1997; (22):119–24.

39. Marshall CJ, Schumann GB, Ward JH, et al. Cytologic identification of clinically occult proliferative breast disease in women with a family history of breast cancer. Ann Pathol 1991;95: 157–65.

40. McKittrick R, Fabian C, Kamel S, et al. Dysplasia and other biomarker abnormalities as potential surrogate endpoint biomarkers in breast chemoprevention trials [abstract]. Proc Am Soc Clin Oncol 1995;14:A348.

41. Alpers CE, Wellings SR. The prevalence of carcinoma in situ in normal and cancer-associated breast. Hum Pathol 1985;16:796–807.

42. Frykberg ER, Bland KI. In situ breast carcinoma. Adv Surg 1993;26:29–72.

43. Eriksson ET, Schimmelpenning H, Aspenblad U, et al. Immunohistochemical expression of the mutant p53 protein and nuclear DNA content during the transition from benign to malignant breast disease. Hum Pathol 1994;25: 1228–33.

44. Rohan TE, Hartwick W, Miller AB, Kandel RA. Immunohistochemical detection of c-erbB-2 and p53 in benign breast disease and breast cancer risk. J Natl Cancer Inst 1998;90:126–9.

45. Beatson GT. On the treatment of inoperable cases of carcinoma of the mamma: suggestions for a new method of treatment with illustrative cases. Lancet 1986;2:104–7.

46. Kelsey JL, Gammon MD. The epidemiology of breast cancer. CA Cancer J Clin 1991;41:147–65.

47. Hulka BS, Liu ET, Lininger RA. Steroid hormones and risk of breast cancer. Cancer 1994; 74:1111–24.

48. Russo J, Tay LK, Russo IH. Differentiation of the mammary gland and susceptibility to carcinogenesis. Breast Cancer Res Treat 1982;2:5–73.

49. Henderson BE, Ross R, Bernstein L. Estrogens as a cause of human cancer: the Richard and Hilda Rosenthal Foundation Award Lecture. Cancer Res 1988;48:246–53.

50. Pike MC, Spicer DV, Dahmoush L, Press MF. Estrogens, progestogens, normal breast cell proliferation, and breast cancer risk. Epidemiol Rev 1993;15:17–35.

51. Spicer DV, Pike MC. Breast cancer prevention through modulation of endogenous hormones. Breast Cancer Res Treat 1993;28:179–93.

52. Dickson RB, Thompson EW, Lippman ME. Regulation of proliferation, invasion, and growth factor synthesis in breast cancer by steroids. J Steroid Biochem Mol Biol 1990;37:305–16.

53. Cauley JA, Gutal JP, Kuller LH, et al. The epidemiology of serum sex hormones in postmenopausal women. Am J Epidemiol 1989;129:1120–31.

54. Moore M. Male breast cancer. In: Harris JR, Lippman ME, Morrow M, Hellman S, editors. Diseases of the breast. Philadelphia: Lippincott-Raven; 1996. p. 859.

55. Committee on the Relationship Between Oral Contraceptives and Breast Cancer. Institute of Medicine, Division of Health Promotion and Disease Prevention. Oral contraceptives and breast cancer. Washington, D.C.: National Academy Press; 1991.

56. Pike MC, Henderson BE, Krailo MD, et al. Breast cancer in young women and use of oral contraceptives: possible modifying effect of formulation and age at use. Lancet 1983;2:926–9.

57. The Centers for Disease Control Cancer and Steroid Hormone Study. Long-term oral contraceptive use and the risk of breast cancer. JAMA 1983;249:1591–5.

58. Stadel BV, Rubin GL, Webster LA, et al. Oral con-

traceptives and breast cancer in young women. Lancet 1985;2:970–3.

59. Miller DR, Rosenberg L, Kaufman DW, et al. Breast cancer risk in relation to early contraceptive use. Obstet Gynecol 1986;68:863–8.

60. Jick SS, Walker AM, Stergachis A, Jick H. Oral contraceptives and breast cancer. Br J Cancer 1989;59:618–21.

61. Romieu I, Willett WC, Colditz GA, et al. Prospective study of oral contraceptive use and risk of breast cancer in women. J Natl Cancer Inst 1989;81:1313–21.

62. Hankinson SE, Colditz GA, Manson JE, et al. A prospective study of oral contraceptive use and risk of breast cancer (Nurses' Health Study, United States). Cancer Causes Control 1997;8: 65–72.

63. Weinstein AL, Mahoney MC, Nasca PC, et al. Breast cancer risk and oral contraceptive use: results from a large case-control study. Epidemiology 1991;2:353–8.

64. Wingo PA, Lee NC, Ory HW, et al. Age-specific differences in the relationship between oral contraceptive use and breast cancer. Obstet Gynecol 1991;78:161–70.

65. Collaborative Group on Hormonal Factors in Breast Cancer. Breast cancer and hormonal contraceptives. Collaborative reanalysis of individual data on 53,297 women with breast cancer and 100,239 women without breast cancer from 54 epidemiological studies. Lancet 1996;347:1713–27.

66. Smith HO, Kammerer-Doak DN, Barbo DM, Sarto GE. Hormone replacement therapy in the menopause: a pro opinion. CA Cancer J Clin 1996;46:343–63.

67. Consensus Conference. Osteoporosis. JAMA 1984;252:799–802.

68. Bhatia NN, Bergman A, Karram MM. Effects of estrogen on urethral function in women with urinary incontinence. Am J Obstet Gynecol 1989;160:176–81.

69. Campbell S, Whitehead M. Oestrogen therapy and the menopausal syndrome. Clin Obstet Gynecol 1977;4:31–47.

70. Sherwin BB. Estrogen and cognitive function in women. Proc Soc Exper Biol Med 1998;217:17.

71. The Writing Group for the PEPI Trial. Effects of estrogen or estrogen/progestin regimens on heart disease risk factors in postmenopausal women: the Postmenopausal Estrogen/Progestin Interventions (PEPI) trial. JAMA 1995; 273:199–208.

72. Stampfer MJ, Colditz GA. Estrogen replacement therapy and coronary heart disease: a quantitative assessment of the epidemiologic evidence. Prev Med 1991;20:47–63.

73. Wenger NK, Speroff L, Packard B. Cardiovascular health and disease in women. N Engl J Med 1993;329:247–56.

74. Grady D, Rubin SM, Petitti DB, et al. Hormone therapy to prevent disease and prolong life in postmenopausal women. Ann Intern Med 1992;117:1016–37.

75. Lindsay R. Estrogen therapy in the prevention and management of osteoporosis. Am J Obstet Gynecol 1987;156:1347–51.

76. Weiss NS, Ufe CL, Ballard JH, et al. Decreased risk of fractures of the hip and lower forearm with postmenopausal use of estrogen. N Engl J Med 1980;303:1195–8.

77. Mack TM, Pike MC, Henderson BE, Pfeffer RI. Estrogens and endometrial cancer in a retirement community. N Engl J Med 1976;294:1261–2.

78. Boring JE, Bain CJ, Ehrmann RL. Conjugated estrogen use and risk of endometrial cancer. Am J Epidemiol 1986;124:434–41.

79. Antunes CM, Stolley PD, Rosenshein NB, et al. Endometrial cancer and estrogen use: report of a large case-control study. N Engl J Med 1979; 300:9–13.

80. Hoover R, Gray LA, Cole P, MacMahon B. Menopausal estrogens and breast cancer. N Engl J Med 1976;295:401–5.

81. Gambrell RD, Maier RC, Sanders BI. Decreased incidence of breast cancer in postmenopausal estrogen-progestogen users. Obstet Gynecol 1983;62:435–43.

82. Hunt K, Vessey M, McPherson K, Coleman M. Long-term surveillance of mortality and cancer incidence in women receiving hormone replacement therapy. Br J Obstet Gynecol 1987;94:620–35.

83. Bergkvist L, Adami H-O, Persson I, et al. The risk of breast cancer after estrogen and estrogen-progestin replacement. N Engl J Med 1989; 321:293–7.

84. Mills PK, Beeson L, Phillips RL, Fraser GE. Prospective study of exogenous hormone use and breast cancer in Seventh-Day Adventists. Cancer 1989;64:591–7.

85. Colditz GA, Hankinson SE, Hunter DJ, et al. The use of estrogens and progestins and the risk of breast cancer in postmenopausal women. N Engl J Med 1995;332:1589–93.

86. Grodstein F, Stampfer MJ, Colditz GA, et al. Post-

menopausal hormone therapy and mortality. N Engl J Med 1997;336:1769–75.

87. Colditz GA. Relationship between estrogen levels, use of hormone replacement therapy, and breast cancer. J Natl Cancer Inst 1998;90(11):814–23.

88. Fornander T, Rutqvist LE, Cedermark B, et al. Adjuvant tamoxifen in early breast cancer: occurrence of new primary cancers. Lancet 1989;1:117–20.

89. Andersson M, Storm HH, Mouridsen HT. Incidence of new primary cancers after adjuvant tamoxifen therapy and radiotherapy for early breast cancer. J Natl Cancer Inst 1991;83:1013–7.

90. Rutqvist LE, Johansson H, Signomklao T, et al. Adjuvant tamoxifen therapy for early stage breast cancer and second primary malignancies. J Natl Cancer Inst 1995;87:645–51.

91. Chang J, Powles TJ, Ashley SE, et al. The effect of tamoxifen and hormone replacement therapy on serum cholesterol, bone mineral density and coagulation factors in healthy postmenopausal women participating in a randomized, controlled tamoxifen prevention study. Ann Oncol 1996;7(7):671–5.

92. Powles TJ, Hickish T, Kanis JA, et al. Effect of tamoxifen on bone mineral density measured by dual-energy x-ray absorptiometry in healthy premenopausal and postmenopausal women. J Clin Oncol 1996;14(1):78–84.

93. Powles TJ, Jones AL, Ashley SE, et al. The Royal Marsden Hospital pilot tamoxifen chemoprevention trial. Breast Cancer Res Treat 1994;31:73–82.

94. Fisher B, Joseph P, Costantino D, et al., and other NSABP investigators. Tamoxifen for prevention of breast cancer: report of the National Surgical Adjuvant Breast and Bowel Project P-1 study. J Natl Cancer Inst 1998;90:1371–88.

95. Early Breast Cancer Trialists' Collaborative Group. Tamoxifen for early breast cancer: an overview of the randomized trials. Lancet 1998;351:1451–67.

96. Veronesi U, Maisonneuve P, Costa A, et al. Prevention of breast cancer with tamoxifen: preliminary findings from the Italian randomized trial among hysterectomised women. Italian Tamoxifen Prevention Study. Lancet 1998;352:93–7.

97. Anzano MA, Peer CW, Smith JM, et al. Chemoprevention of mammary carcinogenesis in the rat: combined use of raloxifene and 9-cis-retinoic acid. J Natl Cancer Inst 1996;88:123–5.

98. Gradishar WJ, Jordan VC. Clinical potential of new antiestrogens. J Clin Oncol 1997;15(2):840–52.

99. Boss SM, Huster WJ, Neild JA, et al. Effects of raloxifene hydrochloride on the endometrium of postmenopausal women. Am J Obstet Gynecol 1997;177:1458–64.

100. Cummings SR, Norton L, Eckert S, et al. Raloxifene reduces the risk of breast cancer and may decrease the risk of endometrial cancer in postmenopausal women. Two-year findings from the multiple outcomes of raloxifene evaluation (MORE) trial [abstract 3]. Proc Am Soc Clin Oncol 1998;17:2a.

101. Jordan VC, Glusman JE, Eckert S, et al. Incident primary breast cancers are reduced by raloxifene: integrated data from multicenter, double-blind, randomized trials in ~ 12,000 postmenopausal women [abstract 466]. Proc Am Soc Clin Oncol 1998;17:122a.

102. Valavaara R. Phase II trials with toremifene in advanced breast cancer: a review. Breast Cancer Res Treat 1990;16:S31–5.

103. Brunning PF. Droloxifene, a new anti-oestrogen in postmenopausal advanced breast cancer: preliminary results of a double blind dose finding phase II trial. Eur J Cancer 1992;28A:1404–7.

104. Sato M, Turner CH, Wang T, et al. LY353381.HC1: a novel raloxifene analog with improved SERM potency and efficacy in vivo. J Pharmacol Exp Ther 1998;287(1):1–7.

105. Toko T, Saito H, Fujioka A, et al. Antitumor activity of miproxifene phosphate (TAT-59) against human mammary carcinoma. Gan to Kagaku Ryoho 1998;25(6):829–38.

106. Sporn MB, Roberts AB. Role of retinoids in differentiation and carcinogenesis. Cancer Res 1983;43:3034–40.

107. Lotan R. Retinoids and apoptosis: implications for cancer chemoprevention and therapy. J Natl Cancer Inst 1995;87:1655–7.

108. Delia D, Aillo A, Formelli F, et al. Regulation of apoptosis induced by the retinoid N-(4-hydroxyphenyl) retinamide and effect of deregulated bcl-2. Blood 1995;85:359–67.

109. Mangelsdorf DJ, Umesono K, Evans RM. The retinoid receptors. In: Sporn MB, Roberts AB, Goodman DS, editors. The retinoids: biology, chemistry, and medicine. 2nd ed. New York: Raven Press; 1994. p. 319–49.

110. Toma S, Isnardi L, Raffo P, et al. Effects of ALL-trans-retinoic acid and 13-cis-retinoic acid on breast-cancer cell lines: growth inhibition and apoptosis induction. Int J Cancer 1997;70:619–27.

111. Bishoff ED, Gottardis MM, Moon TE, et al. Beyond tamoxifen: the retinoid X receptor-selective ligand LGD1069 (TARGRETIN) causes complete regression of mammary carcinoma. Cancer Res 1998;53:479–84.

112. De Palo G, Camerini T, Marubini E, et al. Chemoprevention trial of contralateral breast cancer with fenretinimide. Rationale, design, methodology, organization, data management, statistics and accrual. Tumori 1997;83:884–94.

113. De Palo G, Veronesi U, Camerini T, et al. Can fenretinide protect women against ovarian cancer? J Natl Cancer Inst 1995;87:146–7.

114. Cancer incidence in five continents. Age-standardized incidence rates, four-digit rubrics, and age-standardized and cumulative incidence rates, three-digit rubrics. IARC Sci Publ 1992;120:871–1011.

115. Dhingra K. A phase II chemoprevention trial designed to identify surrogate endpoint biomarkers in breast cancer. J Cell Biochem 1995;23Suppl:19–24.

116. Mariani L, Formelli F, De Palo G, et al. Chemoprevention of breast cancer with fenretinide (4-HPR): study of long-term visual and ophthalmologic tolerability. Tumori 1996;82:444–9.

117. National Cancer Institute. Annual Cancer Statistics Review including Cancer Trends: 1950-1985. Bethesda, MD: U.S. Department of Health and Human Services; 1988.

118. Wynder EL, Cohen LA, Muscat JE, et al. Breast cancer: weighing the evidence for a promoting role of dietary fat. J Natl Cancer Inst 1997;89:766–75.

119. Rose DP, Connolly JM, Liu XH. Dietary fatty acids and human breast cancer cell growth, invasion, and metastasis. Adv Exper Med Biol 1994;364:83–91.

120. Bagga D, Capone S, Wang HJ, et al. Dietary modulation of omega-3/omega-6 polyunsaturated fatty acid ratios in patients with breast cancer. J Natl Cancer Inst 1997;89:1123–31.

121. Zheng W, Gustafson DR, Sinha R, et al. Well-done meat intake and the risk of breast cancer. J Natl Cancer Inst 1998;90:1724–9.

122. Boyd NF, Greenberg C, Lockwood G, et al. Effects at two years of a low-fat, high-carbohydrate diet on radiologic features of the breast: results from a randomized trial. J Natl Cancer Inst 1997;89:488–96.

123. Chlebowski RT, Blackburn GL, Buzzard JM, et al. Adherence to a dietary fat intake reduction program in postmenopausal women receiving therapy for early breast cancer. The Women's Intervention Nutrition Study. J Clin Oncol 1993;11:2072–80.

124. Willett WC, Stampfer MJ. Sobering data on alcohol and breast cancer. Epidemiology 1997;8(3):225–7.

125. Mezzetti M, La Vecchia C, Decarli A, et al. Population attributable risk for breast cancer: diet, nutrition, and physical exercise. J Natl Cancer Inst 1998;90(5):389–94.

126. Jirtle RL, Haag JD, Ariazi EA, Gould M. Increased mannose 6-phosphate/insulin-like growth factor II receptor and transforming growth factor β-1 levels during monoterpene-induced regression of mammary tumors. Cancer Res 1993;53:3849–52.

127. Messina MJ, Pensky V, Setchell KD, Barnes S. Soy intake and cancer risk: a review of the in vitro and in vivo data. Nutr Cancer 1994;21:113–31.

128. Bardon S, Picard K, Martel P. Monoterpenes inhibit cell growth, cell cycle progression. Nutr Cancer 1998;32(1):1–7.

129. Lamartiniere CA, Zhang JX, Cotroneo MS. Genistein studies in rats: potential for breast cancer prevention and reproductive and developmental toxicity. Am J Clin Nutr 1998;68(6 Suppl):1400S–5S.

130. Temple WJ, Lindsay RL, Magi E, Urbanski SJ. Technical considerations for prophylactic mastectomy in patients at high risk for breast cancer. Am J Surg 1991;161:413–5.

131. Wong JH, Jackson CF, Swanson JS, et al. Analysis of the risk reduction of prophylactic partial mastectomy in Sprague-Dawley rats with 7,12-dimethylbenzanthracene-induced breast cancer. Surgery 1986;90:67–71.

132. Nelson H, Miller SH, Buck D, et al. Effectiveness of prophylactic mastectomy in the prevention of breast tumors in C3H mice. Plast Reconstr Surg 1989;83:662–9.

133. Pennisi VR, Capozzi A. Subcutaneous mastectomy data: a final statistical analysis of 1500 patients. Plast Surg 1989;13:15–21.

134. Woods JE, Meland NB. Conservative management in full-thickness nipple-areolar necrosis after subcutaneous mastectomy. Plast Reconstr Surg 1989;84:258–64.

135. Schrag D, Kuntz KM, Garber JE, Weeks JC. Decision analysis: effects of prophylactic mastectomy and oophorectomy on life expectancy among women with BRCA1 or BRCA2 mutations. N Engl J Med 1997;336:1465–71.

136. Lynch HT, Lemon SJ, Durham C, et al. A descrip-

tive study of BRCA1 testing and reactions to disclosure of test results. Cancer 1997;79:2219–28.

137. Willemsen HW, Kaas R, Peterse JH, Rutgers EJ. Breast carcinoma in residual breast tissue after bilateral subcutaneous mastectomy. Eur J Surg Oncol 1998;24:331–8.

138. Ziegler LD, Kroll SS. Primary breast cancer after prophylactic mastectomy. Am J Clin Oncol 1991;14:451–4.

139. Jameson MB, Roberts E, Nixon J, et al. Metastatic breast cancer 42 years after bilateral subcutaneous mastectomies. Clin Oncol 1997;9:119–21.

140. Goodnight JE, Quagliana JM, Morton DL. Failure of subcutaneous mastectomy to prevent development of breast cancer. J Surg Oncol 1984; 26:198–201.

141. Eldar S, Meguid MM, Beatty JD. Cancer of the breast after prophylactic subcutaneous mastectomy. Am J Surg 1984;148:692–3.

142. Hartmann LC, Schaid DJ, Woods JE, et al. Efficacy of bilateral prophylactic mastectomy in women with a family history of breast cancer. N Engl J Med 1999;340:77–84.

143. Singletary SE, Taylor SH, Guinee VF. Occurrence and prognosis of contralateral carcinoma of the breast. J Am Coll Surg 1994;178:390–6.

144. Bilimoria MM, Morrow M. The woman at increased risk for breast cancer: evaluation and management strategies. CA Cancer J Clin 1995;45:263–78.

145. Kroll SS, Miller MJ, Schusterman MA, et al. Rationale for elective contralateral mastectomy with immediate bilateral reconstruction. Ann Surg Oncol 1994;1:457–61.

146. Schairer C, Persson I, Falkeborn M, et al. Breast cancer risk associated with gynecologic surgery and indications for such surgery. Obstet Gynecol 1997;70:150–4.

147. Parazzini F, Braga C, LaVecchia C, et al. Hysterectomy, oophorectomy in premenopause, and risk of breast cancer. Obstet Gynecol 1997;90:453–6.

3

Screening and Diagnostic Imaging

JAN M. JESKE, MD
JOEL R. BERNSTEIN, MD
MARGARET A. STULL, MD

Mammography is currently the best available screening modality for early detection and diagnosis of breast cancer. Periodic examination of asymptomatic females with mammography has been shown to reduce breast cancer mortality.[1] In accordance with the American Cancer Society recommendations, the available scientific data suggest a benefit from annual mammographic screening of all women beginning at the age of 40 years, combined with annual physical examination and monthly breast self examination.[2] For women between 20 and 39 years of age, the ACS recommends a breast physical exam every three years and monthly breast self exam. Patients with a first-degree premenopausal relative diagnosed with breast cancer may consider beginning annual screening examinations 10 years prior to the age at which the relative was diagnosed, in an attempt to benefit from early detection.[3]

Screening mammography evaluates asymptomatic women with the goal of discovering unsuspected breast cancer at an early and potentially curable stage. The routine screening mammogram is comprised of a craniocaudal (CC) and mediolateral oblique (MLO) image of each breast. Abnormalities detected on the screening exam are further evaluated with a diagnostic mammogram.

Diagnostic mammography is performed on patients presenting with signs or symptoms of potential breast pathology. The request for a diagnostic mammogram should be considered a consultation to provide evaluation of the patient's symptoms or mammographic findings and make further management recommendations. Tailored mammographic images, physical examination, and breast ultrasound are frequently used to further investigate and explain a particular clinical or radiographic concern. Alternative projections and magnification views often supplement the standard mammogram. Spot compression views of a particular site of concern can improve visualization of an underlying lesion and allow for more accurate assessment of lesion margins. Magnification mammography is best suited for enhanced characterization and visualization of microcalcifications.

It is well known that mammography is unable to detect every breast cancer. The false negative rate of mammography ranges from four to thirty-four percent.[4] The diagnosis of breast cancer therefore, is not excluded by a negative mammogram. Patient management should take into account the clinical assessment, despite a negative mammogram.

When appropriate, the diagnostic exam includes ultrasonography of a mammographic finding, palpable abnormality, or site of pain. Breast sonography aids in the characterization of mammographically detected masses and can confirm equivocal radiographic findings. Breast ultrasound is the initial imaging modality of choice for evaluating palpable masses in women < 30 years of age and in lactating and pregnant women, as per the American College of Radiology standards.[5]

BREAST IMAGING REPORTING AND DATA SYSTEMS

To improve the quality of mammography reporting and early breast cancer detection, a consortium of medical experts has developed the Breast Imaging Reporting Data System (BIRADS).[6] The American College of Radiology (ACR), in collaboration with the National Cancer Institute, the Centers for Disease Control and Prevention, the Food and Drug Administration, the American Medical Association, the American College of Surgeons, and the College of American Pathologists, created BIRADS to standardize communication of mammographic results, reduce ambiguous breast imaging reports, and facilitate the collection and analysis of medical audit data at individual mammography practices as well as at the national level.

There are four main sections in BIRADS: breast imaging lexicon, reporting system, follow-up and outcome monitoring, and ACR National Mammography Database (NMD). The lexicon provides standardized language for lesion characterization. It also provides descriptive terms for masses, calcifications, architectural distortion, and associated findings of skin and nipple retraction as well as trabecular thickening and axillary adenopathy.

The reporting system uses a standardized format for the mammographic report, noting available comparison films, breast tissue composition, a concise description of any significant findings, and a final assessment with appropriate recommendations. The mammographic study is classified by BIRADS according to one of the following decision categories:

1. Category 0: incomplete. Needs additional imaging evaluation. This category typically arises after a screening mammography, when the patient must be recalled for additional evaluation before a final assessment can be made.
2. Category 1: negative. The study is normal.
3. Category 2: benign finding. There is a benign finding described and no evidence of malignancy.
4. Category 3: probably benign finding—short interval follow-up suggested. Lesions in this category have imaging characteristics that are most likely benign. Follow-up is performed at a 6-month interval to establish stability of a lesion with low probability of cancer and detect those few cancers that initially present with benign morphology. Ninety-eight percent of these lesions subsequently prove to be benign.[7] This approach limits unnecessary tissue sampling.
5. Category 4: suspicious abnormality—biopsy should be considered. Lesions in this category have a 30 percent positive predictive value for being malignant; therefore, biopsy is recommended.[7]
6. Category 5: highly suggestive of malignancy—appropriate action should be taken. These lesions have morphologic features characteristic of cancer. Intervention is required. The positive predictive value for category 5 lesions is 97 percent.[7]

These assessment categories are consistent with those mandated by the final regulations under the Mammography Quality Standard Act (MQSA).[8] These categories are not intended to replace clinical evaluation of the breast. Clinical assessment directs the ultimate course of action when the mammogram is "negative" and there is concern about a clinically suspicious abnormality.

The BIRADS section on follow-up and outcome monitoring enables an individual radiologist to assess his or her overall mammography interpretation skills by performing a mammography audit. There is a detailed description of the necessary core data to be collected and calculated for a comprehensive medical audit. The ACR BIRADS committee is encouraging mammography practices to participate in the National Mammography Database. The program will enable evaluation of mammographic screening in the diagnosis of clinically occult breast cancer at the national level.

MAMMOGRAPHIC APPEARANCE OF BREAST CANCER

Breast cancer has numerous clinical and imaging presentations. The classic mammographic appearance of infiltrating breast cancer is an irregular mass, often with ill-defined or spiculated margins. In addition to a discrete mass, the invasive tumor can also present as a subtle asymmetric density or an architectural distortion. Clustered pleomorphic calcifications are the common presentation of in situ carcinoma that may or may not be associated with invasive disease.

Secondary signs of malignancy, often associated with advanced stages of breast cancer, are detectable clinically and radiographically as areas of skin thickening or dimpling, nipple retraction, and axillary adenopathy. Diffuse skin thickening and breast edema manifested as increased mammographic density are associated with lymphangitic spread of cancer involving the dermal lymphatics with inflammatory cancer. The underlying primary tumor is often obscured by the diffuse breast edema. These findings must be differentiated from mastitis. Typically, the diagnosis of inflammatory cancer is made clinically and by biopsy. Isolated nipple and areolar thickening can occur in patients with Paget's disease of the nipple.

Mammographic Analysis of Masses

The mammographic mass is a space-occupying lesion seen in two different projections. Mammographic analysis of the mass is based on its shape, margins, and density. Round or oval shaped masses are typically associated with a benign etiology, most commonly a cyst or fibroadenoma. Increasing lobulations, irregular shapes, and spiculations increase the probability of malignancy.

Assessment of the lesion margin adds important distinguishing information. Circumscribed lesions with sharp, distinct margins are almost always benign (Figure 3–1). Poorly defined margins reflect the irregular interface of the cancer cells invading the surrounding breast tissue. Due to superimposed normal fibroglandular tissue, lesion margins can occasionally be obscured and difficult to accurately assess. Spot compression views and ultrasonography allow for further characterization of lesion margins, particularly in dense breast tissue.

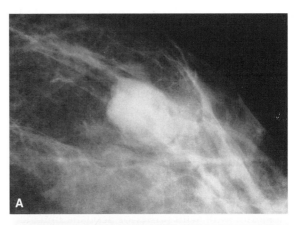

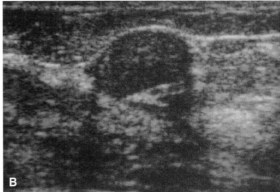

Figure 3–1. *A,* Mammographic image reveals the circumscribed and gently lobulated margins of this fibroadenoma. *B,* Corresponding ultrasound shows the solid nature of this benign tumor as evidenced by the homogenous hypoechoic internal architecture.

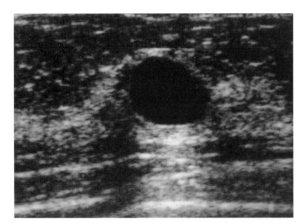

Figure 3–2. Sonographic depiction of a simple cyst. Note the lack of internal echoes and increased echogenicity deep to the fluid (posterior acoustic enhancement).

Most breast cancers are mammographically dense (more radio-opaque) relative to an equal volume of normal fibroglandular tissue. The presence of radiolucent fat within a lesion is characteristic of a benign etiology. Fat containing lesions include hamartoma (fibroadenolipoma), lipoma, galactocele, fat necrosis, and lymph nodes.

Sonographic Evaluation of Masses

Sonograpraphy is an excellent method for distinguishing a simple cyst from a solid, circumscribed tumor. On sonography, the simple cyst has smooth, rounded, or oval margins, contains no internal echoes, and has a sharply defined posterior wall with posterior acoustic enhance-

ment (Figure 3–2). The complex cystic structure containing internal echoes or an intracystic mass requires further evaluation so as to not overlook pathology such as papillary carcinoma or a necrotic neoplasm (see Figure 3–8). Thorough sonographic evaluation of all lesion margins and internal architecture is necessary to detect subtle signs of malignancy. Subtle margin irregularity and internal heterogeneity may be the only findings to suggest a malignant process. Sonographic features associated with breast malignancy include marked hypoechogenicity, irregular margins, and shadowing.[9] Malignant lesion margins visualized with ultrasound are often poorly defined, with an angulated, microlobulated, or branching pattern.

Imaging Specific Types of Infiltrating Breast Cancer

Approximately 85 percent of breast carcinomas arise from ductal structures, with the remaining 15 percent arising from lobular structures. Infiltrating ductal carcinoma accounts for the largest group of breast cancers, representing 65 to 80 percent of cases.[10] The classic mammographic presentation of infiltrating ductal carcinoma is a high-density mass with spiculated margins (Figure 3–3A). Sonographically, this lesion is typically seen as a shadowing, hypoechoic mass with irregular margins (Figure 3–3B). The presentation of infiltrating ductal car-

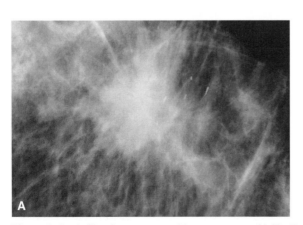
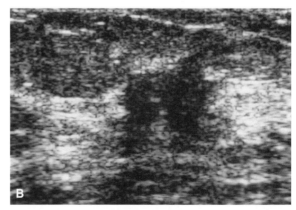

Figure 3–3. *A,* Classic mammographic appearance of infiltrating ductal carcinoma demonstrating irregular, spiculated margins. *B,* Sonographic visualization of the same infiltrating ductal carcinoma illustrating a hypoechogenic mass with irregular margins.

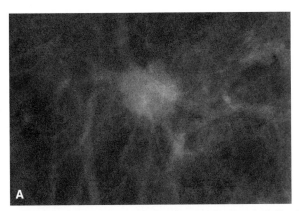
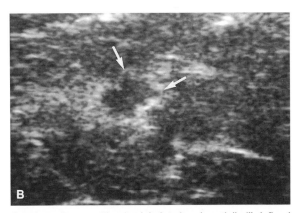

Figure 3–4. *A,* Mammographic spot view of a 0.8 cm infiltrating ductal carcinoma with microlobulated and partially ill-defined margins. *B,* Sonographic image of the same infiltrating ductal carcinoma demonstrating the marked irregularity of the tumor margins (*arrows*), despite the small size.

cinoma, however, can mimic a benign lesion with partially circumscribed margins (Figure 3–4).

Infiltrating lobular carcinoma is the second most common type of invasive breast cancer, representing approximately 15 percent of cases.[10] It has a higher rate of multicentricity and bilaterality than infiltrating ductal carcinoma.[11] Infiltrating lobular carcinoma is known for its insidious nature, delaying clinical and mammographic diagnosis. The subtle nature of infiltrating lobular carcinoma is thought to be due to its pattern of single-file cellular infiltration and lack of associated desmoplastic reaction.[12] This tumor often presents as an evolving asymmetric density, or, less often, a spiculated mass on mammography (Figure 3–5A).[13,14] Despite its elusive appearance on mammography, infiltrating lobular carcinoma appears sonographically indistinguishable from infiltrating ductal carcinoma (Figure 3–5B).[3]

Medullary, colloid, and papillary carcinomas often present as partially circumscribed mammographic masses. Medullary carcinoma, accounting for approximately six percent of breast carcinomas, typically presents in patients < 50 years of age and can be mistaken for a fibroadenoma (Figure 3–6). The slow growing colloid carcinoma, also known as mucinous carcinoma, comprises only two percent of all breast cancers and is more common in older females (Figure 3–7). Papillary carcinoma represents less than one percent of all breast cancers and is associated with spontaneous serosanguinous nipple discharge. An

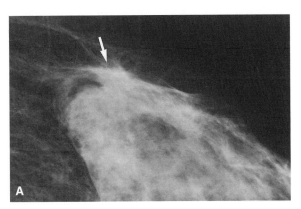
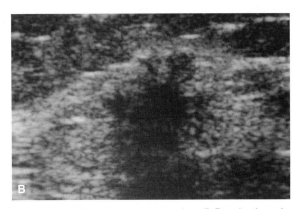

Figure 3–5. *A,* The arrow identifies a vague, developing asymmetric density on this spot compression view. *B,* Despite the subtle mammographic appearance, the ultrasound image clearly visualizes this infiltrating lobular carcinoma revealing the markedly jagged margins.

intracystic mass or intraductal lesion depicted by sonography raises concern for a papillary neoplasm (Figure 3–8).

Tubular carcinoma accounts for less than two percent of breast cancers. Due to its very slow growth, this tumor is typically small at the time of detection. Tubular carcinoma often presents as a small spiculated mass on mammog-

raphy, indistinguishable from infiltrating ductal carcinoma (Figure 3–9). Tubular carcinoma can be confused or associated with a radial scar (sclerosing papillomatosis), a benign entity (Figure 3–10).

Phyllodes tumor, once termed "cystosarcoma phyllodes," comprises less than one percent of breast tumors. Approximately ten percent of

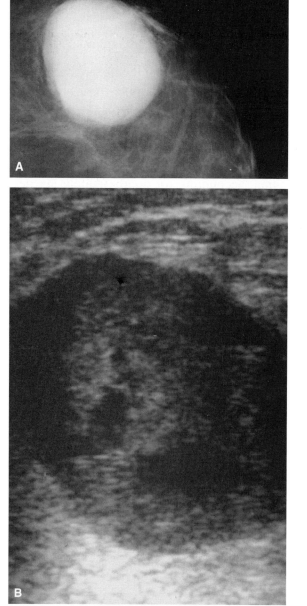

Figure 3–6. *A,* Mammographic image of a 6 cm circumscribed medullary carcinoma. *B,* Ultrasound reveals the heterogeneous hypoechoic nature of this medullary carcinoma.

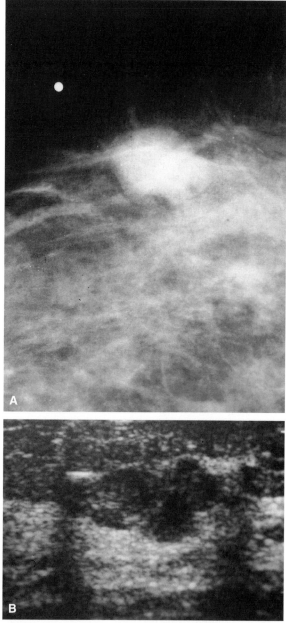

Figure 3–7. *A,* This partially circumscribed mammographic nodule represents a colloid (mucinous) carcinoma. *B,* The heterogeneous hypoechoic and lobulated appearance of this colloid carcinoma is easily visualized with ultrasound.

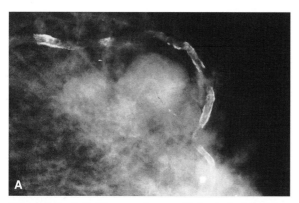 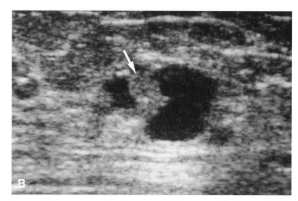

Figure 3–8. *A,* Papillary carcinoma with the typical appearance of a partially circumscribed mass. *B,* Sonographic image of the same papillary neoplasm reveals the intracystic mass (*arrow*).

phyllodes tumors are malignant. This tumor can present as a rapidly growing palpable mass. Breast imaging usually shows a large rounded or lobulated circumscribed mass. Cystic spaces can be seen by sonography (Figure 3–11).

Metastasis to the breast, although uncommon, can occur from a variety of primary malignancies, including melanoma, lymphoma, lung cancer, and contralateral breast carcinoma. Mammographically, the metastatic lesions tend to be round and lack spiculations (Figure 3–12).

BREAST CALCIFICATIONS

The presence of suspicious microcalcifications on a mammogram can make possible the early diagnosis of clinically occult breast cancer. Since the description of calcifications on radiographs of breast cancer by Leborgne in 1951[15] there have been substantial improvements in the mammo-

graphic detail of this finding as well as greater awareness of its importance. Current mammographic techniques can detect calcification in as many as 50 percent of all breast cancers.[16] Screening studies have shown that 90 percent of all cases of nonpalpable ductal carcinoma in situ (DCIS)[17] and 70 percent of minimal carcinomas[18] were detected on the basis of microcalcifications. Many women, however, have some form of calcification in their breasts, the great majority of which are benign. Thus, we are challenged to both detect and analyze calcifications seen on mammograms to accurately diagnose breast cancer without incurring consequences of a false positive or false negative study.

Detection

Nowhere in medical imaging are fine detail images as vital as they are in the detection and

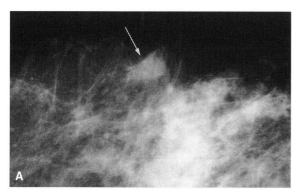 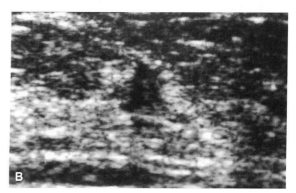

Figure 3–9. *A and B,* Mammographic and sonographic images demonstrating the irregular shape and spiculated margins of this 0.5 cm tubular carcinoma (*arrow*).

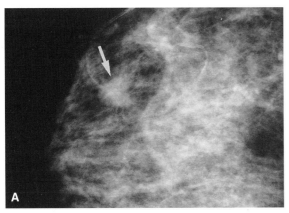
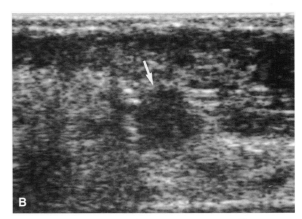

Figure 3–10. *A and B,* The imaging appearance of this benign radial scar (arrow) mimics the tubular carcinoma in Figure 3–9.

evaluation of breast microcalcifications, which may be as small as 0.1 mm. It is necessary to optimize the technique in all stages of production of the mammographic image to yield high contrast, high resolution, and motion-free films. Viewing conditions, including the routine use of a hand magnifying lens to systematically search each film, are also important. Magnification radiography in the study of breast calcifications, although at the cost of a higher radiation dose (2×), provides greater resolution than that achieved with a hand lens.

Analysis

Due to the frequency of calcifications on mammograms, careful analysis is needed to recognize clearly benign calcifications and allow follow-up of low suspicion calcifications. While some calcifications have classically benign or malignant features that allow the mammographer to easily characterize them for appropriate action, there is a sizable intermediate or indeterminate group that requires thorough analysis to assess the likelihood of malignancy. The characteristics most useful in evaluating calcifications include size, number, form, distribution, and location.

Size

Calcifications associated with malignancy are often as small as 0.1 to 0.3 mm in diameter and usually < 0.5 mm. However, larger granular forms, up to 2 mm, and longer fine linear forms of calcification, may occasionally be seen. The individual calcifications in cancer often vary in

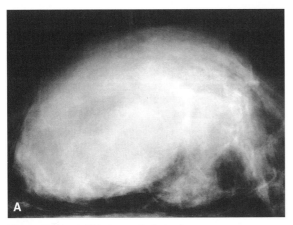
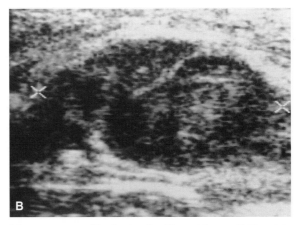

Figure 3–11. *A,* This large phyllodes tumor encompasses much of the mammographically visualized breast tissue. *B,* Sonography confirms the solid nature of this mass, heterogeneous and hypoechoic.

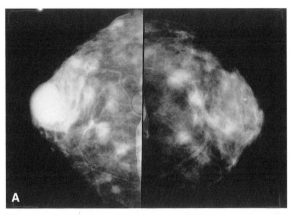 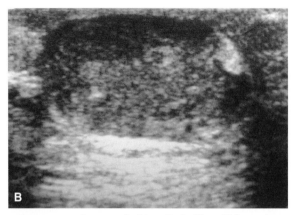

Figure 3–12. *A,* Bilateral craniocaudal (CC) images demonstrating numerous round masses in this patient with multiple myeloma metastasis. *B,* Sonographic image of the largest metastatic lesion in the right breast, depicting the heterogeneous hypoechoic nature.

size. In a group of mixed-size calcifications, the degree of suspicion should relate to the smallest forms.

Number

The presence of a focal group of five heterogeneous microcalcifications in a volume of 1 cm^3 of tissue has been accepted as suspicious.[19] Biopsy of fewer calcifications may be performed if new, pleomorphic, or fine linear or branching calcifications have developed since a prior mammogram. Generally, the greater the number of suspicious calcifications grouped in a small area, the higher the chance of malignancy.[20,21] Magnification studies are used to more accurately determine the number of calcifications present. The pathologist invariably finds more calcifications than are visible on the mammogram.

Shape

Small round to oval dense punctate calcifications located in cystically dilated acini are considered benign lobular calcifications. Malignant calcifications are typically ductal in origin, forming in ductal cellular secretions or necrotic cellular debris. Fine linear and branching ductal calcifications or pleomorphic calcifications grouped to form a cast of the duct are most typical of malignancy, often comedo car-

cinoma, but are not the most common presentation. Irregular granular forms are more frequently seen, often differing in size and varying from jagged "fractured crystal" shapes to round punctate dots similar to lobular calcifications. It is this overlap of benign and malignant shapes of granular calcifications that results in the large indeterminate group of microcalcifications requiring biopsy. Magnification studies are invaluable in characterizing these calcifications, allowing elimination of some typically lobular forms from consideration for biopsy.

Distribution

Bilateral diffusely scattered calcifications are almost always benign and are often associated with adenosis. However, the calcifications of adenosis or sclerosing adenosis may be focal and indistinguishable from malignancy. Malignant calcifications are usually found as a focal cluster involving a small area of one breast but can be more extensive, presenting as one or several clusters in the distribution of the ductal system of one lobe, or virtually an entire breast. While some benign masses contain coarse calcifications, the presence of fine or pleomorphic calcifications associated with a mass increases the likelihood of malignancy and may suggest a related extensive intraductal component.

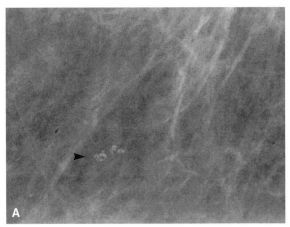
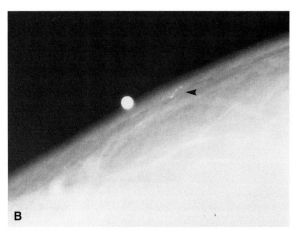

Figure 3–13. Skin calcification. *A,* Lucent centered sebaceous gland calcification (*arrow*) appears intramammary on standard projection. *B,* Tangential view confirms location of calcium in the skin (*arrow*).

Location

Calcifications must be proven to be within the breast to accurately evaluate their significance. Mimics of breast parenchymal calcification include skin calcium, artifacts, and pseudocalcifications.

Benign Calcifications

Analysis of breast calcifications by an experienced mammographer will allow accurate diagnosis of characteristically benign calcifications. The various types are described below.

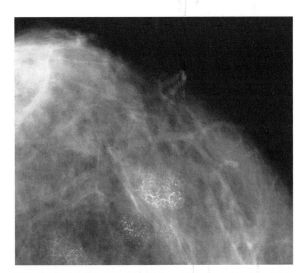

Figure 3–14. Pseudocalcification. Talc powder in moles beneath breast mimics parenchymal calcification.

Skin Calcification and Pseudocalcification

Skin calcification is commonly related to sebaceous glands and appears as lucent, centered rings in a peripheral location (Figure 3–13A). Skin calcification may be punctate or irregular, and may appear to lie within the breast parenchyma on standard views. Therefore, a tangential view skin localization study (Figure 3–13B) may be necessary to prove a cutaneous location. Calcium in warts, moles, scars, and dermal lesions as well as pseudocalcifications due to tattoos, talc, deodorant, or film artifacts can be misleading (Figure 3–14).

Vascular Calcifications

Calcification caused by atherosclerosis in arterial walls is usually easy to recognize due to the typical continuous linear tubular pattern (Figure 3–15A). Early changes of short segment calcifications appearing as discontinuous deposits in one wall may have a granular or fine linear appearance that can arouse suspicion (Figure 3–15B). Magnification views in alternate projections will usually allow a correct diagnosis.

Calcium in Cysts

Thin, curvilinear calcifications defining the margin of a mass are seen with cyst wall calci-

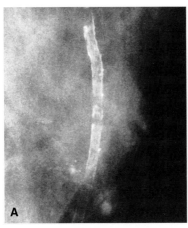
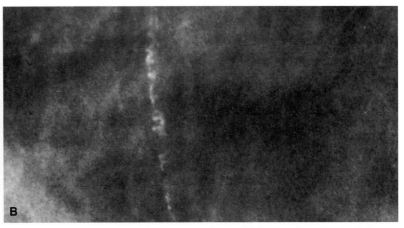

Figure 3–15. Vascular calcification. *A,* Typical tubular arterial calcification. *B,* Irregular linear calcification, due to incomplete arterial wall involvement, can appear suspicious.

fications. Intracystic calcium particles suspended in fluid, known as "milk of calcium," may appear in multiple tiny cysts or a single larger cyst. This diagnosis is best proven with a 90-degree lateral film showing a meniscus or teacup shape of layered calcium in a cyst (Figure 3–16). These calcifications may be difficult to see when viewed en face in the CC view.

Fibroadenoma

Calcifications appear in fibroadenomas as a result of involution which may be due to myxoid degeneration, hyalinization, or infarction. Early calcifications may occur in the periphery of the mass and progress to large, geographic areas of calcium the appearance of which has been compared to popcorn (Figure 3–17). Eventually, the soft-tissue component may be completely replaced by a dense conglomerate of calcifications. However, when this classic pattern is not followed, an involuted fibroadenoma may appear as fine pleomorphic calcifications without a visible mass and biopsy may be required for diagnosis.

Secretory Calcification

Inspissated ductal secretions in normal or dilated ducts may calcify to form solid, coarse, and linear ductal casts involving one or more ducts diffusely and often bilaterally. Large, tubular periductal calcifications can appear in plasma-cell mastitis (Figure 3–18). Increased density of the subareolar parenchyma may be found. These large, rod-like secretory calcifications are usually easily differentiated from malignant calcifications by their large size and greater length.

Fat Necrosis

Calcifications due to fat necrosis are often seen as fine-rim calcifications surrounding a lucent center, varying in size from a few millimeters to

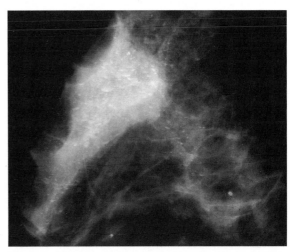

Figure 3–16. Milk of calcium. Layered sedimented calcium in microcysts appears curvilinear or teacup-shaped on horizontal beam lateral film.

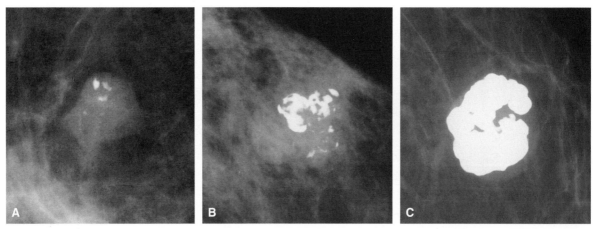

Figure 3–17. Fibroadenoma. *A,* Few early coarse peripheral calcifications. *B,* Classic popcorn calcification. *C,* Large dense calcification nearly replaces mass.

several centimeters. Small ring forms, usually < 5 mm in diameter, are often idiopathic (Figure 3–19A). Dystrophic calcifications deposited after trauma, hemorrhage, surgical biopsy, and radiation may appear as larger and less regular calcifications surrounding an oil cyst (Figure 3–19B). It is important to note that this type of calcium may appear several years after a lumpectomy and breast radiation. In its early stages, it can be difficult to differentiate from recurrent malignant calcifications.

Lobular Calcifications: Adenosis/Sclerosing Adenosis

Lobular calcifications form in the acini in association with such entities as adenosis, sclerosing adenosis, atypical lobular hyperplasia, and cystic hyperplasia. Characteristically, these calcifications are small, dense, and round (Figure 3–20A). If a lobule is distorted by surrounding sclerosis, the individual forms may be more irregular. The distribution of calcifications in adenosis and sclerosing adenosis is often bilateral, diffuse, and inhomogeneous due to variable involvement of individual lobules. These characteristic findings indicate a benign process. Alternatively, the calcifications can be more focal, presenting as unilateral loosely grouped calcifications, regional calcifications, or a solitary small cluster (Figure 3–20B). In

these situations, careful analysis of the calcifications with magnification views may allow periodic follow-up, but biopsy will often be necessary to exclude carcinoma.

Malignant and Indeterminate Calcifications

Microcalcifications are present in as many as 50 percent of all breast cancers and in an even higher percentage of stage 0 and stage 1 breast cancers.[16–18] The presence of clustered microcalcifications may be the only indication of early preinvasive malignancy. Mammographic

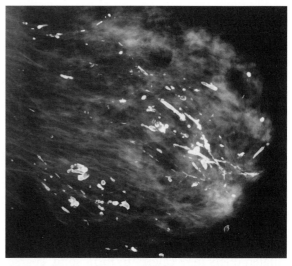

Figure 3–18. Secretory calcification. Large, solid rod-like and tubular calcifications appear in a ductal orientation.

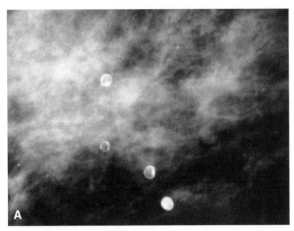

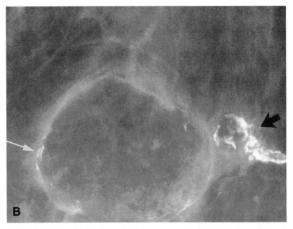

Figure 3–19. Fat necrosis. *A,* Dense round lucent-centered calcifications caused by idiopathic fat necrosis. *B,* Postoperative oil cysts with thin eggshell (*white arrow*) and course rim calcification (*black arrow*).

detection of microcalcifications in patients with DCIS accounts for this entity rising from a small percentage of lesions found at biopsy to the current rate of 20 to 40 percent for biopsies for clinically occult lesions.[22] Stomper and colleagues,[23] in a group of 100 patients with DCIS, reported that 84 percent of cases presented with microcalcifications, either alone (72%) or as calcifications associated with a soft-tissue density (12%).

Classic malignant calcifications are typically associated with comedo carcinoma but are also present in other histologic subtypes of DCIS. Characteristic malignant calcifications occur as fine, pleomorphic, linear, and branching calcifications (Figure 3–21) or multiple irregular granules forming castings arranged in a ductal distribution (Figure 3–22). The extent of involvement may vary from < 1 cm to an entire lobule or even a whole breast (Figure 3–23). Holland observed a significant discrepancy between the estimated mammographic and actual histopathologic extent of DCIS.[24] This discrepancy is most pronounced for low grade DCIS. Mammography underestimates the histopathologic extent by 16 percent for high grade DCIS and 47 percent for low grade DCIS.[24]

Clustered irregular granular calcifications,

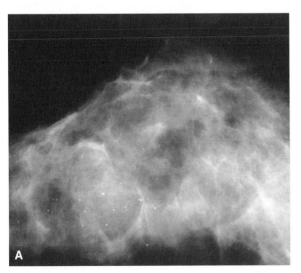

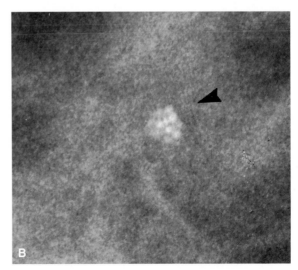

Figure 3–20. Lobular calcification. *A,* Punctate, round, scattered calcifications (were bilateral) due to adenosis. *B,* Small group of round clustered calcifications (*arrow*), likely acinar, in a dilated lobule.

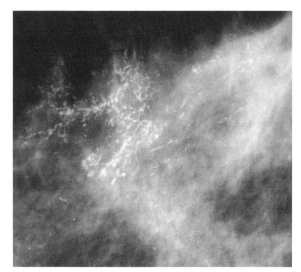

Figure 3–21. Linear and branching calcifications typical of comedo type ductal carcinoma in situ.

not clearly ductal in distribution, or mixed forms of granular and casting calcifications, are a more common presentation of DCIS (65%) compared to the classic pure casting and linear forms (35%).[23] These granular calcifications are seen more frequently in low-grade, noncomedo carcinoma, although there is enough overlap that one cannot reliably subtype DCIS based on the mammographic morphology. It is also this group, because of the variability of the granular

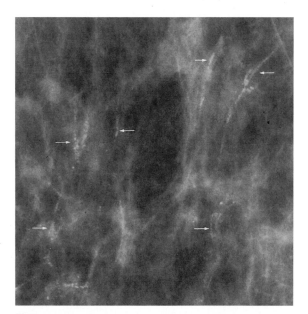

Figure 3–22. Granular calcifications forming ductal casts (*arrows*) in comedo type ductal carcinoma in situ.

calcifications (Figure 3–24), that may have the most similarity to benign forms of calcium and thus require the greatest scrutiny. Invasive breast cancer associated with DCIS involving

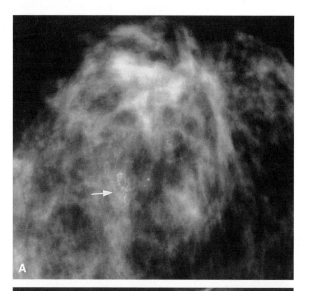

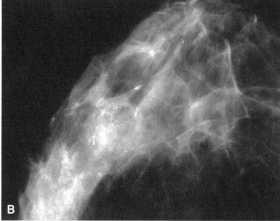

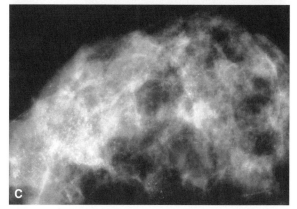

Figure 3–23. Distribution of microcalcifications in ductal carcinoma in situ. *A,* focal (*arrow*); *B,* segmental; *C,* diffuse (whole breast).

25 percent or more of the area of the tumor is classified as an extensive intraductal component (EIC) (Figure 3–25). Magnification mammography is helpful in defining the extent of the in

situ component and defining the margins of the resection. Magnification mammography is needed to accurately determine the number, shape, and distribution of calcifications. However, even after careful study, clustered granular calcifications are often considered indeterminate and biopsy is performed, resulting in a yield for malignancy of 20 to 33 percent.[20,21,25,26]

GALACTOGRAPHY

Galactography or ductography may be used to evaluate patients presenting with spontaneous isolated bloody or clear nipple discharge. Numerous studies document a 10 to 15 percent incidence of carcinoma in women with spontaneous unilateral discharge from a single duct.[27–29] The incidence of carcinoma in patients with bloody versus serous discharge is similar.[27] Other types of discharge, including green, yellow, or milky discharges, have not been associated with carcinoma.[12]

Galactography is not indicated in pregnant or lactating women or when the discharge occurs from multiple bilateral ducts. Galactography

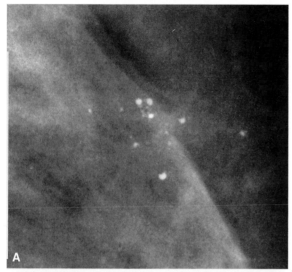
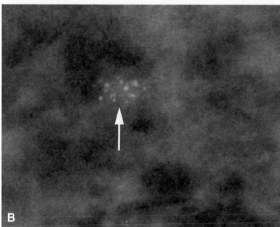
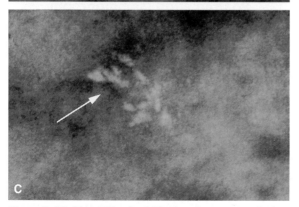

Figure 3–24. Variability of calcifications in non-comedo ductal carcinoma in situ. *A,* round, punctate granules; *B,* pleomorphic granules (*arrow*) which vary in size; *V,* "fractured crystal," highly irregular granules (*arrow*).

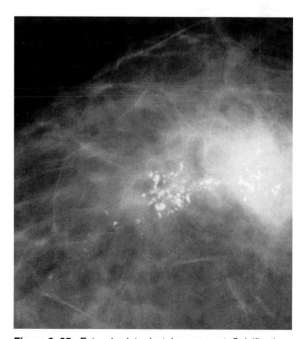

Figure 3–25. Extensive intraductal component. Calcifications within a tumor mass and extention into surrounding tissue.

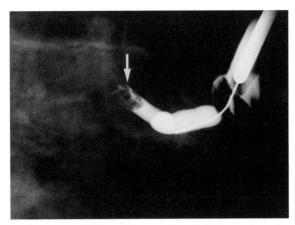

Figure 3–26. Galactographic image demonstrating the abrupt duct termination due to an intraductal filling defect (*arrow*), in this case, a benign intraductal papilloma.

should not be performed on a patient with active mastitis because it may worsen the inflammation.

Evaluation of women with bloody or serous nipple discharge should begin with mammography. If the mammogram is unrevealing, ductography can be performed by painlessly cannulating the discharging duct and gently injecting radiographic contrast material. Postinjection mammographic images reveal intraductal filling defects or abrupt duct termination when pathology is present (Figure 3–26). The benign intraductal papilloma is the most common cause of spontaneous serosanguinous nipple discharge. Benign duct ectasia may also cause nipple discharge.

Prior to surgical excision of the ductal lesion, preoperative galactography can be performed with a mixture of iodinated contrast material and methylene blue dye to enable intraoperative localization of the involved duct. It has been suggested that this technique can allow a more accurate and limited resection.[27]

EVALUATION OF THE CONSERVATIVELY TREATED BREAST

Mammography is an essential tool for monitoring conservatively treated breast cancer patients. Recognizing the distinctions between mammographic appearance of the expected postsurgical, postradiation developments and that of recurrent carcinoma is critical for patient care.

Postexcision Mammography

Magnification mammography is useful after surgery to ensure complete excision of the malignant lesion. If the targeted lesion and all tumor-related calcifications are not clearly included on the specimen radiograph, or if there is discordance between the pathology results and the preoperative diagnosis, magnifications mammography can reveal the retained primary lesion or residual malignant calcifications. Postoperative magnification mammography is useful prior to radiation to ensure complete excision of the calcium-containing tumor. Unfortunately, mammography cannot definitively predict the histologic extent of tumors.

Mammography performed within the first few weeks after tumorectomy is often limited by the patient's discomfort, breast edema, postsurgical architectural distortion, and the presence of postoperative fluid collections (ie, seromas and hematomas) (Figure 3–27A). Postexcision changes frequently result in increased density that can obscure subtle residual malignant calcifications (Figure 3–27B).

Although these alterations regress and stabilize with time, they are accentuated and prolonged by subsequent radiation therapy.[30,31]

Postradiation Mammography and Long-Term Follow-up

Mammography is important for long-term monitoring to evaluate for recurrent disease or new lesions in either breast. This should commence with a post-treatment baseline mammogram being performed within 3 to 9 months following tumor excision and completion of radiation therapy. Standard views may be supplemented with special projections to fully define post-therapy changes. Magnification mammography is particularly important when evaluating the breast for retained or recurrent malignant microcalcifications. Subsequent annual or more frequent mammograms should be obtained as indicated by clinical or radiographic evaluation. Comparison of the post-treatment mammograms to preceding studies is necessary to accurately assess radiographic changes following completion of therapy. Among the most common post-therapy changes are breast edema, skin thickening, postoperative fluid collections, scarring, fat necrosis, and calcifications.

The mammographic findings of skin thickening, irregular breast parenchyma, and breast edema following surgery and radiation are most prominent on the post-treatment baseline study and typically diminish over 2 to 3 years following conservative therapy.[30,32] Once mammographic stability of the breast has been established, any increase in the architectural distortion or enlargement of the dense scar at the surgical site suggests the presence of recurrent tumor. Interrupted lymphatic drainage after extensive axillary node dissection may produce chronic breast edema. Recurrent edema with erythema may be a manifestation of infection (mastitis), inflammatory breast carcinoma, or recurrent breast cancer with lymphatic involvement. Postoperative fluid collections, such as hematomas or seromas at the lumpectomy site, present mammographically as high-density oval masses that may have ill-defined or spiculated margins (see Figure 3–27). These diminish in size as the fluid is resorbed over a period of 6 to 18 months.[30,31] If the fluid collection is enlarging or an abscess is suspected, ultrasonography can be used to evaluate the process further and to guide diagnostic needle aspiration.

Coarse, benign, dystrophic calcifications can develop several years after radiation and surgery. These calcifications frequently represent fat necrosis or occasionally calcified suture material in the surgical bed. Sometimes the developing benign calcifications have an indeterminate appearance necessitating tissue sampling. Occasionally fat necrosis can present as an irregular mass-like lesion that may simulate tumor recurrence.

Recurrent Breast Cancer

The mammographic indications of tumor recurrence at the surgical site frequently develop between 2 to 3 years following conservative breast surgery.[33] The development of increased

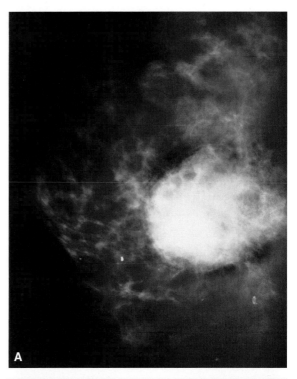

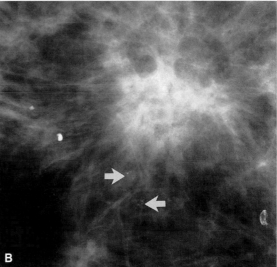

Figure 3–27. Postoperative fluid collection obscuring residual malignant microcalcifications. *A,* The large high density oval mass with ill-defined margins represents the postsurgical fluid collection. *B,* Magnification view 2 months later shows postsurgical scar with resorption of the seroma and adjacent subtle residual malignant calcifications (*arrows*).

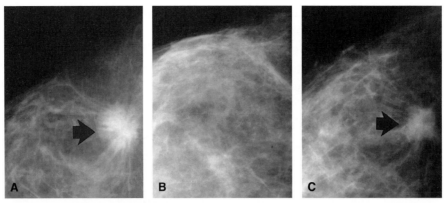

Figure 3–28. Recurrent infiltrating ductal carcinoma. Sequential views of the right breast show *A*, the spiculated primary tumor (*arrow*) in the lateral breast; *B*, post-lumpectomy changes; and *C*, recurrent invasive disease (*arrow*) in the surgical bed.

skin thickening, progressive architectural distortion, enlargement of the surgical scar, a new soft-tissue mass, or new pleomorphic microcalcifications raise the suspicion of recurrent disease (Figures 3–28 and 3–29). Calcifications associated with recurrent DCIS frequently resemble the mammographic appearance of the original tumor.[34] Contrast-enhanced MR imaging may help distinguish scar tissue from recurrent disease.[35] Computed tomography (CT) scanning can be used to assess extensive local breast disease (Figure 3–30), revealing direct chest-wall invasion or tumor recurrence in the chest wall. Computed tomography is also useful in assessing regional and distant metastatic disease.

EVALUATION OF THE AUGMENTED BREAST

The presence of breast implants causes technical problems that impair the ability to detect breast cancer by mammography. The radiopaque implant blocks x-ray transmission, which limits the imaging of breast tissue. Implants compress breast tissue against the skin which can obscure a significant amount of anterior breast tissue on conventional mammographic images. Implants also diminish the compressibility of the breast, particularly if there is capsular contracture.

Improved visualization of the anterior breast tissue is provided by implant displacement

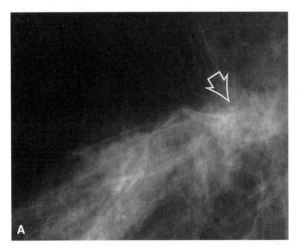
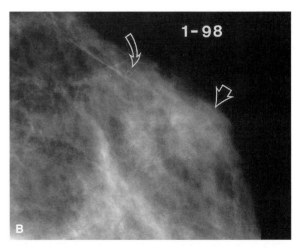

Figure 3–29. Recurrent DCIS and invasive ductal carcinoma developing 3 years after breast conservation therapy. *A*, Image on 12/96 shows architectural distortion at the lumpectomy site (*arrow*). *B*, Spot magnification view demonstrates faint microcalcifications (*curved arrow*) adjacent to enlargement of the surgical scar representing DCIS associated with invasive tumor (*straight arrow*).

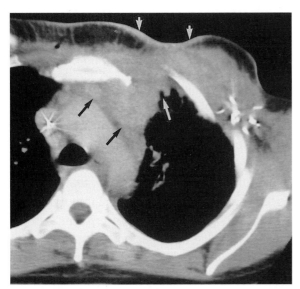

Figure 3–30. Recurrent infiltrating ductal carcinoma after left mastectomy and radiation therapy. CT scan shows dermal involvement (*short white arrows*), left chest wall and axillary recurrence with direct invasion into the mediastinum and subpleural space (*long white arrow*). Confluent pathologic mediastinal adenopathy (*black arrows*) is present. Tumor surrounds the left axillary clips.

views (Figure 3–31). This modified positioning technique supplements the standard views in women with cosmetic augmentation. Unfortunately, breast tissue near the chest wall is not completely imaged with either standard or modified views.

Breast cancer has the same mammographic features in women with or without implants

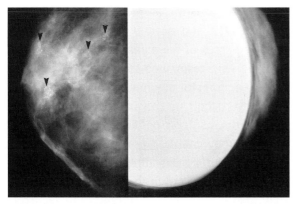

Figure 3–31. Multicentric DCIS in a woman with subpectoral implants. Implant displacement and standard MLO view (photographed back to back for comparison) show multiple groups of pleomorphic microcalcifications (*arrows*). The malignant calcifications are more conspicuous on the implant displacement image.

(Figure 3–32). Lesions are usually more conspicuous on the implant displacement views (see Figure 3–31). Patients with cosmetic augmentation or reconstruction with implants may develop parenchymal scarring that should not be confused with a malignant process. Dystrophic calcifications and calcifications associated with the fibrous capsule surrounding the implant can occur but are usually clearly benign in appearance.

Ultrasonography of the augmented breast assists in the evaluation of palpable and mammographically detected masses (Figure 3–33). Ultrasound can identify a palpable implant valve and distinguish a focal implant herniation or contained implant rupture from a breast parenchymal abnormality, eliminating the need

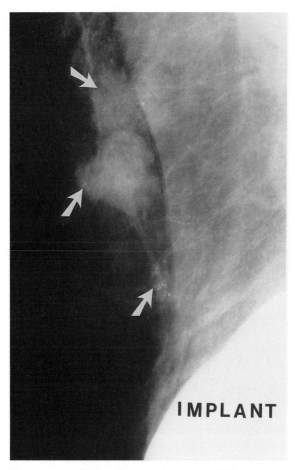

IMPLANT

Figure 3–32. Multifocal invasive disease with EIC adjacent to implant. Mammographic image reveals three irregular masses (*arrows*) with bridging spicules and pleomorphic malignant calcifications in the right axillary tail and inferior axilla.

for tissue sampling.[30,36] If a suspicious or indeterminate parenchymal abnormality is confirmed, ultrasound guided fine-needle aspiration or core biopsy limits the risk of implant rupture.

Magnetic resonance imaging is widely used to evaluate prosthetic implant integrity and can aid in differentiating an implant complication from an intramammary lesion.[37,38] Dynamic, contrast-enhanced MR imaging shows promise for improved detection and monitoring of breast cancer in certain women with cosmetic breast augmentation or breast reconstruction using prosthetic implants.[36]

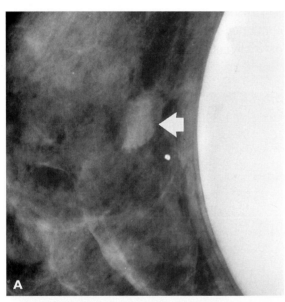
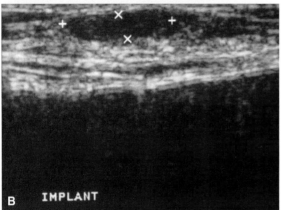

Figure 3–33. Stromal fibrosis presenting as an indeterminate mass. *A,* Implant displacement view shows the oval lesion (*arrow*) with partially defined margins located superficial to the implant. *B,* Ultrasound demonstrates the oval hypoechoic mass directly subjacent to the dermis. The anterior aspect of the intact hypoechoic implant is seen deep to the breast tissue.

MAGNETIC RESONANCE IMAGING OF THE BREAST

High–spatial–resolution MR imaging of the breast is evolving as an important adjunctive diagnostic tool for the detection, characterization, staging, and monitoring of breast cancer. Contrast-enhanced MR imaging may allow more accurate preoperative evaluation of primary malignant breast lesions that may be underestimated or not seen on mammography or by ultrasonography. Magnetic resonance imaging has revealed unsuspected multifocal, multicentric, diffuse, and bilateral disease in patients with a solitary mammographic lesion.[39–41]

The sensitivity of contrast-enhanced MR imaging approaches 100 percent in the detection of invasive breast cancer when compared to mammography and physical examination.[35,39,41] The specificity of breast MR imaging ranges from 37 to 97 percent.[39,41,42] This wide range is attributed to the overlap in contrast enhancement of benign and malignant lesions. Higher specificity for breast MR imaging can be achieved using a dynamic contrast-enhanced technique with three-dimensional imaging. On dynamic contrast-enhanced studies, malignant lesions typically exhibit rapid enhancement, whereas benign lesions show slower or no enhancement. False-positive enhancing lesions include fibroadenomas, sclerosing adenosis, radial scars, mastitis, atypical hyperplasia, lobular neoplasia and normal breast tissue during various phases of the menstrual cycle.[35–37]

Magnetic resonance imaging is also capable of demonstrating mammographically and clinically occult in situ carcinoma.[39–46] High-resolution contrast-enhanced dynamic MR imaging may enable more accurate evaluation of tumors in dense fibroglandular tissue and assist in screening of high-risk patients.[35,39–41] It may also be useful in differentiating recurrent carcinoma from scarring and in evaluating the response to neoadjuvant chemotherapy.[39]

Limitations of MR imaging include the high cost of the examination, limited availability of dedicated imaging equipment, and significant overlap in the enhancement patterns of benign and malignant lesions. Additional large multi-institutional studies will help define the clinical usefulness and cost effectiveness of MR imaging in the assessment of breast cancer.

NUCLEAR MEDICINE TECHNIQUES FOR BREAST IMAGING

Scintigraphic imaging of the breast frequently uses the single-gamma radiotracer technetium-99m (Tc-99m) sestamibi. Studies have indicated 95 to 97 percent sensitivity for breast tumors > 1 cm.[47] The sensitivity, however, is poor for small, nonpalpable or medially located lesions, ranging from 26 percent for lesions < 0.5 cm to 56 percent for lesions between 0.5 cm and 1 cm.[47] The specificity for Tc-99m sestamibi imaging ranges from 73 to 90 percent.[47,48]

Breast cancer imaging has also been performed using positron emission tomography (PET) imaging of a structural analog of glucose, fluorodeoxyglucose (FDG). The sensitivity and specificity for PET scanning of the breast range from 70 to 90 percent and 85 to 95 percent, respectively.[47,48] As with scintigraphic imaging, lesions < 1 cm are not reliably detected with PET imaging. Improvements in the ability to detect small lesions will be necessary before clinical utility of scintigraphy and PET can be proven.

COMPUTER-AIDED DIAGNOSIS

Computer-aided detection and diagnosis (CAD) is an evolving technology that functions as a "second reader" of the mammographic films.[49] Current CAD requires digitizing the mammography films to allow computer analysis. The computer program identifies areas of the breast that match certain prescribed tissue patterns, densities, or calcifications for further review by the interpreting radiologist. Limitations of CAD include the increased film handling time and high start-up costs. Prospective clinical studies are needed to determine the efficacy of the CAD methods.

CONCLUSION

Increased public awareness of the importance of breast cancer screening and continued technical advances in breast imaging will enhance patient care by allowing early detection, staging, and monitoring of the disease. Recognition of the diverse imaging presentations of breast cancer is crucial for early diagnosis and proper management.

REFERENCES

1. Breast cancer screening for women ages 40–49. NIH Consens Statement. 1997;Jan 21–23; 15(1):1–35.
2. Feig SA, D'Orsi CJ, Hendrick RE, et al. American College of Radiology Guidelines for Breast Cancer Screening. Am J Roentgenol 1998;171: 29–33.
3. Kopans DB. Breast imaging. Philadelphia: Lippincott-Raven Publishers; 1998.
4. Huynh PT, Jarolimek, AM, Daye S. The false-negative mammogram. Radiographics 1998; 18:1137–54.
5. American College of Radiology (ACR). 1998 Standards. Reston (VA): American College of Radiology; 1998. p. 317.
6. American College of Radiology (ACR). Breast imaging reporting and data system (BIRAD-STM). 3rd ed. Reston (VA): American College of Radiology;1998.
7. Orel SG, Kay N, Reynolds C, et al. BI-RADS categorization as a predictor of malignancy. Radiology 1999;211:845–50.
8. Federal Register, Part II, Department of Health and Human Services, 1997, October 28.
9. Stavros AT, Thickman D, Rapp CL, et al. Solid breast nodules: use of sonography to distinguish between benign and malignant lesions. Radiology 1995;196:123–34.
10. Adler DD. Imaging evaluation of spiculated masses. In: Friedrich M, Sickles EA, editors. Radiological diagnosis of breast diseases. Berlin: Springer-Verlag; 1997.
11. Fisher ER. What is early breast cancer? In: Zander J, Baltzer J, editors. Early breast cancer; histopathology, diagnosis, treatment. New York: Springer;1985.

12. Bassett LW, Jackson VP, Johan R, et al. Diagnosis of diseases of the breast. Philadelphia: W. B. Saunders Company; 1997.

13. Mendelson EB, Harris KM, Doshi N, et al. Infiltrating lobular carcinoma: mammographic patterns with pathologic correlation. Am J Roentgenol 1985;153:265–71.

14. Newstead GM, Baute PB, Toth HK. Invasive lobular and ductal carcinoma: mammographic findings and stage at diagnosis. Radiology 1992;184:623–7.

15. Leborgne R. Diagnosis of tumor of the breast by simple roentgenography: calcification in carcinoma. Am J Roentgenol 1951;65:1–11.

16. Miller RR, Davis R, Stacey AJ. The detection and significance of calcification in the breast. A radiological and pathological study. Br J Radiol 1976;49:12–26.

17. Feig SA, Shaber GS, Patchefsky A. Analysis of clinically occult and mammographically occult breast tumors. Am J Roentgenol 1977;128:403–8.

18. Moskowitz M. The predictive value of certain mammographic signs in screening for breast cancer. Cancer 1983;51:1007–11.

19. Sickles EA. Mammographic features of early breast cancer. Am J Roentgenol 1984;143:461–4.

20. Egan RL, McSweeney MD, Sewell CW. Intramammary calcification without an associated mass in benign and malignant disease. Radiology 1980;137:1–7.

21. Muir BB, Lamb J, Anderson TS, Kirkpatrick AE. Microcalcification and its relationship to cancer of the breast: experience in a screening clinic. Clin Radiol 1983;34:193–200.

22. Rebner M, Rajic V. Noninvasive breast cancer. Radiology 1994;190:623–31.

23. Stomper PC, Connolly JL, Meyer JE, Harris JR. Clinically occult ductal carcinoma in situ detected with mammography: analysis of 100 cases with radiographic-pathologic correlation. Radiology 1989;172:235–41.

24. Holland R, Hednriks JH, Verbeek AL, et al. Extent, distribution and mammographic/histological correlations of breast ductal carcinoma in situ. Lancet 1990;335:519–22.

25. Meyer JE, Kopans DB, Stomper PC, Lindfors KK. Occult breast abnormalities: percutaneous preoperative needle localization. Radiology 1984;150:335–7.

26. Feig SA. Mammographic evaluation of calcifications. In: Kopans DB, Mendelson EB, editors. Syllabus: a categorical course in breast imaging. Radiol Soc North Am; 1995.

27. Van Zee KJ, Perez GO, Minnard E, et al. Preoperative galactography increases the diagnostic yield of major duct excision for nipple discharge. Cancer 1998;82:1874–80.

28. Tabar L, Dean PB, Pentek Z. Galactography: the diagnostic procedure of choice for nipple discharge. Radiology 1983;149:31–8.

29. Leis HP. Management of nipple discharge. World J Surg 1989;13:736–42.

30. Mendelson EB. Evaluation of the postoperative breast. Radiol Clin North Am 1992;30:107–38.

31. Kopans DB. The altered breast: pregnancy, lactation, biopsy, mastectomy, radiation, and implants. In: Kopans DB. Breast imaging. 2nd ed. Philadelphia: Lippincott-Raven; 1997. p. 445–96.

32. Brenner RJ, Pfaff JM. Mammographic features after conservative therapy for malignant breast disease: serial findings standardized by regression analysis. Am J Roentgenol 1996;167:171–8.

33. Mendelson EB, Tobin CE. Imaging the breast after surgery and radiation therapy. In: Syllabus: a categorical course in breast imaging. Radiological Society of North America; 1995. p. 175–84.

34. Liberman L, Van Zee KJ, Dershaw DD, et al. Mammographic features of local recurrence in women who have undergone breast-conserving therapy for ductal carcinoma in situ. Am J Roentgenol 1997;168:489–93.

35. Viehweg P, Paprosch I, Strassinopoulou M, et al. Contrast-enhanced magnetic resonance imaging of the breast: interpretation guidelines. Top Magn Reson Imaging 1998;9:17–43.

36. Brenner RJ. Tumor detection in the augmented breast. In: Gorczyca DP, Brenner RJ, editors. The augmented breast: radiologic and clinical perspectives. New York: Thieme; 1997. p. 154–69.

37. Gorczyca DP. Magnetic resonance imaging of the failing implant. In: Gorczyca DP, Brenner RJ, editors. The augmented breast: radiologic and clinical perspectives. New York: Thieme; 1997. p. 121–43.

38. Reynolds HE. Evaluation of the augmented breast. Radiol Clin North Am 1995;33:1131–45.

39. Orel SG, Schnall MD, Powel, et al. Staging of suspected breast cancer: effect of MR imaging and MR-guided biopsy. Radiology 1995;196:115–22.

40. Mumtaz H, Hall-Craggs M, Davidson T, et al. Staging of symptomatic primary breast cancer with MR imaging. Am J Roentgenol 1997;169:417–24.

41. Nunes LW, Schnall MD, Orel SG, et al. Breast MR

imaging: interpretation model. Radiology 1997;202:833–41.

42. Hulka CA, Smith BL, Sgroi DC, et al. Benign and malignant breast lesions: differentiation with echo-planar MR imaging. Radiology 1995; 197:33–8.

43. Orel SG, Reynolds C, Schnall MD, et al. Breast carcinoma: MR imaging before re-excisional biopsy. Radiology 1997;205:429–36.

44. Stompre PC, Herman S, Klippenstein DL, et al. Suspect breast lesions: findings at dynamic gadolinium-enhanced MR imaging correlated with mammographic and pathologic features. Radiology 1995;197:387–95.

45. Muller-Schimpfle M, Ohmenhauser K, Stoll P, et al.

Menstrual cycle and age: influence on parenchymal contrast medium enhancement in MR imaging of the breast. Radiology 1997;203:145–9.

46. Soderstrom CE, Harms SE, Copit DS, et al. Three-dimensional RODEO breast MR imaging of lesions containing ductal carcinoma in situ. Radiology 1996;201:427–32.

47. Williams MB, Pisano ED, Schnall MD, et al. Future directions in imaging of breast diseases. Radiology 1998;206:297–300.

48. Wahl RL. Nuclear medicine techniques in breast imaging. Sem Ultrasound CT MRI 1996;17: 494–505.

49. Feig SA, Yaffe MJ. Digital mammography. Radiographics 1998;18:893–901.

4

Image-Directed Breast Biopsy

RICHARD E. FINE, MD

The recent increase in the detection of nonpalpable breast abnormalities requiring further evaluation is thought to be the direct result of more favorable participation in mammography screening. Appropriate diagnostic work-up will lead to a relative increase in lesions that are of sufficient risk to warrant a biopsy. In fact, it has been estimated that approximately 1.2 million breast biopsies are performed per year in the United States. Unfortunately, an average positive predictive value for mammography of 20 percent (range 15 to 35%) will yield a significant number of biopsies performed for benign disease.[1-4] If 5 women are identified on the mammogram to have a lesion requiring biopsy, only 1 of these 5 women will be found to have breast cancer. Therefore, if traditional methods for histologic confirmation are used, all 5 women would proceed to the operating room for an open surgical biopsy after first having had wire localization in the radiology suite. Image-guided percutaneous breast biopsy, an effective alternative, has recently gained favor. Image-guided percutaneous breast biopsy would provide a secondary level of screening for these five women in a less invasive, cost-effective manner as well as a histologic diagnosis without sacrificing accuracy.[5-9] The patient with breast cancer may then proceed to definitive surgical management and the other four women with a benign diagnosis may be placed in an appropriate follow-up protocol. It is with this concept in mind that we review the state-of-the-art in image-guided percutaneous breast biopsy.

NEEDLE LOCALIZATION BREAST BIOPSY

The gold standard with which image-guided percutaneous breast biopsy is compared is the needle or wire localization open surgical breast biopsy. However, this traditional management of a suspicious nonpalpable breast abnormality is not without its own error rate. The inability to successfully remove the appropriate lesion ranges from 0.5 to 17 percent.[10-15] Some of the reasons given for unsuccessful biopsies include (1) poor radiologic placement of the localization wire, (2) preoperative and intraoperative dislodgment of the wire, (3) surgical inaccuracy and inadequacy in excising the appropriate tissue, (4) failure to obtain a specimen radiograph, and (5) the pathologist missing the focus of disease when searching through a larger tissue sample provided by the surgeon.

The needle localization and open surgical breast biopsy is typically more invasive. Although a surgeon may discount the importance of a scar on the breast, women frequently have a great concern over even a one- to two-inch scar, especially on the superior aspect of the breast. The possibility of altered breast shape associated with tissue removal is also important. This fear is thought to be responsible for women failing to participate in recommended screening.

In addition to cutaneous scarring, parenchymal scarring may also complicate future mammographic follow-up.[6] Kopans has suggested that significant parenchymal scarring is rarely associated with a properly performed needle localization breast biopsy.[12] However, surgeons are frequently faced with mammographic reports indicating architectural distortion at the site of a prior biopsy that might mimic the changes associated with a malignancy.

Despite the potential advantages of image-guided percutaneous breast biopsy, there are still reasons why a standard needle localization open surgical biopsy may be chosen for histologic diagnosis. Some patients desire complete surgical removal of a breast abnormality and will not be satisfied with a "sampling procedure." Certain facilities and insurance plans do not provide access to facilities where image-guided procedures (ie, stereotactic) are performed. There are also certain lesion characteristics, patient characteristics, and potential pathologic entities that may render image-guided breast biopsy difficult or inappropriate.

The essentials for a properly performed wire localization breast biopsy include accurate localization, a comfortable, confident patient, and appropriate surgical planning and technique.[10,12–15] The radiologist most often localizes the lesion with orthogonal mammography.[12,16] Increasingly, stereotaxis and ultrasonography are used to identify the location of a nonpalpable lesion.[17,18] Whichever technique is used, it is important to have the wire within 1 cm of the lesion for the localization to be considered accurate and to limit the potential for error.[19]

The majority of these procedures are performed under local anesthesia with or without intravenous sedation.[12,14,20] Appropriate instillation of local anesthesia for both image-guided percutaneous biopsies and open surgical procedures is important for gaining the patient's confidence in the earliest aspect of the procedure. This will ensure a calmer patient through the remainder of the procedure. A skin wheal is raised using a small (27- or 30-gauge) needle with 1 percent Xylocaine ™ (lidocaine). Deeper local anesthetic should be placed (25-gauge needle) as a block around the potential dissection site. Despite the added cost, some have found sedation or general anesthesia to lessen the discomfort while improving the technical ease and success of removing the lesion with a needle localization and open surgical breast biopsy.[10]

While planning the incision site, cosmesis should be taken into consideration without ignoring cancer surgery principles.[18] If a lesion has a relatively low probability of malignancy and is within a reasonable distance from the nipple-areolar complex, a circumareolar incision should be considered. Regardless of the wire insertion site, localization mammography should be used to estimate the location of the lesion within the breast.[21] The breast incision does not necessarily require inclusion of the guide wire insertion site. In addition to using localization mammography, familiarity with the localization wire lengths and inherent markings may aid in a more accurate estimation of lesion location (Figures 4–1A to 4–1C).[19–21]

Once the lesion location is determined, the incision is planned to avoid tunneling of a more suspicious lesion through benign breast tissue.[22] The incision is carried straight down through the subcutaneous layer without the development of any flaps until the body of the wire is encountered and can be brought into the confines of the biopsy cavity. This is designed to maintain more support during closure and to avoid potential indentation.[18,19] On the basis of the relationship of the lesion to the tip of the wire, the excision is performed.

If the needle localization biopsy is being performed as a follow-up to an abnormal lesion on image-guided percutaneous breast biopsy or a presumed malignancy, it is then performed as a needle localization lumpectomy.[23] Margin assessment becomes crucial to the success of the procedure. A technique of assisting the pathologist with margin assessment involves intraoperative inking of the margins by the surgeon using the Davidson™ multicolor inking system. The anterior, 12, 3, 6, and 9 o'clock positions as well as the deep margins may be marked with corresponding colors (red, green, blue, black, yellow, and orange), using a cotton-tipped applicator (Figure 4–2). The specimen is then dipped into 3

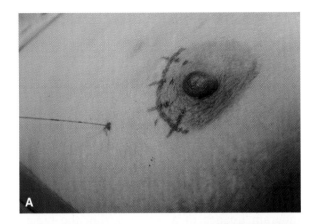

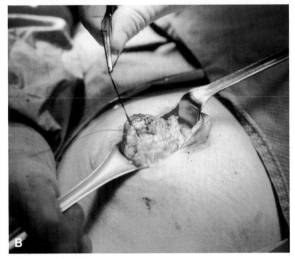

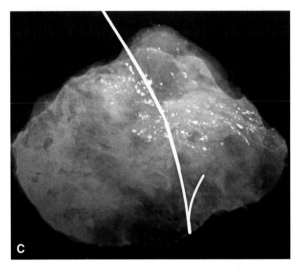

Figure 4–1. *A,* Based on the wire length, angle of insertion, and the localization mammograms, the position of the wire tip and lesion are determined and the incision planned. *B,* The incision is carried down through subcutaneous tissue, the wire is brought into the confines of the cavity and then a 2-0 silk suture is used for traction, and dissection is carried out around the course and tip of the wire. *C,* The specimen radiograph maybe magnified to determine the completeness of excision of microcalcifications.

percent acetic acid (vinegar) to set the colors. Subsequently, the specimen is sent to the radiology department for a specimen radiograph and then on to the pathology department. The specimen is sent dry so as to allow further stabilization of the ink prior to pathology sectioning.

When the probability of malignancy is high or already confirmed, a technique to ensure adequate margins may be instituted, especially when the procedure is for a potential multifocal process, such as ductal carcinoma in situ (DCIS). Once the main biopsy/lumpectomy specimen is removed, random additional margins may be taken from the walls of the biopsy cavity (12, 3, 6, 9 o'clock, and deep positions). The thickness of the additional margins is approximately 5 to 10 mm. The multicolor inking system is used to mark the side of the specimen representing the new margin of resection.

If there is focal margin involvement of the main specimen, the resection is felt to be adequate, if the additional margins are clear.

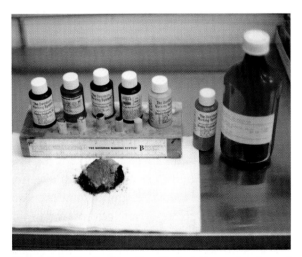

Figure 4–2. The Davidson™ multicolor inking system is used to identify margins of resection.

After hemostasis is obtained with electrocautery, the wound is closed. Closure consists only of reapproximating the subcuticular and dermal layers. There is neither draining nor reconstruction of the deep aspect of the biopsy cavity. If postoperative radiation therapy is a probability for the patient, small hemoclips are placed in the walls and base of the cavity. This will assist the radiation oncologist in planning therapy (especially the boost therapy required for close margins or used as a standard treatment in many centers). A clear, waterproof, Tegaderm™ dressing is applied, which allows the patient to shower or bathe in the immediate postoperative period.

The patient returns to the office during the following week for wound assessment, to discuss the pathology, and to plan future follow-up. A baseline mammogram of the biopsied breast is obtained after 6 months to look for any parenchymal scarring and to evaluate for appropriate and adequate biopsy. If the preoperative mammogram contained suspicious calcifications at the site of the biopsy, a baseline mammogram should be obtained prior to the initiation of radiotherapy.

IMAGE-GUIDED BREAST BIOPSY

The physician will have several concerns about instituting an image-guided breast biopsy program. Will patients accept sampling rather than excision? What will be the false-negative rate? Will we maintain the proper indications, and who should perform the image-guided breast biopsy—radiologists or surgeons?

While the physicians deal with these concerns, the patient is exposed to media headlines such as "The Needle Replaces the Knife." It does not take a very sophisticated patient-consumer to understand that a needle is less invasive than a knife. In addition to the media deluge, patients are also exposed to corporate-driven advertisement of new breast biopsy devices. Acceptance of a new technology, in the face of physician reluctance, is now being influenced by outside sources.

Stereotactic Breast Biopsy: Equipment

Percutaneous breast biopsy for nonpalpable disease requires imaging. The two main imaging modalities are stereotaxis and ultrasonography. These modalities are complementary to one another and therefore knowledge of both is required to provide the physician with the full range of options. Stereotactic breast biopsy is performed using specialized mammography equipment. The equipment obtains stereo mammogram images of a lesion within the breast and then relies on computerized triangulation of the targeted lesion to calculate the three-dimensional position of this lesion.[5,24] There are two main types of stereotactic equipment, the upright add-on and the dedicated prone.[25–27] Add-on stereotactic equipment uses standard upright mammography with an attachable platform to perform targeting and biopsy (Figure 4–3). Add-on stereotactic units provide the advantage of maximum use of the equipment, which has dual capabilities: screening or diagnostic mammography and stereotactic breast biopsy. This can provide considerable cost savings by avoiding not only dedicated equipment but also dedicated space within a breast diagnostic facility. Despite these potential advan-

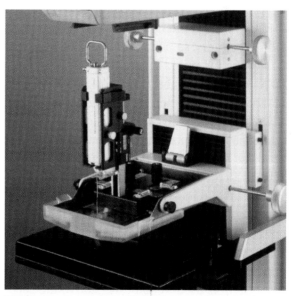

Figure 4–3. The StereoLoc™ is the upright add-on stereotactic guidance system used with the Lorad™ mammography unit.

tages, add-on stereotactic breast biopsy units traditionally have been less popular than dedicated prone stereotactic tables. Because of the upright patient position and patient visualization of the procedure, there is the potential for an increase in syncopal episodes.[5,28] In addition, the upright units provide minimal work space and limited access to the breast. Dedicated prone stereotactic tables are more costly and require dedicated space for performing stereotactic breast biopsy. These disadvantages appear to be outweighed by several advantages. The prone position allows gravity to aid the technologist in reaching more posterior lesions. A greatly enhanced work space underneath the table and out of the patient's view allows for the addition of more advanced breast biopsy devices.

There are two dedicated prone systems available, the Mammotest/Mammovision™ (Fischer Imaging, Denver, Colorado) and the Lorad Stereoguide™ (Lorad, a division of Trex Medical, Danbury, Connecticut) (Figures 4–4A and 4–4B).

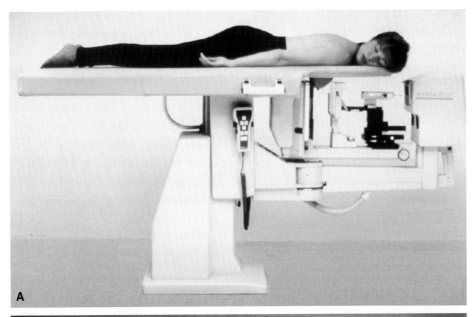

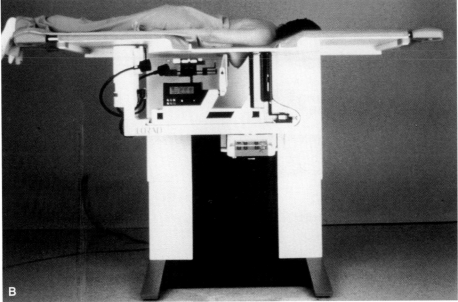

Figure 4–4. *A*, Fischer Mammotest/Mammovision™. *B*, Lorad Stereoguide™.

The Stereoguide™ table has, until recently, also been distributed as the ABBI™ table by the U.S. Surgical Corporation. The Fischer Mammotest/Mammovision™ is a unidirectional patient-positioning table, with the aperture for the patient's breast located at one end of the table. Access around the breast is approximately 180° to 210° with rotation of the C-arm and mammography tube head. Special software features increase the angle of access to the breast up to 240° with "target on scout" and close to 360° with the "lateral arm." The Lorad Stereoguide™ is a bidirectional patient-positioning table with the aperture for the breast in the center of the table and a foot extension at either end. With the facility to rotate the patient 180° and the addition of the 180° rotation of the C-arm, there is a true 360° access to the breast.

Specimen Acquisition Devices

The stereotactic biopsy equipment is amenable to the addition of a number of different devices that are used in specimen acquisition. These include fine-needle aspiration (FNA), automated Tru-cut needle core, and vacuum-assisted biopsy devices (Mammotome™, MIBB™) (Figure 4–5). Breast biopsy acquisition devices (ABBI™, Site-Select™) have larger cannula type tools and are designed for an image-guided excision of tissue as a substitute for traditional surgical biopsy.

Fine-needle aspiration using stereotactic guidance was the first minimally invasive biopsy technique used for nonpalpable lesions and is preferred by some to this day. In 1989, *Lancet* published a classic article from the Karolinski Institute, which evaluated the stereotactic fine needle biopsy of 2,594 mammographically detected, nonpalpable lesions from 1983 to 1987.[29] Of the 2,005 (77.3%) cases judged to be benign, only 1 turned out to be malignant 14 months later. Of the 576 cases (21.9%) selected for needle localization followed by open breast biopsy on the basis of cytologic and/or mammographic interpretation, cancer was identified in 429 (75.7%). Dowlatshahi and colleagues published 528 cases of stereotactic FNA, in corroboration with the University of Kiel from the Federal Republic of Germany.[17] In their report stereotactic guidance with 23-gauge FNA had a sensitivity of 95 per-

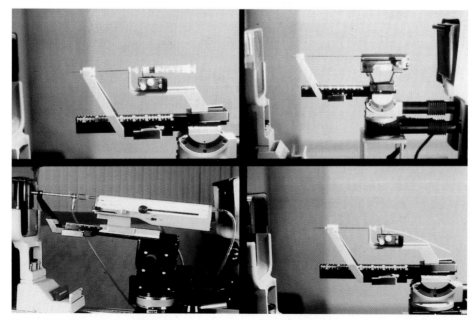

Figure 4–5. Prone stereotactic tables can perform fine-needle aspiration, needle core biopsy, vacuum-assisted biopsy, and wire localization procedures.

cent and accuracy of 92 percent. Furthermore, this article confirmed the accuracy of stereotactic localization by imaging the tip of the needle within 2-mm of the center of the lesion in 96 percent of the cases.

Acceptance of FNA as a standard technique for the performance of stereotactic biopsy had limited success, especially in the United States. Fine-needle aspiration has long been recognized to have several potential pitfalls. This includes insufficient sampling as high as 38 percent, a low ranging sensitivity ranging between 68 and 93 percent, and specificity varying between 88 and 100 percent.[30] The broad range of sensitivity and specificity is dependent on a number of factors, including the type of lesion to be sampled, the individual performing the aspiration, and the individual interpreting the cytologic specimen. Finally, cytology rarely provides a specific benign diagnosis.

Automated Tru-cut™ Type Biopsy

In the late 1980s, Parker (Radiology Imaging Associates, Englewood, Colorado) and others began working with the automated Tru-cut Biopsy™ instrument (Bard Urologic, Covington, Georgia) designed for biopsy of the prostate. He combined this technology on the prone Fischer™ stereotactic table for performing large-core stereotactic breast biopsy. In 1991, Parker published a case series of 102 patients, where every patient had a stereotactic-guided, large-core needle biopsy, followed by traditional surgical excision of the lesion.[5] There was agreement of histologic results in 98 cases (96%). One cancer missed with a core was determined to be a very difficult lesion to localize because of its posterior position. This article set the stage for the standardization of stereotactic biopsy techniques, which is still being followed today. In addition to the use of dedicated prone stereotactic equipment, he also advocated the use of "long throw" biopsy needle devices. The longer excursion of the inner and outer sheaths of the needle provided a con-

sistently larger tissue sample. The standard use of the 14-gauge needle eliminated the issue of insufficient sampling. Several different gauge needles for automated Tru-cut™ biopsy have been evaluated. The lower rate of insufficient sampling and increased sensitivity, without increased complications, have led to the minimum 14-gauge size becoming the standard.[31,32] Another principle identified to increase the accuracy is the routine use of pre- and postfire stereotactic imaging. Prefire stereo images assess the appropriate alignment of the needle to the lesion, and postfire stereo images document the penetration of the needle through the lesion. Tru-cut™-type core-needle biopsy with stereotactic localization was demonstrated by Parker and others to be a cost-effective procedure, which was less invasive and reduced patient anxiety. It has a lower false-negative rate when compared with FNA.[5–8] Furthermore, the need for cytologic expertise is avoided, which is important in the community setting where expert cytopathologist interpretation may not be available.

Initial experience with stereotactic breast biopsy was based on film screen technology until 1993, when the charged coupled device (CCD) camera replaced the film cassette image receptor. This facilitated digital recreation of the breast lesion on a computer monitor. Several advantages for digital image acquisition were immediately recognized. As the software improved, image acquisition time decreased. This significantly reduced procedure time, which, in turn, increased patient comfort. A more comfortable patient was less likely to move and as a result the breast and target lesion remained stationary for improved targeting accuracy. A critical difference between digital image acquisition and film screen image acquisition involves postprocessing of the image. Once a film is developed, the characteristics of the lesion on the film cannot be changed. When a digital image is acquired, the lesion can be enhanced, magnified, and even inverted to appear black on a white background. These postprocessing features are especially helpful when evaluating small clusters of microcalcifications. An additional bonus for patients included lower radiation with each procedure, related to a narrow field of view. Digital imaging for stereotactic biopsy is not full field (ie, the entire breast is not imaged). The area of the breast imaged is limited to a square area of 5 × 5 cm. The true learning curve in performing stereotactic breast biopsy revolves around this narrow field of view. The lesion for which the biopsy is to be performed requires prior identification on a high-quality, film-screen diagnostic mammogram. The physician must recognize and transfer the appearance of the lesion to a digital image. The digital image is at least four times magnified, is dependent on monitor resolution, and the lesion is not seen in association with the full anatomic image of the breast.

Performing Stereotactic Breast Biopsy

After review of the mammogram, the general approach to the breast is chosen. The shortest skin-to-lesion distance and the ability to visualize the lesion are both factors in choosing the approach.[33] Also important is assuring enough tissue beyond the lesion to account for the excursion ("throw") of the biopsy needle during sampling. A lesion in the lower inner aspect of the breast may be approached from the mediolateral position. A lesion in the most inferior six o'clock position of the breast may be approached from the mediolateral or lateromedial position on the Fischer Mammotest™ table. The "lateral arm" may be attached to access the lesion through the noncompressed portion of the breast. The six o'clock lesion may also be approached from the caudal cranial position (ie, from below) on the Lorad Stereoguide™ table. The mammography technologist is responsible for positioning the patient for the desired approach. Other responsibilities of the technologist include calibration and maintenance of the equipment and quality assurance.

The first digital image to be taken is the zero-degree scout image. No matter what approach to the breast is taken, the scout image is perpendicular to the plane of the skin. Once the appropriate lesion is identified, it is positioned in the middle third of the scout image, from left to the right. A set of stereo images are obtained by rotating the mammography tube head to a +15° and −15° to yield an arc of separation between the two stereo images of 30° (Figure 4–6). When targeting for an automated Tru-cut instrument, a central target is chosen on the lesion in image number one, and a corresponding target is chosen on the lesion in image number two. Additional targets or offsets are chosen around the center of the lesion, for example, at 12, 3, 6, and 9 o'clock positions (Figure 4–7). With the appropriate targets entered into the system, the software determines the horizontal, parallax shift of the lesion from stereo image number one to stereo image number two. The vertical coordinate is unchanged. A trigonometric formula then calculates the horizontal, vertical, and depth coordinates of the lesion's center within the breast.

With the three-dimensional coordinates of the lesion calculated, the puncture device or stage, which houses the biopsy instrumentation, is motor driven to the calculated horizontal and vertical positions. The biopsy device is advanced toward the skin, and the site for insertion is identified. A local anesthetic is injected to raise an appropriate skin wheal. Additional local anesthetic may be judiciously injected into the deeper aspects of the breast. This is done in a radial manner to avoid placing too much local anesthetic in any one area for fear of moving the targeted lesion, or placing too much local anesthetic in front of the lesion for fear of limiting its visualization. An 11-blade scalpel is used to make a vertical-oriented skin incision of 2 to 4 mm in length. The needle is advanced into the breast to a position several millimeters short of the center of the calculated depth of the lesion. On the basis of the mechanics of the biopsy instruments in use

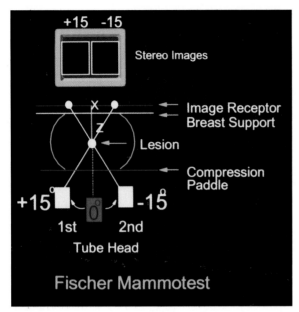

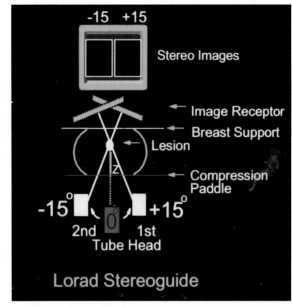

Figure 4–6. Viewing the stereotactic tables from above. The diagram illustrates the movement of the tube head for acquiring stereo images and the resultant z-value determination.

(dead space at needle tip, sample notch size, excursion or throw of instrument), a precalculated pull-back is determined by each biopsy instrument manufacturer. The depth chosen is the calculated depth minus this predetermined pull-back depth. By using the pull-back depth, the sampling notch will be positioned for more adequate, fuller sampling of the lesion (Figure 4–8).

Prefire stereo digital images are acquired to assess the alignment of the needle tip in rela-

tionship to the lesion to be biopsied. There must be symmetry of alignment between the two stereo images. If the alignment is satisfactory, the automated Tru-cut instrument is fired and the first sample from the center of the lesion is obtained. Prior to removing the needle from the breast, it is important to document symmetrical penetration of the needle through the center of the lesion by taking stereo postfire images of the lesion (Figures 4–9A, 4–9B). The needle is withdrawn from the breast, the speci-

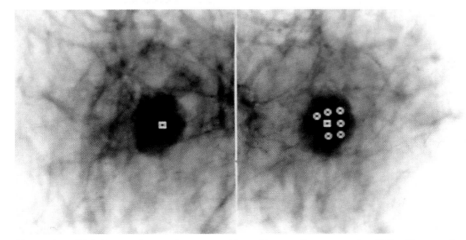

Figure 4–7. Digital stereo images in reverse video with central targets and multiple offsets on the Fischer™ system.

men is placed on moistened gauze, and the biopsy instrument is recocked and reinserted into the breast through the same skin incision to acquire the next target or offset sample. The same process is repeated until all samples are obtained. The average number of needle core biopsy samples for a nodular density is five or six (Figure 4–10). When biopsies of microcalcifications are performed, a greater sampling is required. Even in open biopsy surgical literature, pathologic assessment has identified atypical hyperplasia and DCIS at a "distance" from the targeted microcalcifications.[34] Lieberman from Memorial Sloan Kettering Hospital discussed the issue of how many core biopsy specimens are needed.[35] In her report, biopsies of 145 lesions were performed; 92 were nodular densities and 53 were microcalcifications. Five cores yielded diagnosis in 99 percent of the biopsies for nodular densities. Five cores yielded a diagnosis in only 87 percent of the patients presenting with microcalcifications; six or more cores yielded a diagnosis in 92 percent of the cases. When the targeted samples have been obtained, a set of postprocedure dig-

ital images are acquired. The purpose of these images is to document the removal of the microcalcifications and to verify the presence of residual calcifications. A specimen radiograph of the tissue documents the inclusion of microcalcifications within the core samples.[36,37] Frequently, only a few calcifications are evident on specimen radiography. Increasingly, the literature has begun to support concern over insufficient sampling of core biopsy for microcalcifications. Israel and Fine reported a series of 500 consecutive core-needle biopsies with a sensitivity of 97.8 percent and a false-negative rate of 1.5 percent. However, upgrading of diagnosis on open surgical excision was evident in 33 percent of the cases, where atypical ductal hyperplasia was identified on core-needle biopsy, and DCIS was identified on excision.[38] The presentation for the upgrading of diagnosis was microcalcifications, where the average core sampling was between 9 and 12 samples. Not surprisingly, atypical ductal hyperplasia diagnosed at stereotactic core-needle biopsy has been called an indication for open surgical biopsy.[39,40] Consis-

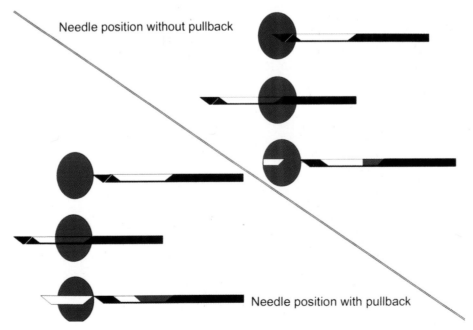

Needle position without pullback

Needle position with pullback

Figure 4–8. Positioning the needle at the lesion center will result in failure to sample the front half of the lesion. With a 5-mm pull-back to the front of the lesion, the entire length of the lesion will be sampled.

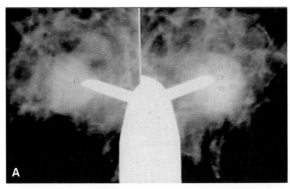
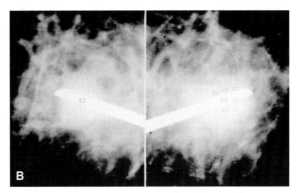

Figure 4–9. *A,* Prefire alignment; the relation of the tip of the needle to the lesion must be symmetrical. *B,* Postfire alignment; the relation of the tip of the needle to the lesion must be symmetrical.

tent with the reporting of others, Liberman reported a series of 25 cases of atypical ductal hyperplasia identified on stereotactic core-needle biopsy, with significant upgrading (52%) to carcinoma on open surgical excision.[41]

Vacuum-Assisted Biopsy Devices

A solution to decrease the upgrading of diagnosis is to increase tissue sampling. Tissue sampling can be increased by increasing the number of samples taken, increasing the size of the tissue sample taken, and/or the manner in which the tissue samples are obtained. A vacuum-assisted biopsy satisfies these requirements.[25,42] Not only is the sample size larger, but the samples may be taken in a circumferencial, contiguous manner to allow reconstruction of the histologic architecture of the area of the biopsy. The Mammotome™ consists of a driver, which may be housed on either of the dedicated prone stereotactic systems. Inside the driver, there is a biopsy probe that consists of three parts. The probe body has a sampling notch with several holes connected to a vacuum. The second part of the probe is a rotating cutter lumen that fits inside the probe body and is rotated by a circular gear mechanism in the driver. The third and last component of the probe is the knockout pin, which fits inside the cutter lumen and is attached to the rear vacuum to assist in retrieving tissue samples from the probe body. The probe is manufactured in two sizes: 14- and 11-

gauge.[43] The Mammotome™ system is ideally suited for taking biopsy specimens of microcalcifications under stereotactic guidance. Once the calcifications have been imaged stereotactically, they are targeted on the computer monitor. By changing the position of the sampling notch, multiple tissue samples can be obtained using only a single target probe insertion. The target may be centered in the cluster of microcalcifications or preferentially placed at the cluster's edge so that the overlying probe will not obscure a small cluster of microcalcifications when digital images are obtained. When the three-dimensional coordinates are calculated by the stereotactic system software, the driver and probe are positioned at the corresponding horizontal and vertical coordinates. The driver and probe are advanced toward the breast, where local anesthetic is injected. The probe is inserted through a vertical skin incision to the appropriate

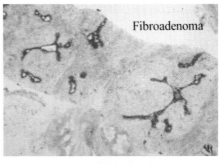
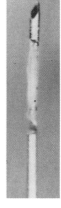

Fibroadenoma

Figure 4–10. 14-gauge needle core biopsy sample with histologic confirmation of fibroadenoma.

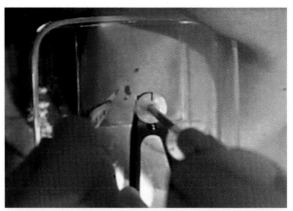

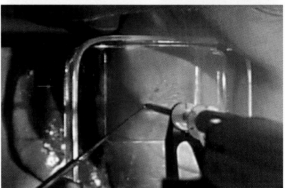

Figure 4–11. Local anesthetic injection, skin incision with an 11-blade scalpel followed by insertion of vacuum-assisted probe into the skin, in preparation for biopsy.

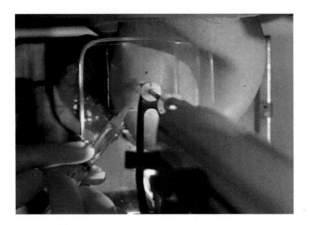

depth (Figure 4–11). Prefire stereo images assess the alignment of the probe with the microcalcifications. The driver is designed with a spring-loaded mechanism to permit automated advancement of the probe through the breast tissue. The sampling notch may be positioned within the breast by the automated forward movement of the probe, or it can be manually aligned with the lesion by taking the driver to the appropriate depth with the probe already in its full excursion. The alignment of the sampling notch with

the lesion is confirmed with postfire (alignment) stereo images (Figure 4–12). A vacuum pulls breast tissue into the sampling notch, and the cutter is advanced across the sampling notch, cutting the tissue free from inside the breast. The tissue sample is removed from the specimen retrieval chamber. The entire process is then repeated. The number of biopsy samples taken is based on the size of the lesion and the volume of tissue desired. On average, approximately 12 to 16 tissue samples are obtained for a small cluster of microcalcifications, frequently resulting in removal of the entire mammographic evidence of the lesion. The vacuum assistance provides several advantages. It eliminates the need for pinpoint accuracy required with automated Tru-cut biopsy instruments and facilitates removal of multiple tissue samples without removal of the biopsy probe.[42] In addition, the notch may be positioned for specific directional sampling, on the basis of the alignment of the probe notch with the lesion. The larger tissue samples provide a greater chance

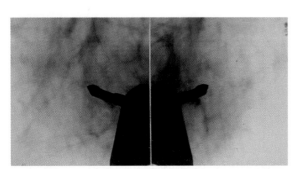

Figure 4–12. The vacuum assisted probe may be used for directional sampling. In this example, the majority of samples will be taken between 3:00 and 9:00 through the 6:00 position.

of lesion removal and a greater percentage of positive specimen radiographs (Figure 4–13). Burbank and Jackman have demonstrated that the improved accuracy with the directional vacuum-assisted biopsy device decreases the upgrading of diagnosis seen with core-needle biopsy.[44,45] Burbank showed that the 14-gauge device provided no upgrading of atypical ductal hyperplasia to carcinoma at open biopsy. Jackman compared 14-gauge vacuum-assisted device to 14-gauge core-needle biopsy and illustrated a reduction of upgrading of atypical ductal hyperplasia from 48 to 18 percent. Postprocedure imaging yields a well-defined air-contrast cavity in the majority of cases. The 11-gauge core probe also allows a marker clip to be placed in the wall of the biopsy cavity to assist in the localization of the area in the future when all evidence of the lesion has been eliminated.[46] This marker clip and/or the residual cavity may be localized if the diagnosis requires further surgical management. The complication rate for the device is less than 1 percent, which is comparable to core-needle biopsy.[7,42] Ecchymosis of the skin at the insertion site is common as well as intraparenchymal hemorrhage localized to the biopsy cavity, but clinically significant hematomas that interfere or complicate subsequent surgery or follow-up are rare.

DIFFICULTIES IN STEREOTACTIC BREAST BIOPSIES

It is important for the physician to anticipate that some patients and some lesions will be difficult for obtaining biopsy specimens. Certain lesion characteristics, such as low-density nodules, faint or nonclustered microcalcifications, or vague asymmetric densities, may be difficult to visualize with digital imaging despite postprocessing features. The position of certain lesions, such as those that are very superficial, those against the chest wall, or those in the axillary tail of the breast, may require innovative positioning by the experienced technologist. However, some lesions may be inaccessible. It

is essential that the physician be able to recognize and correct for targeting errors (Figures 4–14A to 4–14C). Certain patient characteristics will interfere with the success of a stereotactic breast biopsy. Patients with neurologic or musculoskeletal conditions may not tolerate positioning on the stereotactic table. Patients that are coughing because of an acute or chronic respiratory condition will increase breast motion and lesion movement, which may interfere with accurate targeting. Patients with a high level of anxiety, especially those suffering from claustrophobia or agoraphobia, may require sedation. As any biopsy has the potential for bleeding complications, those patients with a history of bleeding abnormalities or who are taking anticoagulants will require correction prior to biopsy. The small or ptotic breast creates one of the most common difficulties in stereotactic breast biopsy. A breast that flattens to a marginal thickness in compression may lead to "stroke margin problems." The stroke margin is defined as the distance in millimeters from the postfired biopsy needle/probe to the back of the breast or the rear image receptor. The stroke margin must be greater than zero on the Lorad Stereoguide™ system or greater than a positive 4 mm on the Fischer Mammotest™ table (Figure 4–15). When a breast is very thin, or the lesion is more posteriorly positioned, a negative stroke margin may be encountered. This situation will result in the biopsy needle or probe striking the rear image receptor and piercing the back of the patient's breast skin.

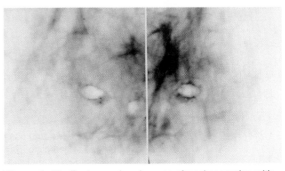

Figure 4–13. Postprocedure images after six samples with the vacuum-assisted device illustrated the air-contrast cavity and the majority of calcifications removed.

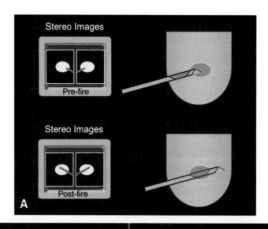

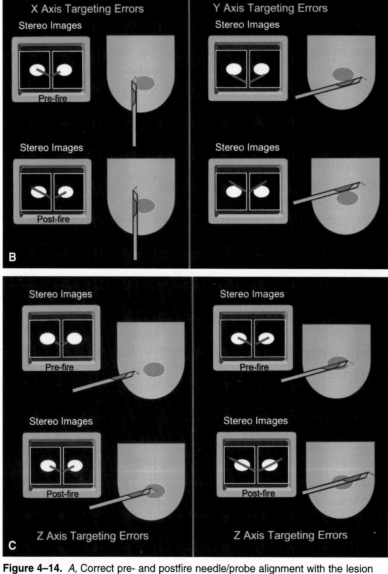

Figure 4–14. *A,* Correct pre- and postfire needle/probe alignment with the lesion result in favorable tissue sampling. *B,* An "X" targeting error will result in the needle/probe being off to one side of the lesion. A "Y" targeting error will result in the needle/probe being above or below the lesion. *C,* A "Z" axis targeting error will illustrate the needle/probe being too far in front or too far past the lesion. All three targeting errors become less important with the vacuum-assisted device.

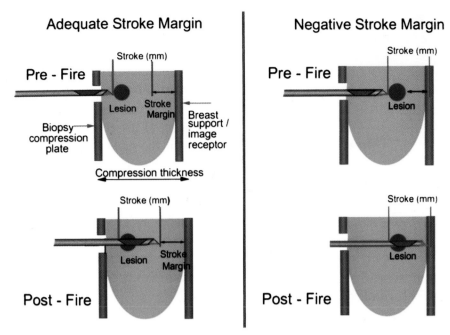

Figure 4–15. With an adequate stroke margin, the back of the breast and image receptor are protected. Ignoring a negative stroke margin will result in patient discomfort and damage to the image receptor.

Several mechanisms for correcting stroke margins are available. The most commonly employed is pulling back the prefire position of the needle/probe several millimeters until the calculated stroke margin is adequate (Figure 4–16). Other methods for dealing with stroke margin difficulties include, but are not limited to, taking a different approach to the breast lesion, using a shorter "throw" biopsy instrument, manual insertion of the Mammotome™ probe, use of the lateral arm, and implementation of a double-paddle technique.

BREAST ULTRASONOGRAPHY

Breast ultrasonography is an effective diagnostic tool when used in the proper clinical setting. Appropriate indications for breast ultrasonog-

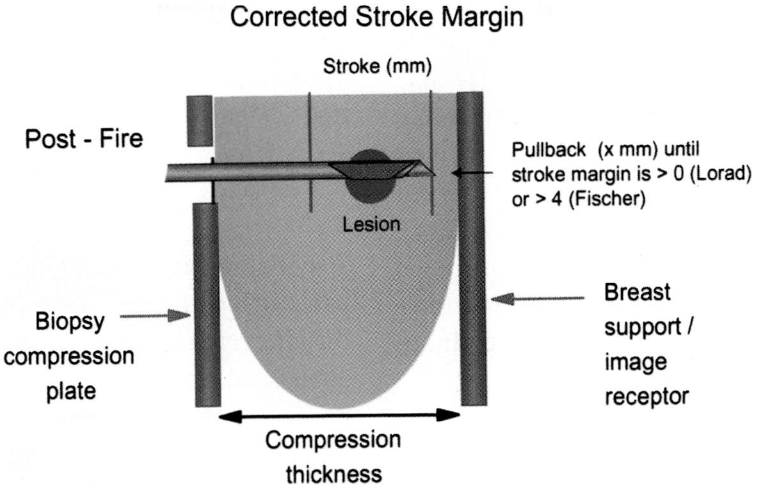

Figure 4–16. The most common method for correcting for an inadequate stroke margin involves reducing the depth of the needle/probe by "x" mm.

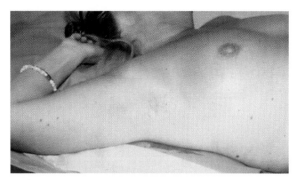

Figure 4–17. The patient is positioned supine, with the ipsilateral arm raised for ultrasound scanning. The position may be altered by rolling the patient and/or propping the patient with a pillow to allow scanning through the thinner portions of the breast.

raphy have been somewhat controversial. A lower comfort level with hands-on breast ultrasonography and a heavy reliance on ultrasonographers has, until recently, minimized the importance of breast ultrasonography. The availability of computer-enhanced imaging and high-frequency transducers have allowed the indications for breast ultrasonography to move well beyond distinguishing cystic from solid lesions.[47,48]

Diagnostic breast ultrasonography may be used to evaluate palpable abnormalities, especially in a radiographically dense breast. Mammographically indeterminate lesions will not only be evaluated for cystic versus solid nature, but the sonographic characteristics may assist in distinguishing a lesion's benign or malignant nature. Diagnostic breast ultrasonography will assist the clinician in evaluating the patient that is pregnant or lactating. Postoperative follow-up for both benign and malignant disease may be enhanced with ultrasonography, including monitoring and management of seromas and hematomas. The chest wall and the conserved breast can be assessed for recurrent disease. The axilla may be scanned for preoperative staging. Associated with every diagnostic indication is the ability to use ultrasonography to guide interventional procedures.

The goals of diagnostic breast ultrasonography are to reduce the number of benign biopsies by recognizing simple cysts and areas of fibroglandular tissue, which may clinically pre-

sent as a "thickening" or a mammographic asymmetry. When a focal abnormality is identified, an ultrasound-guided percutaneous biopsy will provide an efficient and cost-effective diagnosis.

Breast ultrasonography can easily be integrated into the surgeon's practice as a direct extension of his clinical breast evaluation. The patient in the supine position with the ipsilateral arm raised, much like the clinical breast examination, is ready for ultrasound examination (Figure 4–17). The 7.5- to 10-MHz linear array transducer is used for a targeted diagnostic ultrasound examination of a clinical abnormality. Whole breast ultrasound is usually done for two reasons:

1. In the patient with a suspected breast cancer to look for other areas of involvement;
2. High-risk patient with a clinically difficult breast and normal or non-specific mammogram to look for an occult lesion.

The scanning techniques commonly used include the radial scan, transverse sweeping scan, and tangential scan of the nipple. The axilla may also be scanned, especially in association with a known malignancy. The normal sonographic anatomy of the female breast that can be routinely imaged includes skin, subcutaneous fat, breast parenchyma, Cooper's ligament, retromammary fat, pectoral muscle and fascia, ribs, and pleura.[49] Diagnosis of ultrasound abnormalities is dependent on familiarity with the normal sonographic breast anatomy and the recognition of patterns of different breast types (Figure 4–18).

Indications for Intervention

A symptomatic or enlarging cyst, whether palpable or nonpalpable, is a common indication for intervention. Typically, a symptomatic, palpable cyst is aspirated by inserting a needle under palpation guidance and withdrawing fluid until the lesion is no longer palpable. Ultrasound guidance for aspiration may be just as appropriate for the palpable lesion as it is

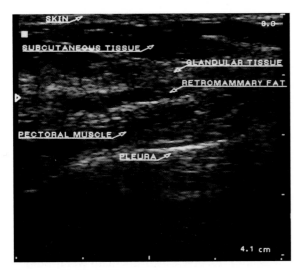

Figure 4–18. Normal breast anatomy.

obtained in a cost-effective, efficient manner in the office setting.

Ultrasound-guided aspiration and/or biopsy will assist in the management of postoperative complications, such as seromas or hematomas. With the increasing use of breast conservation therapy, the architectural distortion identified at the lumpectomy site may be ideally suited for further evaluation with image-guided breast biopsy. Ultrasound-guided FNA of clinical

necessary for the nonpalpable lesion.[50,51] Ultrasound guidance may assist in getting the needle into a thick-walled cyst, documenting any cyst wall irregularities and confirming total cyst collapse (Figures 4–19A, 4–19B).

Cysts not meeting the criteria for a simple cyst require aspiration. A lesion with a mixed internal echo pattern and posterior enhancement suggests the presence of fluid versus a solid lesion, and an aspiration may be attempted prior to a core-needle biopsy.[52] The aspiration of thick, paste-like material, frequently found with mammary duct ectasia, might require a local anesthetic and the use of a larger-gauge (18 g) needle.

The presence of a nonpalpable, solid lesion is an indication for an ultrasound-guided core-needle biopsy to obtain a histologic diagnosis.[53] Once again, ultrasound guidance is advantageous for guiding a core-needle biopsy for the palpable solid lesion as well as the nonpalpable lesion. Ultrasound visualization and documentation of the needle within the biopsy lesion enhances the accuracy. For the solid lesion with smooth margins, a homogeneous internal echo pattern and ellipsoid shape, such as a fibroadenoma, core-needle biopsy will achieve a specific benign diagnosis. For the more suspicious lesion with jagged edges, nonhomogeneous and irregular shadowing considered to be suspicious for carcinoma, the diagnosis may be

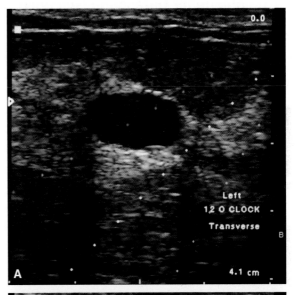

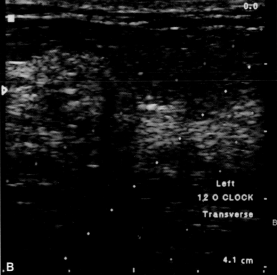

Figure 4–19. *A,* This anechoic, smooth-walled lesion with reverberation artifact is being prepared for aspiration, using an attachable needle guide. The lesion is aligned with the puncture lines on the ultrasound monitor. *B,* Postcyst aspiration documenting complete resolution.

adenopathy may assist in staging or evaluation of recurrent disease. With image-guided aspiration and drainage, frequently a part of the surgical management of intracavitary abscesses, it only makes sense that a more conservative approach should be considered for breast abscess. Ultrasound guidance is advantageous for the aspiration of pus or the insertion of a catheter for drainage and also to monitor the resolving abscess.

Technique for Ultrasound Guidance

Whether guiding a 25-gauge needle for the aspiration of a simple cyst, a needle for the insertion of a local anesthetic, a wire for localization, or a 14-gauge needle for core-needle biopsy, the principles for ultrasound-guided biopsy remain the same. It must be remembered that an ultrasound image visualized on the ultrasound monitor represents a "slice" of the breast of approximately 1.5 mm in thickness. When scanning brings the lesion requiring intervention into focus, we once again are only seeing a 1.5-mm

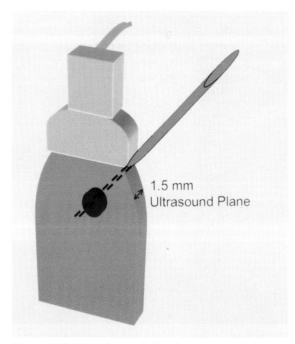

Figure 4–20. The ultrasound plane is approximately 1 to 1.5 mm thick. The biopsy needle must remain within this thin ultrasound plane at the same time that the lesion is maintained within that same plane to confirm accurate biopsy.

thick slice of this lesion in its location within the breast. This ultrasound plane is parallel to the long axis of the ultrasound transducer. Therefore, the intervening instrument must be guided along the long axis of the transducer. When the tip of the needle is seen advancing toward the lesion and penetrates that lesion, we know that the needle is in the same 1.5-mm plane as the slice of the lesion being visualized and therefore within the lesion (Figure 4–20).[54–56]

To aspirate an enlarging or symptomatic cyst, one simply wipes the skin with an alcohol preparation and inserts a small needle (25-, 22-, 20-gauge); feedback is immediate when fluid is seen in the syringe. When using a larger-gauge needle for aspiration of a complex cyst, a local anesthetic may be injected with a small-gauge needle (30-, 27-, 25-gauge) and aspiration performed with an 18-gauge needle. Cytologic evaluation of the aspirated fluid is reserved for bloody fluid or lack of cyst resolution.[55]

Ultrasound core-needle biopsy for histologic diagnosis requires more planning. When the lesion requiring a core-needle biopsy is identified, the skin is marked at the edge of the transducer for the proposed insertion site of the needle. The optimal insertion site and approach to the lesion is the shortest skin-to-lesion distance. For best cosmesis, care should be taken to avoid placing the scar of the insertion site near the inner portion of the breast. At this point, the breast is prepared with an appropriate antiseptic solution. The transducer is likewise prepared, or a sterile sleeve may be placed over the transducer. Sterile ultrasound gel is available in individual packets. The local anesthetic is then injected under direct ultrasound visualization. The skin is anesthetized as well as the track leading to the lesion. In addition, the local anesthetic is applied above, below, and to the opposite side of the lesion. The use of ultrasound visualization limits obscuring the lesion with the administration of too much local anesthesia in any one area. A small skin incision is made at the transducer edge using an 11-blade scalpel. The core biopsy needle is then inserted

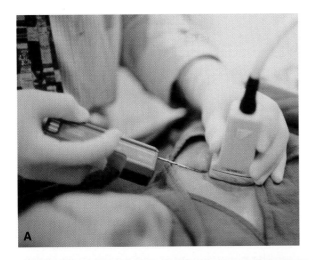

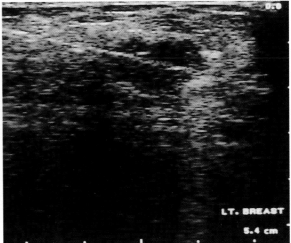

Figure 4–21. *A,* With the ultrasound transducer and breast stabilized with the nondominant hand, the biopsy instrument is advanced forward through a small skin incision maintaining orientation of the needle in the long axis of the transducer. *B,* Documenting alignment and penetration under real-time ultrasound guidance.

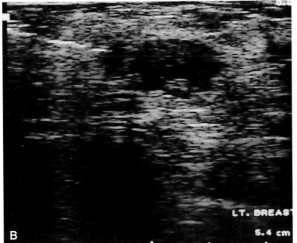

into the breast, and the lesion is approached with ultrasound guidance. The needle may be guided freehand or directed by an attachable needle guide that is available from certain ultrasound manufactures.[49,53,54] The attachable needle guides assist the neophyte in maintaining the proper needle alignment within the narrow ultrasound plane to ensure accurate lesion sampling. Visualization is maximized by keeping the needle at a more shallow angle and therefore parallel to the sole of the transducer. The shallow angle of the needle will also minimize the chance of penetrating the chest wall and subsequently the pleura. The freehand method of biopsy allows greater flexibility in the needle insertion site and angle of approach of the needle to the breast lesion. With either method, the needle is observed and the information docu-

mented as it approaches the lesion. When the position of the needle is confirmed at the front of the lesion, the needle/gun combination is fired.[53,57,58] There are several needle/gun combinations available, some of which are disposable and others that use disposable needles within a more permanent housing (gun). The mechanism of tissue acquisition is similar with the automated movement of an inner sheath that contains a sampling notch followed immediately by an outer sheath that cuts the tissue free. This action is accomplished under direct ultrasound visualization (Figure 4–21). The needle is then withdrawn, and the specimen is transferred onto a moistened telfa pad. Additional tissue samples are taken in the same manner through the existing incision until the lesion is adequately sampled. Approximately three to five tissue samples are obtained, depending on the quality of the samples and the confirmation of the needle penetrating the lesion. When adequate sampling is achieved, manual compression is applied. The incision may be approximated with a Steri-strip™, and a Tegaderm™ dressing is applied (Figure 4–22).

The accuracy of ultrasound core-needle biopsy has been widely documented.[53,54,56,59] Staren reviewed his series of more than 1,000 consecutive diagnostic ultrasound scans. Of these, 210 patients underwent ultrasound-guided core biopsy of nonpalpable, mammographically detected lesions using a 14-gauge needle. Symptomatic cysts underwent ultrasound-guided FNA. Lesions characterized as fibroadenoma, indeterminate, or suspicious underwent ultrasound-guided FNA and/or core-needle biopsy. There were no false positives and the false-negative rate was 3.6 percent. Small lesions were noted with ultrasound characteristics that warranted biopsy on diagnostic grounds alone. Staren concluded that ultrasound-guided aspiration and/or biopsy could accurately diagnose nonpalpable, mammographically detected breast masses.

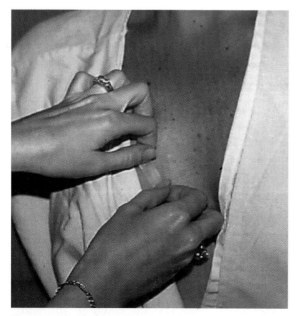

Figure 4–22. The skin incision is re-approximated using a Steri-strip™ after manual compression has been applied for hemostasis. A dressing may then be applied.

SUMMARY

When patients are referred with mammographic abnormalities requiring further evaluation, the mammographic lesion is evaluated to determine if the work-up is complete. When the abnormality is determined to require a biopsy, options are presented to the patient. The options presented should include traditional, open surgical biopsy and percutaneous, image-guided breast biopsy. The option of image-guided breast biopsy must include a discussion of monitoring and follow-up. If this type of breast biopsy is acceptable, then the physician must choose the most appropriate method of imaging to guide the biopsy.

Microcalcifications, which cannot be visualized with the current ultrasound technology, will require stereotactic guidance. Certain nodular densities, architectural distortions, and asymmetric densities without ultrasound findings will also be amenable to stereotactic biopsy.[45,53,54] When both mammography and ultrasonography visualize a lesion, such as a solid nodular density, ultrasonography is the preferable method for image guidance.[52,53,55] The real-time nature of ultrasound imaging provides increased accuracy and is more cost effective. In addition, ultrasound-guided biopsies are more comfortable for the patient. The patient may lie supine, and local anesthetic may be injected under direct visualization. This contrasts with stereotactic breast biopsy, where the patient lies prone on a stereotactic table with her breast in compression for the entire procedure and her neck hyperextended. Also, the ability to guide the injection under direct visualization resolves concerns associated with the liberal use of local anesthesia and the potential for obscuring or moving a lesion undergoing stereotactic core-needle biopsy.

The vast majority of nonpalpable lesions recommended for biopsy are evaluated with percutaneous image-guided breast biopsy. If a benign diagnosis is obtained, no further work-up is recommended, and the patient is placed in a follow-up protocol. A specific benign diagnosis (fibroadenoma) requires only a return to routine screening. With microcalcifications or nodular densities with a less specific benign diagnosis, short-term mammography in 4 to 6 months is recommended.[31]

The obvious indication to proceed with open surgical excision is an image-guided biopsy for malignancy and atypical hyperplasia. Medical judgment or lack of pathologic and radiologic diagnostic concordance would also be sufficient cause for further intervention. The issue of pathologic concordance with a suspicious mammographic lesion has fueled a debate over the indication to perform an image-guided breast biopsy on a highly suspicious lesion. Histologic confirmation assists in patient planning and allows wider excision for clear margins at the first surgical setting. Image-guided breast biopsy of a suspicious lesion may bypass open biopsy altogether for those patients that require a mastectomy and are not candidates for breast conservation. Histologic confirmation of an obvious cancer with image-guided technology leaves a tumor in situ to aid in the successful performance of the sentinel lymph node biopsy procedure.[60] Concerns over potential added cost with image-guided biopsy are exaggerated.

As technology advances and the approach to breast cancer treatment evolves, additional indications for image-guided biopsy of suspicious lesions will emerge. For many, image-guided percutaneous breast biopsy has permanently altered the management of nonpalpable breast disease. Image-guided percutaneous breast biopsy will provide the stage for achieving nonoperative histologic diagnosis and the potential for future therapeutic modalities.

REFERENCES

1. Kopans DS. The positive predictive value of mammography. AJR Am J Roentgenol 1992;158:521–6.
2. Sailors DM, Crabtree JD, Land RL, et al. Needle localization for non-palpable breast lesions. Am Surg 1994;60:186–9.
3. Wilhelm NC, DeParedes ES, Pope RT. The changing mammogram: a primary indication for needle localization biopsy. Arch Surg 1986;121:1311.
4. Miller RS, Adelman RW, Espinosa MH, et al. The early detection of nonpalpable breast carcinoma with needle localization. Experience with 500 patients in a community hospital. Am Surg 1992;58:193–8.
5. Parker SH, Lovin JD, Jobe WE, et al. Nonpalpable breast lesions: stereotactic automated large-core biopsies. Radiology 1991;180:403–7.
6. Elvecrog EL, Lechner MC, Nelson MT. Nonpalpable breast lesions: correlation of stereotaxic large-core needle biopsy and surgical biopsy results. Radiology 1993;188:453–5.
7. Parker SH, Burbank F, Jackman RJ, et al. Percutaneous large-core breast biopsy: a multi-institutional study. Radiology 1994;193:359–64.
8. Dershaw DD, Morris EA, Liberman L, et al. Nondiagnostic stereotaxic core breast biopsy: results of rebiopsy. Radiology 1996;198:323–5.
9. Liberman LL, Fahs MC, Dershaw DD, et al. Impact of stereotaxic core breast biopsy on cost of diagnosis. Radiology 1995;195:633–7.
10. Tinnemans JGM, Wobbes T, Hendricks JHCL, et al. Localization and excision of nonpalpable breast lesions. A surgical evaluation of three methods. Arch Surg 1987;122:802–6.
11. Norton LW, Zeligman BE, Pearlman MD. Accuracy and cost of needle localization breast biopsy. Arch Surg 1988;123:947–50.
12. Kopans DB, Meyer JE, Lindfors KK, McCarthy KA. Spring-hookwire breast lesion localizer: use with rigid compression mammographic systems. Radiology 1985;157:537–8.
13. Bigelow R, Smith R, Goodman PA, Wilson GS. Needle localization of non-palpable breast lesions. Arch Surg 1985;120:565–9.
14. Landercasper J, Gunderson SB, Gunderson AL, et al. Needle localization and biopsy of nonpalpable lesions of the breast. Surg Gynecol Obstet 1987;164:477–81.
15. Homer MJ, Smith TJ, Marchant DJ. Outpatient needle localization and biopsy for nonpalpable breast lesions. JAMA 1984;252:2452–4.
16. Feig SA. Localization of clinically occult breast lesions. Radiol Clin North Am 1983;21:155–71.
17. Dowlatshahi K, Gent HJ, Schmidt R, et al. Nonpalpable breast tumors: diagnosis with stereotaxic localization and fine-needle aspiration. Radiology 1989;170:427–33.

18. Schwartz GF, Goldberg BB, Riften MD, D'Orazio SE. Ultrasonography: an alternative to x-ray guided needle localization of nonpalpable breast masses. Surgery 1988;104:870–3.

19. Kopans DB. Breast Imaging. Philadelphia: Lippincott Williams & Wilkins; 1998.

20. Wilhelm MC, Wanebo HJ. Technique and guidelines for needle localization biopsy of nonpalpable lesions of the breast. Surg Gynecol Obstet 1988;176:439–41.

21. Swann CA, Kopans DB, McCarthy KA, et al. Practical solutions to problems of triangulation and preoperative localization of breast lesions. Radiology 1987;163:577–9.

22. Leeming R, Madden M, Levy L. An improved technique for needle localization biopsies of the breast. Surg Gynecol Obstet 1993;177:85–7.

23. Fisher B. Reappraisal of breast biopsy prompted by the use of lumpectomy. JAMA 1985;253:3585–8.

24. Fine RE, Boyd BA. Stereotactic breast biopsy: a practical approach. Am Surg 1996;62:96–102.

25. Lovin JD, Parker SH, Leuthke JM, Hopper KD. Stereotactic percutaneous breast core biopsy, technical adaptation, and initial experience. Breast Dis 1990;176:741–7.

26. Parker SH, Lovin JD, Jobe WE, et al. Stereotactic breast biopsy with a biopsy gun. Radiology 1990;176:741–7.

27. Caines JS, McPhee MD, Konak GP, Wright BA. Stereotactic needle core biopsy of breast lesions using a regular mammographic table with an adapable stereotaxic device. AJR Am J Roentgenol 1994;163:317–21.

28. Parker SH, Burbank F. State of the art: a practical approach to minimally invasive breast biopsy. Radiology 1996;200:11–20.

29. Azavedo E, Svane G, Auer G. Stereotactic fine-needle biopsy in 2594 mammographically detected non-palpable breast lesions. Lancet 1989;171:373–6.

30. Schmidt RA. Stereotactic breast biopsy. Cancer J Clin 1994;44:172–91.

31. Parker SH. When is a core really a core? Radiology 1992;185:641–2.

32. Dowlatshahi K, Yaremko ML, Kluskens LF, Jokich PM. Nonpalpable breast lesions: findings of stereotaxtic needle-core biopsy and fine-needle aspiration cytology. Radiology 1991;181:745–50.

33. Soo MS. Imaging-guided core biopsies in the breast. South Med J 1998;91:994–1000.

34. Tocino I, Gaargia B, Carter D. Surgical biopsy findings in patients with atypical hyperplasia diagnosed by stereotactic core needle biopsy. Ann Surg Oncol 1996;3(5):482–8.

35. Lieberman LL, Dershaw DD, Rosen PR, et al. Stereotactic 14-gauge breast biopsy: how many core biopsy specimens are needed? Radiology 1994;192:793–5.

36. Lieberman LL, Evans WP, Dershaw DD, et al. Radiography of microcalcifications in stereotaxic mammary core biopsy specimens. Radiology 1994;190:223–5.

37. Meyer JE, Lester SC, Grenna TH, White FV. Occult breast calcifications sampled with large-core biopsy: confirmation with radiography of the specimen. Radiology 1993;188:581–2.

38. Israel PZ, Fine RE. Stereotactic needle core biopsy for occult breast lesions: a minimally invasive alternative. Am Surg 1995;61:87–91.

39. Jackman RJ, Nowels KWW, Shepard MJ, et al. Stereotaxic large-core needle biopsy of 450 non-palpable breast lesions with surgical correlation in lesions with cancer or atypical hyperplasia. Radiology 1994;193:91–5.

40. Liberman L, Dershaw DD, Rosen PP, et al. Stereotaxic core biopsy of breast carcinoma: accuracy of predicting invasion. Radiology 1995;194:379–81.

41. Liberman L, Cohen MA, Dershaw DD, et al. Atypical ductal hyperplasia diagnosed at stereotaxic core biopsy of breast lesions: an indication for surgical biopsy. AJR Am J Roentgenol 1995;164:1111–3.

42. Burbank F, Parker SH, Fogerty TJ. Stereotactic breast biopsy: improved tissue harvesting with the mammotome. Am Surg 1996;62:738–44.

43. Berg WA, Kerbs TL, Campassi C, et al. Evaluation of 14 and 11-gauge directional vacuum-assisted biopsy probes and 14-gauge biopsy guns in a breast parenchymal model. Radiology 1997;205:203–8.

44. Burbank F. Stereotactic breast biopsy of atypical ductal hyperplasia and ductal carcinoma in in situ lesions: improved accuracy with directional vacuum-assisted biopsy. Radiology 1997;202:843–7.

45. Jackman RJ, Burbank SH, Parker SH, et al. Atypical ductal hyperplasia diagnosed at stereotactic breast biopsy: improved reliability with 14-gauge, directional vacuum-assisted biopsy. Radiology 1997;204:485–8.

46. Burbank F, Forcier N. Tissue marking clip for stereotactic breast biopsy: initial placement accuracy, long-term stability and usefulness as a guide for wire localization. Radiology 1997;205:407–15.

47. Dempsy PJ. Breast sonography: historical perspectives, clinical application and image interpretation. Ultrasound Q 1988;6:69.

48. McSweeney MB, Murphy CH. Whole breast sonography. Radiol Clin North Am 1985;23:157–67.

49. Leucht W. Teaching atlas of breast ultrasound. New York: Thieme; 1992.

50. Kopans DB, Meyer JE, Lindfors KK, et al. Breast sonography to guide cyst aspiration and wire localization of occult solid lesions. AJR Am J Roentgenol 1984;143:489–92.

51. Meyer JE, Christian RL, Frenna TH, et al. Image-guided aspiration of solitary occult breast "cysts." Arch Surg 1992;127:433–35.

52. Jackson VP. The role of ultrasound in breast imaging. Radiology 1990;177:305–11.

53. Parker SH, Stavros AS. Interventional breast ultrasound. In: Parker SH, Jobe WE, editors. Percutaneous breast biopsy. New York: Raven; 1993. p. 129.

54. Fornage BD. Interventional ultrasound of the breast. In: McGahan JP, editor. Interventional ultrasound. Baltimore: Williams & Wilkins; 1990. p. 71.

55. Staren ED. Surgical office-based ultrasound of the breast. Am Surg 1995;61:619–26.

56. Fornage BD, Coan JD, David CZ. Ultrasound-guided needle biopsy of the breast and other interventional procedures. Radiol Clin North Am 1992;30:167–85.

57. Staren ED. Ultrasound-guided biopsy of non palpable breast masses by surgeons. Ann Surg Oncol 1996;3:476–82.

58. Parker SH. Needle selection. In: Parker SH, Jobe WE, editors. Percutaneous breast biopsy. New York: Raven; 1993. p. 7.

59. Parker SH, Jobe WE, Dennis MA, et al. Ultrasound-guided automated large-core breast biopsy. Radiology 1993;187:507–11.

60. Pijpers R, Meijer S, Hoekstra OS, et al. Impact of lymphoscintigraphy on sentinel node identification with technitium-99m colloidal albumin in breast cancer. J Nucl Med 1997;38:366–8.

5

Histopathology of Malignant Breast Disease

ROBERT A. GOLDSCHMIDT, MD

The basic classification of malignant breast diseases has remained relatively unchanged since the most recent WHO revision in 1982.[1] These conditions can be broadly divided into epithelial and nonepithelial lesions, with separation of the former into in situ and invasive tumors (Table 5–1). Although recent studies have shed new light onto our understanding of the basic biology and natural history of breast cancer, this traditional classification still retains its relevance for clinicians involved in the diagnosis and treatment of malignant breast disease.

DUCTAL CARCINOMA IN SITU

Since, by definition, ductal carcinoma in situ (DCIS) is an atypical proliferation of cells confined by an intact basement membrane to the ductolobular system of the breast, it cannot cause serious morbidity unless it becomes invasive. Thus, the major goal of any pathologic evaluation of a patient with DCIS should be to determine the level of risk of subsequent invasion so that optimal treatment can be offered and possible over- or undertreatment avoided.

In the premammographic era, pure DCIS was most often seen as a mass lesion of high-grade, comedo type and usually treated, appropriately, by mastectomy. In the current clinical setting, however, the vast majority of DCIS present as a mammographic abnormality or may be entirely incidental to the lesion seen on radiography. As the pattern of the disease has shifted over the years from the bulky mass with a high risk of invasion to minute foci of questionable clinical significance, numerous studies have been undertaken to identify prognostic factors and optimize therapy for the individual patient.

The most important change in our concept of DCIS was from the monolithic view of a single disease highly likely to invade if left untreated to the realization that DCIS represents a nonobligate precursor with variable risk of progression, depending on a combination of factors. These factors include histologic pattern (and by extension histologic grade), lesion size, margin status, and ancillary studies such as proliferation markers and *c-erb*B-b2.

Classification and Grading of Ductal Carcinoma In Situ

Although the traditional classification of DCIS based on architectural pattern is now recog-

Table 5–1. MALIGNANT DISEASES OF THE BREAST: EPITHELIAL TUMORS

In Situ Lesions	Invasive Lesions
Lobular carcinoma in situ (LCIS)	Invasive lobular
Ductal carcinoma in situ (DCIS)	Ductal
comedo	no special type (NST)
micropapillary	tubular
cribriform	mucinous
solid	medullary
papillary	invasive
	cribriform
	papillary

nized to be limited in terms of prognostic value, it remains in use by many pathologists and merits review for that reason. In addition, before prognosis can be assessed, the pathologist must establish a diagnosis by applying criteria to separate DCIS from other atypical or nonatypical proliferations. These criteria are almost purely architectural and include the solid, cribriform, micropapillary, papillary, and intraductal comedocarcinoma variants.

Comedo DCIS is the only type likely to present as a palpable mass and accounts for the majority of cases of DCIS diagnosed before the advent of mammography. As will be seen, it is also the most likely to be high grade and as such, the most likely to be associated with concurrent or subsequent invasion. The histologic features of comedo DCIS are solid growth with central necrosis, often with calcification (Figure 5–1). Marked nuclear atypia is often seen, but a recent consensus conference on the classification of DCIS[2] allows use of the comedo designation in the absence of high nuclear grade. Marked fibrosis and elastosis of the surrounding stroma are frequently present, as is an associated periductal lymphocytic infiltrate. Not infrequently, a question of possible microinvasion arises as small nests of tumor cells are trapped in the fibroinflammatory reaction encircling the affected ducts. Diagnostic criteria for microinvasion are not well established, nor is its clinical significance, but at present it is probably best to limit such a diagnosis to those cases where single tumor cells are clearly evident outside an affected duct.

Micropapillary DCIS, sometimes referred to as "clinging carcinoma," may vary in appearance from a relatively flat proliferation with short projections to a pattern of long, slender epithelial fronds lacking fibrovascular cores (Figure 5–2). Peripheral spaces formed by so-called "Roman bridges" are common and lead some to group micropapillary and cribriform lesions together. Key features of micropapillary carcinoma distinguishing it from proliferations that appear similar but are benign are monomorphism and lack of polarity. Myoepithelial cells should be absent from their usual peripheral location, and the atypical cells should be homogeneous in appearance. Micropapillary carcinoma is usually composed of cells with low-grade nuclei, although cases with high nuclear grade are not rare. Centrally located necrotic debris and microcalcification may be present, especially in cases with high-grade nuclei. There is some evidence that micropapillary DCIS may be more likely to involve multiple quadrants than other forms of DCIS.[3] Further studies will be necessary to establish the clinical significance of this finding.

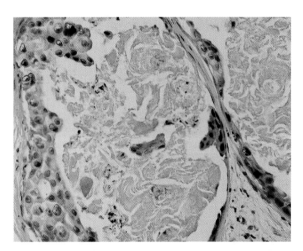

Figure 5–1. DCIS, comedo type, with central necrosis. This would qualify as a high-grade lesion based on nuclear morphology (original magnification x400).

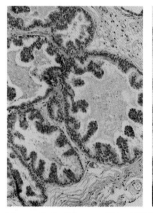 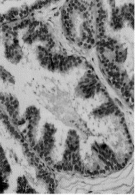

Figure 5–2. Micropapillary DCIS. *Left,* dilated ducts with papillary tufting of the epithelium (original magnification x100). *Right,* the micropapillary structures show stratification and loss of polarity (original magnification x200). This is a low-grade lesion based on nuclear grade and lack of necrosis.

Cribriform DCIS describes a lesion characterized by the formation of secondary microlumens. These lumens tend to be round and uniformly distributed, although some variability is acceptable. The classic term used to describe the monomorphous nature of the cells outlining the spaces is "rigid bridges," referring to the lack of stretched or elongated cells separating glandular spaces (Figure 5–3). Nuclear morphology is typically low grade, although high-grade variants exist. Likewise, necrosis is commonly encountered in cribriform DCIS and may be so prominent as to mimic comedo DCIS. Fortunately, as will be seen in the discussion on grading, this distinction is obviated in current classification systems.

Solid DCIS, as the name implies, consists of a solid proliferation of neoplastic cells filling a ductal structure (Figure 5–4). Nuclear grade may vary widely, and spotty necrosis may be encountered. As in the other forms of DCIS, the monomorphous nature of the cell population is the hallmark of the process.

Papillary DCIS is the least common of the well-described variants and exhibits prominent papillary features with fibrovascular cores but no myoepithelial cell layer (Figure 5–5). As in other variants, a monomorphous cytologic appearance is essential to the diagnosis.

As previously alluded to, DCIS grade has a largely supplanted pattern as the most important guide to clinical behavior and treatment. There have been a variety of different systems proposed, but all include some assessment of nuclear features combined with other factors, typically necrosis or cell polarity, with separation of cases into either two or three grades. Two recent studies[4,5] have compared a number of different grading systems for their interobserver reproducibility. Although none of the systems demonstrated a high degree of agreement among reviewing pathologists, both studies found the Van Nuys system of Silverstein and Lagios[6] to be the most reproducible. This scheme relies on the distinction of three nuclear grades based on size, texture and nucleoli, and

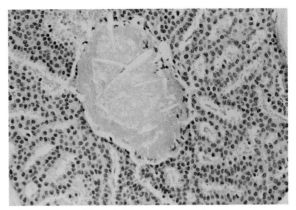

Figure 5–3. Cribriform DCIS with central necrosis (x400). This lesion is intermediate grade based on necrosis and low-grade nuclear features.

on the presence or absence of comedo-type necrosis. Using these parameters, tumors can be divided into three groups. Group 1 (low-grade) includes those tumors with either low- or intermediate-grade nuclei and no necrosis. Group 2 (intermediate-grade) describes those tumors with low- or intermediate-grade nuclei and comedo necrosis, whereas Group 3 (high-grade) encompasses all tumors with high-grade nuclei regardless of necrosis.

Tumor grade has emerged as a significant prognostic factor for risk of recurrence, although other pathologic features may also be important. The Van Nuys grading scheme is part of a prognostic index for DCIS that includes tumor grade, tumor size, and margin width. Evaluation of the latter two factors in DCIS can be problematic,

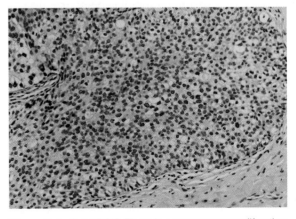

Figure 5–4. Solid DCIS. There is a monotonous proliferation of cells filling the duct (x200). Lack of necrosis and non high-grade nuclear features qualify this as a low-grade lesion.

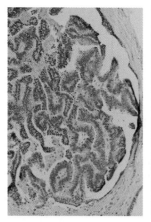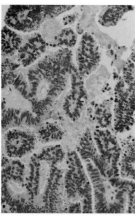

Figure 5–5. Papillary DCIS. *Left,* an intraductal proliferation of papillary structures with fibrovascular cores (original magnification x100). *Right,* high power shows nuclear atypia and stratification (original magnification x200).

however. Since DCIS only rarely forms a grossly visible mass, measurement of lesion size is typically done from microscopic slides. If, as is often the case, tumor is present on more than one slide, the pathologist must be able to reconstruct the specimen to estimate size. This requires that the sections be submitted in an orderly fashion to permit reconstruction. Even so, it is sometimes difficult to know how to report lesion size when small foci of DCIS are scattered throughout a lumpectomy specimen, and such data are not readily available in existing clinical studies.

If tumor size assessment is occasionally a problem, margin width determination is even more of one. The most common approach involves the application of colored ink(s) to the surface of a specimen that has been oriented by the surgeon. The specimen is then submitted for microscopic examination in serial transverse section and the shortest distance between tumor and ink reported as the margin width. Since this method can only examine a tiny fraction of the actual surface area of the specimen, it is a crude measurement at best. Some workers recommend an alternate method in which sections are shaved tangentially from the surface of the specimen to permit wider sampling of the margins. Yet another technique advocated by some surgeons is the separate removal of shaved margins from the biopsy cavity after the specimen has been resected. Ultimately, selection of a

method of margin examination will rely on the experience and preference of the pathologist and surgeon, at least until better clinical studies are available. Since most "recurrences" of DCIS probably represent persistence following incomplete removal, the issue of margins is not of trivial importance. Routine specimen mammography is often helpful in guiding the pathologic sampling by identifying areas of suspicious calcification near resection margins.

A recent study published by Silverstein and Lagios[7] uses a retrospective analysis of DCIS patients to demonstrate that margin width is the only significant risk factor for local recurrence[8]. In their series, there was no difference in recurrence rate between patients who received postoperative radiation and those treated by lumpectomy only, so long as there was an uninvolved margin width of 10mm or more in all directions. In both the radiated and non-radiated groups, the risk of recurrence after 8-year follow-up was 3–4%. Tumor size, nuclear grade, and presence of comedonecrosis did not alter relative risk in these cases. For margin widths of 1-10mm, the recurrence rates were higher (12–20%), but there was still no statistically significant benefit to radiation therapy in this group. Only when final margin width was < 1mm did postoperative radiation show a significant reduction in recurrence rates.

Given the above considerations, the *pathology report* in cases of DCIS must include a large amount of data. Many institutions have found that the use of a template form ensures all vital data is present. Such a form would typically include features such as nuclear grade, pattern, presence of necrosis, distance to margin, lesion size, presence of calcifications, and any other parameters deemed to be important. This type of systematic reporting scheme has the added advantage of making any retrospective clinical studies much easier to perform.

LOBULAR CARCINOMA IN SITU

Lobular carcinoma in situ (LCIS) is, by definition, a microscopic process and as such is almost always an incidental finding seen in association with some other gross or mammographic abnormality. In its most classic form, described by Foote and Stewart in 1941,[8] it is readily identifiable by the general pathologist. The lobular acini are filled and distended by a poorly cohesive proliferation of cells with round, rather bland nuclei, scant cytoplasm, and inconspicuous nucleoli (Figure 5–6). Problems in interpretation of these lesions can arise, however, from variations in qualitative and quantitative aspects of the neoplastic process. For example, the cytologic features of the neoplastic cells may demonstrate more variability, with pleomorphic nuclei and abundant cytoplasm. In such cases, it is often difficult to determine whether one is dealing with lobular carcinoma in situ or so-called "lobular cancerization" by an in situ duct carcinoma. Since there is no reliable marker to distinguish the origin of such a lesion as either lobular or ductal, the distinction must ultimately be made by the pathologist's assessment of the light microscopic features.

The situation may be further complicated by the frequent association of typical ductal carcinoma in situ and LCIS in the same biopsy. The identification, when present, of intracytoplasmic lumens and associated mucin globules in the atypical cells is helpful. The finding of such cells in a proliferative lesion involving the terminal duct/lobular unit is compelling evidence for lobular carcinoma in situ.

Another common feature, seen in up to 75 percent of patients with LCIS, is a pattern of so-called pagetoid spread of atypical cells along small ductules and occasional larger ducts. Typically, this manifests as a proliferation of atypical cells lining the duct, with an overlying layer of intact ductal epithelium. In the atrophic breast of the postmenopausal patient, the latter pattern may be the only evidence of LCIS. Some experts disagree as to whether this appearance represents true ductal involvement rather than an "unfolding" of the lobule yielding a pseudoductular appearance. Recognition of the process, however, is more important than the terminology. The important distinction is between true

LCIS and ductal carcinoma in situ (DCIS) involving lobular units, since the therapeutic implications of these lesions may be quite different. In most cases of in situ duct carcinoma involving the terminal duct/lobular unit in a secondary fashion, there is at least some retention of features suggestive of ductal origin. The presence of large pleomorphic nuclei and/or secondary lumens in such a proliferation would favor DCIS over LCIS. Likewise, as previously mentioned, identification of intracytoplasmic lumens with mucin droplets strongly suggests LCIS. Occasionally, a case will defy classification, even after exhaustive examination of the specimen. If there are foci of coexistent invasive carcinoma or unequivocal DCIS, the distinction becomes one of academic interest only, as treatment would be dictated by those lesions. With a biopsy containing only an in situ lesion of indeterminate etiology, however, communication between the pathologist, surgeon, oncologist, and patient is essential for optimal care.

INVASIVE BREAST CARCINOMA

Invasive (infiltrating) breast carcinoma can be broadly subdivided into ductal and lobular categories, with a number of recognized variants of each. Although current evidence suggests that the majority of invasive cancers arise from cells of the terminal duct lobular unit, their wide variation in appearance and clinical pre-

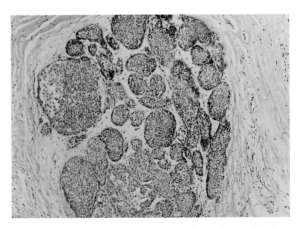

Figure 5–6. Lobular carcinoma in situ. The acini are filled and distended by a monotonous proliferation of small cells with bland nuclear features (original magnification ×100).

sentation continues to make subtyping a useful exercise until some better method of predicting behavior becomes available.

Infiltrating Lobular Carcinoma

Infiltrating lobular carcinoma (ILC) is generally considered to account for up to 16 percent[9] of invasive breast cancers, depending on the study population and the rigidity of diagnostic criteria. It may present as a scirrhous mass grossly and mammographically indistinguishable from infiltrating ductal carcinoma, although it is often more insidious, with only vague gross findings and occasionally negative mammographic appearance. In contrast to invasive ductal carcinoma, invasive lobular cancer presents as a less distinct tumor that is less apparent on physical examination and mammography. As a result, the microscopic extent of disease is often much greater than grossly appreciated, and clear lumpectomy margins are somewhat more difficult to achieve.[10] The classical microscopic description, generally credited to Foote and Stewart,[11] is of a diffusely infiltrative tumor composed of cells with small, round nuclei with minimal pleomorphism or mitotic activity. Intracytoplasmic lumina yielding a signet-ring appearance are often present but are not pathognomonic since they may be seen in ductal carcinomas also. Linear files ("Indian files") of infiltrating tumor cells are the most characteristic pattern of invasion,

often swirling around native ductal structures in a so-called "targetoid" fashion (Figure 5–7).

There are a number of variants of infiltrating lobular carcinoma that have been described, and many tumors show mixtures of two or more types. Most of these variants consist of cells with the same cytologic features as the classical type but different patterns of growth such as alveolar, solid, or tubulolobular. While it is unclear whether identification of these variants has clinical significance, the pleomorphic type does merit separate distinction. This variant consists of cells which infiltrate in the same manner as classical ILC but have high-grade nuclei. Several studies have suggested a more aggressive behavior for these tumors.[12,13]

Infiltrating Ductal Carcinoma

Invasive breast cancers that do not exhibit the features described above for lobular variants are considered to be ductal in origin. While this distinction is somewhat arbitrary, it is firmly embedded in the literature of breast cancer and serves as a useful tool for the recognition and subclassification of malignant breast disease. This large group of tumors accounts for the majority (85 to 95%) of invasive breast cancer cases and can be broadly divided into those of "no special type" or "not otherwise specified" (NST, NOS) and "special type" tumors of distinctive appearance and behavior.

Various studies place the percentage of NST breast carcinomas at 50 to 75 percent of all invasive breast cancers.[13] The tumors within this large group vary widely in appearance and often contain minor components of special type histology. An appreciation of the cytologic features of the tumor cells and of the architectural pattern of the invasive process is useful when studying breast cancer. As will be discussed later, these factors also form the basis for grading NST tumors. In regard to cytology, the nuclei of NST neoplasms can vary from small and rather bland in appearance to those exhibiting marked enlargement and pleomorphism. Mitotic activity can likewise range from mini-

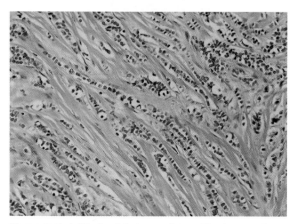

Figure 5–7. Infiltrating lobular carcinoma. The tumor cells infiltrate in typical linear files (original magnification x200).

mal to brisk and generally follows nuclear grade. Architectural patterns are typically described on the basis of degree of gland formation, which may be quite prominent or completely absent. In addition, both cytologic and architectural features may vary widely within a single tumor. Other features, such as extensive necrosis or widespread DCIS, may also have prognostic importance and should be noted.

Ductal carcinomas of special type include a group of tumors distinguished from NST tumors by their unique histologic appearance and often, less aggressive behavior. Within this group are the tubular, mucinous, medullary, invasive cribriform, papillary, and metaplastic variants. Tubular carcinoma has become the most commonly diagnosed special type tumor since the advent of mammography, due to its small size and lack of clinical symptoms. The majority of tubular carcinomas are < 1.0 cm in diameter, accounting for 7 to 21 percent of mammographically detected lesions in various studies.[14,15] Precisely defining tubular carcinoma is elusive, particularly regarding the extent of tubule formation required to make the diagnosis. The basic requirement is the presence of tubular structures lined by a single layer of epithelial cells of low-nuclear grade. The tubule lumens are rounded and/or angulated, and mitosis is rare. The tumor stroma is quite characteristic, consisting of a cellular desmoplastic reaction, often with a central fibrous scar from which the tubules radiate (Figure 5–8). Low-grade DCIS is a frequent accompaniment of tubular carcinoma. As previously alluded to, tumors that are not purely tubular are somewhat controversial. Most authors will accept 90 percent tubular architecture as a minimum criterion for the diagnosis of tubular carcinoma, and many use 75 percent as a cut-off. Lesser degrees of tubular differentiation are generally reported as "tubular features" in an NST tumor. The distinction is not trivial, as several studies have shown prognostic differences related to varying degrees of tubule formation.[16]

Mucinous (colloid) carcinoma of the breast accounts for one to three percent of invasive

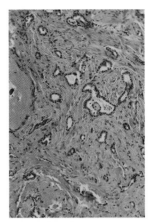
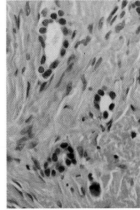

Figure 5–8. Tubular carcinoma. *Left,* the tumor consists of a haphazard arrangement of small tubular structures (original magnification x100). *Right,* the tumor glands are lined by cells with low-grade nuclei (original magnification x400).

breast cancer and has a distinctive gross and microscopic appearance. Such tumors tend to be soft, well-defined, rounded masses with a glistening mucoid surface. The tumor cells show minimal pleomorphism and form tight clusters which float in pools of extracellular mucin (Figure 5–9). As with tubular carcinoma, 90 percent mucinous morphology is the generally accepted minimum for designation as mucinous carcinoma, with its associated favorable prognosis.

Medullary carcinoma is the most controversial of the special-type tumors, both in terms of histologic criteria for diagnosis and subsequent behavior. Poor intraobserver reproducibility, and disagreement over the diagnostic requirements

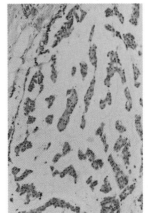
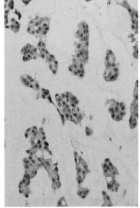

Figure 5–9. Mucinous carcinoma. *Left,* clusters of tumor cells float in a pool of extracellular mucin (original magnification x100). *Right,* in this case, the cells exhibit minimal nuclear atypia (original magnification x200).

for medullary carcinoma, likely account for the reported frequency range of 2 to 10 percent.[17] In our own practice, medullary carcinoma is a distinctly unusual variant. Disclaimers aside, the classic description of medullary is of a soft, fleshy, circumscribed tumor with a homogeneous appearance. Microscopically, the tumor cells have large, often bizarre nuclei, abundant mitoses, and grow in syncytial sheets. Equally important for the diagnosis is the presence of a significant lymphoplasmacytic infiltrate that usually occupies narrow bands of fibrovascular stroma within the tumor and may also surround the periphery of the tumor. Lastly, microscopic circumscription is essential. The tumor must have a smooth, pushing margin without infiltration of surrounding breast tissue or fat by tumor cells (Figure 5–10). Foci of DCIS surrounding the tumor, however, are not uncommon and should not preclude a diagnosis of medullary carcinoma. It is important to adhere to strict diagnostic criteria because the less aggressive behavior ascribed to medullary carcinoma belies its high-grade appearance. Attempts to distinguish an intermediate variant[18] (atypical medullary carcinoma) exhibiting some, but not all, of the classic features and having an intermediate prognosis remain controversial.

Invasive cribriform carcinoma is a relatively infrequent variant in pure form, although combination with tubular carcinoma is not rare. The cribriform designation comes from its resemblance to cribriform DCIS, from which it may occasionally be difficult to distinguish. The histologic appearance is of infiltrating sheets and nests of cells of low-nuclear grade with the typical punched-out spaces seen in its in situ namesake (Figure 5–11). The 90 percent rule for designation as a special-type tumor generally applies for combinations of invasive cribriform carcinoma and NST tumors, while tumors composed entirely of tubular and invasive cribriform structures in any proportion still qualify as special type.

Grading of Invasive Breast Carcinoma

Grading schemes for invasive breast carcinoma originated with the work of Greenhough[19] 60 years ago and have not changed substantially since that time. It is a testament to the power of histological grading of breast cancer that virtually all of the numerous methods and variations proposed over the years correlate to some degree with clinical behavior. While no single system has achieved universal acceptance, all use some combination of nuclear features, mitotic activity, and gland formation. One of the more commonly used methods, and that adopted by the WHO, is the Scarff-Bloom-Richardson system,[20] which assigns a score of one to three points for each of the three above-

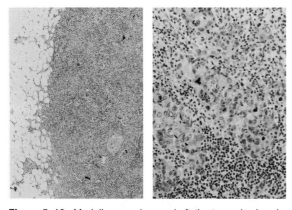

Figure 5–10. Medullary carcinoma. *Left,* the tumor is sharply demarcated from the surrounding fat (original magnification x100). *Right,* the tumor cells are highly pleomorphic with numerous mitoses and a dense lymphoid infiltrate (original magnification x400).

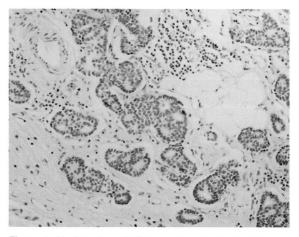

Figure 5–11. Invasive cribriform carcinoma. Nests of tumor with a cribriform configuration infiltrate the stroma (original magnification x200).

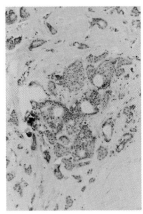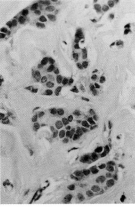

Figure 5–12. Invasive ductal carcinoma, no special type. *Left,* the tumor makes some glandular structures (original magnification x200). *Right,* the nuclei are moderately enlarged with inconspicuous nuclei and no mitoses (original magnification x400). In the Scarff-Bloom-Richardson system, this tumor would score 1 point for architecture, 2 points for nuclei, and 1 point for mitosis, making it grade I.

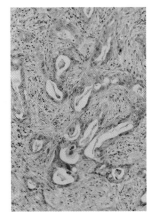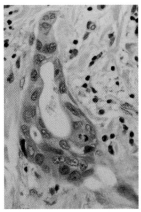

Figure 5–13. Invasive ductal carcinoma, no special type. *Left,* the prominent gland formation scores 1 point for architecture (original magnification x100). *Right,* high nuclear grade and moderate mitotic activity score 3 and 2 points respectively (original magnification x400). The total score of 6 points makes this a grade II tumor.

mentioned parameters. Based on the point total, tumors are assigned to grade I (three to five points), grade II (six to seven points), or grade III (eight to nine points) (Figures 5–12 to 5–14). Further refinement of this method by Elston and Ellis[21] defined specific criteria for nuclear grade, architectural pattern, and mitotic rate, and has resulted in a system showing both strong correlation with outcome and reasonably good interobserver reproducibility.

SPECIMEN HANDLING AND REPORTING

As the surgical approach to breast cancer has changed, so has the pathologist's approach to specimen handling. Many lumpectomy specimens arrive in the pathology lab with a diagnosis already established by fine-needle or stereotactic core biopsy. If the specimen is oriented by the surgeon using sutures or some other method, the margins can then be optimally assessed on permanent section. If the lesion was nonpalpable and removed using stereotactic localization, radiography of the specimen is essential to confirm the adequacy of excision. Hormone receptor assays and other ancillary studies no longer require fresh tumor tissue, thus obviating the need to perform a frozen section, with its atten-

dant problems. Frozen section is entirely appropriate, however, when confirmation of invasive tumor is necessary prior to concurrent axillary dissection or when the surgeon requires intraoperative margin assessment. The popularity of sentinel node techniques using frozen section to determine whether to proceed with axillary dissection is also increasing.

In general, all lumpectomy and re-excision specimens must be assessed, at a minimum, for tumor size, tumor type, and margin width. This requires input from the surgeon as to specimen orientation, and some method for identifying

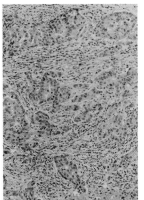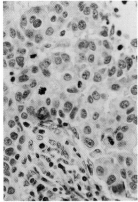

Figure 5–14. Invasive ductal carcinoma, no special type. *Left,* this tumor shows no gland formation (original magnification x100). *Right,* the nuclei are high grade and show numerous mitoses (original magnification x400). The total score of 9 points makes this tumor grade III.

margins on the histologic sections. Typically, this involves the application of colored inks to the surfaces of the specimen prior to sectioning. Adequate fixation prior to processing is of utmost importance in achieving optimal results for histologic examination. Since most breast specimens are fairly fatty, overnight formalin fixation is often necessary. The attendant delay in reporting is more than offset by the quality of the information that can be gleaned from high quality histologic sections.

Because of the large amount of pathologic data entering into breast cancer prognosis and treatment strategy, many pathologists find it helpful to utilize some sort of standardized reporting format as part of the pathology report. As described above for DCIS, we use a breast cancer worksheet to describe relevant features of invasive tumors. Features such as tumor size, grade, subtype, and margin status are described, and this data is included as part of the final report. The design of such a format should include input from clinicians to ensure they receive all information required for optimal patient management as well as any data that may be helpful in future retrospective studies. Standardized forms have been developed by the Association of Directors of Surgical Pathology (ADSP) to serve this purpose.

REFERENCES

1. Azzopardi JG, Chepick OF, Hartmann WH. The World Health Organization histological typing of breast tumors. 2nd ed. Am J Clin Pathol 1982;78:806–16.
2. The Consensus Conference Committee. Consensus conference on the classification of ductal carcinoma in situ. Cancer 1997;80:1798–1802.
3. Bellamy COC, McDonald C, Salter DM, et al. Noninvasive ductal carcinoma of the breast: the relevance of histologic categorization. Hum Pathol 1993;24:16–23.
4. Douglas-Jones AG, Gupta SK, Attanoos RL, et al. A critical appraisal of six modern classifications of ductal carcinoma in situ of the breast (DCIS): correlation with grade of associated invasive tumor. Histopathology 1996;29:397–409.
5. European Commission Working Group on Breast Screening Pathology. Consistency achieved by 23 European pathologists in categorizing ductal carcinoma in situ of the breast using five classifications. Hum Pathol 1998;29:1056–62.
6. Silverstein MJ, Lagios MD, Craig PH, et al. A prognostic index for ductal carcinoma in situ of the breast. Cancer 1996;77:2267–74.
7. Silverstein MJ, Lagios MD, Groshen S, Waisman JR, Lewinsky BS, et al. The influence of margin width on local control of ductal carcinoma in situ of the breast. NEJM 1999;340:1455–61.
7. Foote F, Stewart F. Lobular carcinoma in situ: a rare form of mammary carcinoma. Am J Pathol 1941;17:491–6.
8. Elston CW, Ellis IO. Systemic pathology, Vol.13. The breast. Edinburgh: Churchill Livingstone; 1998.
9. Yeatman TJ, Cantor AB, Smith TJ, et al. Tumor biology of infiltrating lobular carcinoma. Ann Surg 1995;222:549–61.
10. Foote FW, Stewart F. A histologic classification of carcinoma in the breast. Surgery 1946;19:74–9.
11. Eusibi V, Magalhaes F, Azzopardi JG. Pleomorphic lobular carcinoma of the breast: an aggressive tumor showing apocrine differentiation. Hum Pathol 1992;23:655–62.
12. Weidner N, Semple JP. Pleomorphic variant of invasive lobular carcinoma of the breast. Hum Pathol 1992;23:1167–71.
13. Rosen PP. Breast pathology. Philadelphia: Lippincott-Raven; 1997.
14. Cooper HS, Patchefsky AS, Krall RA. Tubular carcinoma of the breast. Cancer 1978;42:2334–42.
15. Parl FF, Richardson LD. The histologic and biologic spectrum of tubular carcinoma of the breast. Hum Pathol 1983;14:694–8.
16. Ridolfi R, Rosen P, Port A, et al. Medullary carcinoma of the breast. A clinicopathologic study with 10 year follow-up. Cancer 1977;40:1365–85.
17. Wargotz ES, Silverberg SG. Medullary carcinoma of the breast. A clinicopathologic study with appraisal of current diagnostic criteria. Hum Pathol 1988;19:1340–46.
18. Greenhough RB. Varying degrees of malignancy in cancer of the breast. J Cancer Res 1925;9:452–63.
19. Bloom HJG, Richardson WW. Histological grading and prognosis in breast cancer. A study of 1409 cases of which 359 have been followed for 15 years. Br J Cancer 1957;11:359–77.
20. Elston CW, Ellis IO. Pathological prognostic factors in breast cancer. I. The value of histological grade in breast cancer: experience from a large study with long-term follow-up. Histopathol 1991;19:403–10.

6

Unusual Breast Pathology

DAVID R. BRENIN, MD
HANINA HIBSHOOSH, MD
DAVID W. KINNE, MD

This chapter reviews clinical and pathologic features of uncommon breast malignancies. The majority of the data used in the course of writing the chapter was obtained from small studies of specific tumor subtypes, or has been gleaned from larger studies that included several types of more common breast cancers. Unfortunately, there is often insufficient information available to draw absolute conclusions regarding therapy and prognosis.

Much of the data cited was collected prior to the widespread use of breast conservation. For this reason, the vast majority of patients studied were treated using mastectomy. The reliance on mastectomy has resulted in a lack of information regarding the natural history and radiosensitivity of many of the tumors presented. Therefore, the risk of local recurrence for patients with rare breast malignancies opting for breast conservation is unclear. There is, however, no reason to suspect a significant difference in the risk of local recurrence in this group of patients compared to patients with more common types of breast cancer. Except where specifically indicated, the clinically appropriate use of breast conservation should be considered in the informed treatment of patients with rare breast malignancies.

PAPILLARY CARCINOMA

Papillary carcinoma accounts for 1 to 2 percent of newly diagnosed breast cancers in women, and a slightly higher proportion in men.[1,2,3] It occurs in both an invasive and noninvasive form. The World Health Organization (WHO) defined papillary carcinoma as follows: "A rare carcinoma whose invasive pattern is predominantly in the form of papillary structures. The same architecture is usually displayed in the metastases. Frequently, foci of intraductal papillary growth are recognizable."[4] Further, the WHO classification states that "papillary carcinoma arising, and limited to a mammary cyst, is [to be] referred to as noninvasive intracystic carcinoma."[4] Invasive carcinoma, however, may be associated with an intracystic carcinoma.[5]

Papillary carcinoma occurs most frequently in the central portion of the breast, and is associated with a malignant nipple discharge in 22 to 34 percent of patients.[1,6] The mean age of diagnosis for papillary carcinoma, 63 to 67 years, is older compared to the more common types of breast cancer.[1,2,7] The tumors tend to grow slowly, not infrequently being present for more than 1 year prior to patients seeking treatment. On physical exam, papillary carcinomas are well-circumscribed, and often lobulated. There may be a bloody nipple discharge. The average clinical size is 2 to 3 cm.[3] Clinically enlarged axillary lymph nodes are not uncommon in patients with larger tumors containing areas of hemorrhagic necrosis. Mammographically, papillary carcinomas typically have sharp margins and are rounded or lobulated. Breast ultrasound may reveal a solid component in a cyst that otherwise appears benign.

The appearance of the gross tumor varies with the proportion of the cystic component. Some fibrosis may be present. The cut surface of the tumor is typically described as tan or gray, and areas of focal hemorrhage and necrosis are not uncommon.[3] Larger tumors may form a large cyst containing partially clotted blood and tumor fragments. Microscopically, the tumors form a predominately frond-like pattern (Figures 6–1 and 6–2). Cystic areas may be present but are not a prerequisite for diagnosis. Distinguishing between benign and malignant papillary tumors can be challenging. Kraus and Neubecker,[8] Lefkowitz and colleagues,[7] and Rosen[3] have attempted to delineate guidelines for diagnosis. Various immunohistochemical markers have been evaluated but have proved to be of little help. Analysis of DNA content, however, has demonstrated significant differences between papillary carcinoma and benign lesions.[9,10]

Papillary carcinoma has a favorable prognosis. Noninvasive papillary carcinoma is a variant of ductal carcinoma in situ (DCIS), and is associated with a less than one percent rate of axillary metastasis.[3,7] To date, there is no significant body of data addressing the use of radiation therapy in the treatment of this lesion. As is the case with DCIS, there are no prospective trials comparing mastectomy to breast preservation with whole breast irradiation in patients with noninvasive papillary carcinoma. The use of breast conservation, however, appears reasonable for these patients, as there is no reason to suspect a significant difference in the risk of local recurrence compared to patients with more common types of noninvasive breast cancer. The low rate of axillary metastasis observed makes elimination of axillary dissection appropriate in patients with noninvasive papillary carcinoma and a clinically negative axilla.

Even less data exists to aid in treatment selection for patients with invasive papillary carcinoma. Fisher and colleagues reported on 35 patients with invasive papillary cancer.[2] Of the 22 patients who underwent axillary dissection, 32 percent were found to have axillary metastases. Of patients with axillary metastases, only two (nine percent) had four or more lymph nodes involved. Life-table plots calculated by Fisher and colleagues showed a favorable prognosis comparable to patients with tubular cancers. At 5-year follow-up, only one patient had died of papillary carcinoma. Recurrences, when they do occur, are typically "late," coming > 5 years after the initial diagnosis.[3] The majority of reports concerning the treatment of invasive papillary carcinoma have addressed patients whose primary therapy consisted of mastectomy with or without axillary dissection. When clinically appropriate, the use of breast conservation,

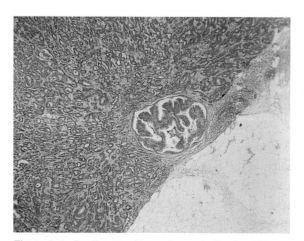

Figure 6–1. Papillary carcinoma demonstrating frond-like pattern (original magnification x400).

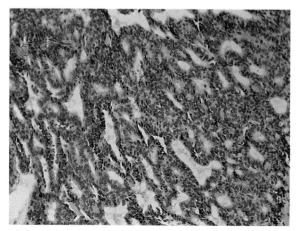

Figure 6–2. Intracystic papillary carcinoma. Note solid cyst wall on periphery (original magnification x400).

whole breast irradiation, and axillary dissection or sentinel node biopsy is a reasonable option.

METAPLASTIC MAMMARY CARCINOMA

Metaplastic mammary carcinoma refers to a classic breast carcinoma containing a variable component exhibiting a nonglandular growth pattern. These tumors constitute fewer than one percent of breast cancers.[11,12] The metaplastic changes typically manifest as squamous cells, spindle cells, and/or as areas of heterologous mesenchymal growth showing cartilaginous or osseous differentiation. The histologic diversity observed in metaplastic mammary carcinoma has led to various subdesignations including spindle-cell carcinoma, carcinoma with osseous metaplasia, carcinoma with pseudosarcomatous metaplasia, squamous cell carcinoma with pseudosarcomatous stroma, and carcinosarcoma. The histogenesis of these carcinomas is assumed to be of ductal origin. Results derived from ultrastructural and immunohistochemical studies suggest that metaplastic mammary carcinomas originate from undifferentiated multipotential cells.[13] Tavassoli suggested that myoepithelial cells are the cell of origin.[11] Although the number of reported cases is small, all of the subtypes appear to have a similar prognosis[14] and will be presented as a single group in this chapter.

Metaplastic mammary carcinoma typically presents as a mass. Skin changes and fixation to underlying tissues have been reported.[15] The gross appearance of the tumor varies with subtype, but most are described as hard with well-circumscribed borders. Cystic degeneration may occur when there is an extensive squamous metaplastic component.[14] Histologically, metaplastic carcinoma is divided broadly into tumors showing squamous and/or heterologous (cartilaginous or osseous) (Figure 6–3) or pseudosarcomatous differentiation. The former appears to be more frequent; however, mixed and transition forms are common. The extent and degree of differentiation varies widely. The histology of carcinoma at metastatic sites may not be predicted by the extent and subtype seen in the breast.

The number of reported patients with metaplastic mammary carcinomas is insufficient to draw accurate conclusions concerning therapy and prognosis. The majority of the data has been obtained from small studies of specific tumor subtypes. Most patients underwent mastectomy. Rosen and Ernsberger reported that in four of seven patients treated with excisional biopsy alone, disease locally recurred between 1 and 3.5 years after diagnosis.[16] There is no information concerning the responsiveness of metaplastic carcinoma to radiation or chemotherapy.[15] When compared to the more common histologies, metaplastic mammary carcinoma has a low rate of axillary lymph node involvement.[17–19] Distant failure, however, is common, with an overall 5-year survival rate reported to be 44 percent.[13] Given the low rate of axillary metastasis and a lack of prognostic information gained by axillary staging in these patients, elimination of axillary lymphadenectomy or the use of sentinel lymph node biopsy alone may be appropriate.

APOCRINE CARCINOMA

Apocrine carcinoma of the breast reportedly accounts for 0.4 percent of new mammary malignancies.[20,21] This tumor derives its name

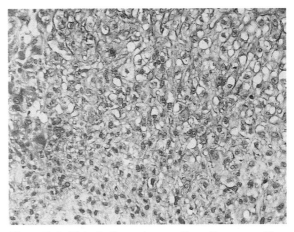

Figure 6–3. Metaplastic carcinoma with cartilagenous differentiation (original magnification x400).

from the apocrine glands normally present in skin. Apocrine carcinomas of the breast, however, do not originate from apocrine glands of the skin. Apocrine carcinomas appear to arise from the apocrine metaplasia commonly found in excised breast tissue.[3] The histologic similarity of apocrine metaplasia commonly found in excised breast tissue, rare carcinomas with apocrine differentiation, and apocrine glands of the skin is due to their common embryological derivation from the epidermis.

Apocrine carcinoma presents in a fashion similar to other, more common breast cancers. The reported age range of affected patients is from 19 to 86 yrs.[22–25] Most patients with infiltrating apocrine carcinoma of the breast present with a palpable mass.[24,25] Abati and colleagues found that approximately one-third of both the intraductal and invasive lesions were detected mammographically.[24] Infiltrating apocrine carcinomas are hard on palpation. Grossly, the lesions are typically gray to white with infiltrating borders.[3] Some tumors are cystic or have a medullary appearance.[3] Microscopically, the cytoplasm is markedly eosinophilic and may be granular or homogeneous. The cellular architecture of both intraductal and invasive apocrine carcinomas is similar to that seen with more common mammary carcinomas. The distinction between atypical apocrine hyperplasia and apocrine intraductal carcinoma can be difficult.[26–28]

The prognosis for patients with apocrine carcinoma of the breast is generally considered to be analogous to patients with similarly staged ductal carcinomas.[23–25] Abati and colleagues identified a 15 percent local recurrence rate in 20 patients with intraductal apocrine carcinomas treated by biopsy alone, but no recurrences in two patients treated with lumpectomy and irradiation.[24] The majority of reported patients with invasive apocrine carcinoma have been treated with mastectomy and some form of axillary dissection. The radiosensitivity of these lesions has yet to be determined, but the use of breast conserving therapy may be appropriate.

ADENOID CYSTIC CARCINOMA

Adenoid cystic carcinoma of the breast, also known as cylindroma, is a rare neoplasm accounting for < 0.1 percent of mammary carcinomas.[29,15] First described in the breast by Geschickter[30] in 1945 and again by Foote and Stewart[5] in 1946, its characteristic histopathologic appearance is identical to like-named tumors arising from the salivary glands. Adenoid cystic carcinomas typically present in the sixth or seventh decade of life. The characteristic presentation is that of a 2 to 3 cm movable tumor which may be tender or painful.[31] The lesions tend to be centrally located in the breast[32] and may exhibit skin changes when superficial. These tumors have a gray to pale yellow cut surface with well-defined margins. Larger lesions have been found to undergo cystic degeneration.[31,33] Adenoid cystic carcinomas of the breast have marked histological heterogeneity, making diagnosis by needle biopsy problematic. Examination of many microscopic fields may be required before the classic cylindromatous and/or cribriform growth pattern is identified. Ro and colleagues divided adenoid cystic carcinomas of the breast into three histologic grades based on the proportion of solid growth to the overall tumor size.[34] Tumors with no solid component were classified as grade I, those with < 30 percent solid component were grade II, and tumors consisting of > 30 percent solid component were grade III. Ro noted that tumors with a solid component were more likely to be larger, recur, or metastasize.

Adenoid cystic carcinoma of the breast has an excellent prognosis. The rate of axillary metastasis is low, less than one percent.[31,34] Distant metastasis is rare.[31] When systemic recurrence does occur, it is typically pulmonary. Metastases to bone,[34] liver,[34] brain,[35] and kidney[36] have also been reported. Distant metastases typically occurr in patients who had negative axillary dissections.[31] There is no prospective data to support one therapeutic modality over another in the treatment of this disease. Reported data on prognosis has been gathered mostly from patients treated with modified radical or radical mastectomy. The use of breast conservation, however, appears reasonable for these patients, as there is no reason to suspect a significant difference in the risk of local recurrence compared to patients with more common types of breast cancer.[37] The low rate of axillary metastasis observed, combined with a lack of prognostic information gained from axillary staging, makes elimination of axillary dissection appropriate in patients with adenoid cystic carcinoma and a clinically negative axilla.

SQUAMOUS CELL CARCINOMA

Squamous cell carcinoma of the breast is an extremely rare form of metaplastic carcinoma consisting of a lesion entirely, or nearly entirely, composed of keratinizing squamous cell carcinoma. Typically, lesions composed of > 90 percent keratinizing squamous carcinoma have been placed in this group. One must be careful to exclude a metastatic squamous cell carcinoma or skin carcinoma involving the breast prior to accepting squamous cell carcinoma as a primary breast tumor. The usual precursor of this cancer is thought to be squamous metaplasia, which occurs in a wide variety of settings including fibroadenoma, cystic lesions, phyllodes tumors, gynecomastia, mammary duct hyperplasia, papillomatosis, subareolar abscesses, and areas of inflammation.[3] In some cases squamous cell carcinoma may represent a variant of metaplastic carcinoma in which the adenocarcinomatous component has been overgrown by the squamous component.[15]

The mean age at diagnosis of patients with squamous cell carcinoma of the breast is similar to that seen with more common breast cancers.[38,39] The lesions are usually palpable, and fixation to the chest wall as well as skin involvement have been observed. Calcifications may be seen on mammography.[40] Grossly, the tumors frequently undergo cystic degeneration producing a cavity filled with necrotic squamous debris. Microscopically, squamous cell carcinomas of the breast resemble similar tumors arising in other sites. Keratin pearls and keratohyaline granules may be present.[3]

As squamous cell carcinoma is a very rare lesion, information on prognosis and treatment is limited. The majority of patients reported in the literature have been treated by mastectomy with axillary dissection. Radiosensitivity of this tumor has not been defined.

SECRETORY CARCINOMA

Secretory carcinoma is a rare tumor affecting both adults and children. In 1966, McDivitt and Stewart described a series of seven young patients with this tumor, referring to it as juvenile carcinoma.[41] It soon became apparent, however, that most patients found to have this tumor were not juveniles. Tavassoli and Norris, reporting on a series of 19 patients, found the median age at the time of diagnosis to be 25 years, with six patients being > 30 years of age.[42] As it became obvious that the majority of patients with "juvenile carcinoma of the breast" were adults, it was redesignated "secretory carcinoma."

Secretory carcinoma has been described in patients from the first to the eighth decade of life. Typically, these lesions are palpable and present as painless, well-circumscribed masses. Grossly, secretory carcinomas are white to gray or tan to yellow in color and may be lobulated.[3] The margins are usually well-circumscribed and rarely infiltrative. Microscopically, the cells are filled with secretory material which is pale pink or amphophilic when stained with hematoxylin and eosin (Figure 6–4).[3,41,42]

Secretory carcinoma is considered a low-grade carcinoma with an excellent prognosis. Axillary metastasis has been identified in approximately 20 percent of cases, but very few patients have been reported to have distant metastasis.[42–44] There is, however, a risk of late local recurrence.[43,45] Wide local excision is preferred in children, with an attempt to preserve the breast bud. In adults, breast conservation is

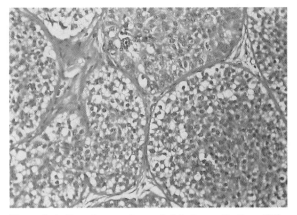

Figure 6–4. Secretory carcinoma (original magnification x400).

appropriate. Axillary lymphadenectomy should be performed selectively based on physical examination or with the identification of metastases on sentinel node biopsy. Radiosensitivity of this tumor has not been defined, and the majority of reported patients treated using breast conservation have not received postoperative radiation therapy.[45]

CARCINOMA OF THE BREAST WITH ENDOCRINE DIFFERENTIATION

Rarely, tumors of the breast may undergo endocrine metaplasia and have the ability to produce ectopic hormones such as human chorionic gonadotropin (HCG), calcitonin, adrenocorticotropin, and epinephrine. Endocrine differentiation may arise in the setting of ductal carcinoma in situ, small-cell undifferentiated carcinoma, mucinous carcinoma, lobular carcinoma, and infiltrating ductal carcinoma.[3,46] Rarely, the microscopic architecture of a breast cancer with endocrine differentiation may mimic the histologic structure of nonmammary tissue that contains the ectopic hormone being produced.

The clinical presentation of patients with carcinomas of the breast with endocrine differentiation is similar to patients with more common mammary neoplasms. Systemic symptoms attributable to the ectopic hormone produced are absent in nearly all cases. However, rare reports of systemic manifestations ascribed to ectopic hormones do exist.[47–49] Most of these

tumors are palpable.[3] Grossly, there are no features specifically associated with endocrine differentiation. Microscopically, most carcinomas of the breast with endocrine differentiation contain argyrophilic cytoplasmic granules. Rarely, choriocarcinomatous differentiation may occur, resulting in tumors that are microscopically similar to syncytiotrophoblast and cytotrophoblast and are strongly reactive for HCG.[3]

There is general agreement that patients with carcinomas of the breast with endocrine differentiation have a similar prognosis to those with like-staged more common mammary cancers.[3,46] Treatment selection should be based on conventional clinical and pathologic criteria.

PHYLLODES TUMOR

First characterized by Muller[50] in 1838, phyllodes tumors are fibroepithelial neoplasms accounting for approximately 0.3 to 0.5 percent of breast tumors in women.[51,52] This tumor's other name, cystosarcoma phyllodes, is used less often and considered by some as misleading for a lesion that is more often benign than malignant. These tumors may be locally aggressive but have minimal capability for metastasis. Phyllodes tumors have been the subject of many reports, but their optimal management has yet to be clearly defined.

Patients typically present with firm, discrete, mobile masses often clinically indistinguishable from fibroadenomas. Palpable axillary lymph nodes may be present in as many as 20 percent of patients but they are infrequently involved by tumor.[3,53] The median age at presentation in the majority of published series is the fourth or fifth decade, with a range of 10 to 86 years.[3,53,54] It is important to note, however, that the mean age of presentation for patients with a fibroadenoma, approximately 30 years, is significantly lower than that for phyllodes tumors.[55] The occurrence of phyllodes tumors in patients < 30 years is rare.[3] Bernstein and colleagues identified race-specific differences in the incidence and mean age of diagnosis of patients in Los Angeles

County with phyllodes tumors.[56] The average annual age-adjusted incidence rate for all racial-ethnic groups combined was 2.1 per 1 million women in the population. Latina whites had the highest incidence rate (2.8 per 1 million population) followed by non-Latina whites, Asians, and African Americans, respectively.[56] Bernstein and colleagues found that the mean age of diagnosis for non-Latina whites was 53.7 years, for Latina whites 45.8 years, African Americans 48.7 years, and Asians 32.9 years. Clinically, tumors that exhibit rapid growth, are > 4 cm, or previously stable tumors that suddenly increase in size, should arouse suspicion. Mammographically, these lesions are smooth and lobulated. With locally invasive disease, margin irregularity may be present. Ultrasound typically reveals a solid mass with no posterior shadowing. Cysts may be present within the lesion.

Grossly, phyllodes tumors are well circumscribed and firm. On sectioning, the tumors are gray to tan and bulging (Figure 6–5). Focal cystic necrosis may be present. Microscopically, phyllodes tumors can be difficult to differentiate from benign cellular fibroadenomas. Typically, an increased cellularity of the stromal component is present. Long epithelial-lined clefts (intracanalicular pattern) are a prominent feature and may help differentiate these tumors from fibroadenomas (Figure 6–6). Mixoid changes may be present. Some degree of epithelial hyperplasia is common, with as many as 10 percent of tumors containing squamous metaplasia.[57] Histologically, these tumors are divided into three groups: benign, low-grade malignant (borderline), and high-grade malignant (Table 6–1). Benign phyllodes tumors are characterized by having < 1 mitosis per 10 high-power fields (HPF). The stromal expansion is uniform throughout the lesion, and the cellularity is modest in extent with mild cellular atypia. Low-grade malignant tumors typically have microscopically invasive borders, moderate heterogeneously distributed stromal expansion, and < 5 mitoses per 10 HPF. High-grade malignant phyllodes tumors have marked

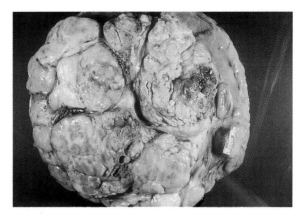

Figure 6–5. Cut surface of phyllodes tumor.

hypercellular stromal overgrowth. Cellular pleomorphism is common, with typically > 5 mitoses per 10 HPF.[3] Although the proportion of patients with clinically enlarged axillary lymph nodes approaches 20 percent,[3,54] the rate of pathologically confirmed axillary metastasis is well under 5 percent.[53,58,59]

The likelihood that a phyllodes tumor will metastasize and/or locally recur depends on its histologic classification. Histologically, benign lesions have a local recurrence rate of six to ten percent.[54,60,61] and minimal risk of systemic metastasis.[3,62] Low-grade malignant phyllodes tumors locally recur in 25 percent to 32 percent of cases[3,57] and have a reported incidence of distant metastasis of under 5 percent.[3] Tumors with a malignant histologic classification have a high rate of local recurrence and a 25 percent risk of systemic metastasis.[3,57,62]

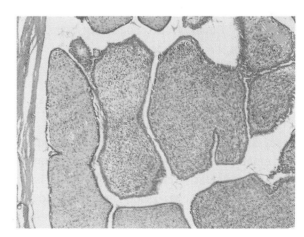

Figure 6–6. Phyllodes tumor (original magnification x100).

Table 6–1. DIFFERENTIATION OF BENIGN, BORDERLINE, AND MALIGNANT PHYLLODES TUMORS

	Benign	Borderline	Malignant
Borders	Pushing	Mostly pushing	Infiltrating
Atypia	Slight	Moderate	Marked
Mitoses/10HPF	<1	1–4	≥ 5
Stromal overgrowth	Rare	Occasional	Frequent

HPF = high-power field

Primary therapy of phyllodes tumors is aimed at reducing the risk of local recurrence. These tumors must be excised to clear surgical margins. The magnitude of the negative margin must be dictated by the histologic features of the tumor and the size of the breast. Excision with negative margins up to 2 cm has been suggested by some authors.[3,15,53,54,62] Mastectomy may be indicated if the lesion cannot be completely excised in a cosmetically acceptable wide local excision. Axillary dissection is not required. Clinically suspicious nodes are invariably hyperplastic and should be individually biopsied. Locally recurrent phyllodes tumor does not mandate mastectomy. Complete excision to wide negative margins is acceptable.[15]

The role of radiotherapy in the treatment of patients with phyllodes tumor remains unclear. There are multiple reports of insensitivity to radiation when used for palliation.[63–65] Two investigators, however, describe the use of postoperative whole breast irradiation following breast-preserving surgery for phyllodes tumor.[66,67] Local recurrence rates were not reported in these studies.

PRIMARY BREAST LYMPHOMA

Primary lymphoma of the breast is a rare disease, accounting for < 1.0 percent of all breast malignancies.[68–70] The origin of this tumor remains unclear. Several investigators have suggested that mucosa-associated lymphoid tissue (MALT) may play a role in its development.[71–73] In 1972, Wiseman and Liao defined the lesion and established the following criteria: (1) a close association between breast tissue and the infiltrating lymphoma, (2) no history of extramammary lymphoma, and (3) the breast must be the primary clinical site.

Patients with primary breast lymphoma typically present with a palpable, sometimes tender, breast mass.[74–76] Rapid growth of the tumor is common.[75,76] Diffuse infiltration, skin changes, and clinically palpable axillary nodes have been described.[75–77] Lymphoma "B" type symptoms are rare.[3,74–76,78] Bilateral involvement has been reported in up to 25 percent of patients.[74,78,79] The majority of patients present in their sixth decade of life, but a bimodal age distribution with peaks in the mid-30s and mid-60s has been reported.[3,74–76,78–80] Mammography and ultrasound of patients with primary breast lymphoma demonstrates a solitary mass in the majority of cases. The imaging characteristics of this lesion are nonpathognomonic.[81]

Grossly, these tumors have a gray-white cut surface, are well circumscribed, fleshy, and may be nodular.[3] The majority of primary breast lymphomas are classified as, mixed, or large cell with diffuse architecture and a B-cell phenotype.[3,75,76,78,79] T-cell tumors are rare.[74,78] In some cases, the linear arrangement of lymphoma cells in the stroma may mimic invasive lobular carcinoma. Immunostains for epithelial and lymphoid markers may be required to differentiate between the two.[3]

Patients with primary breast lymphoma must be staged in a manner similar to other lymphoma patients. Local excision followed by radiation therapy provides excellent local control.[70,75,82,83] Negative margins are not required. Most patients who fail therapy will recur at distant sites or in the other breast.[3] As primary therapy appears to have little impact on survival, radical surgery is rarely required in the treatment of patients with primary breast lymphoma. Patients with stage I disease and those with histologically low-grade tumors have the most favorable prognosis.[69] Systemic therapy should be considered in all cases.[3]

BREAST SARCOMA

First described in 1828 by Chelius,[84] breast sarcoma accounts for less than one percent of all breast malignancies,[85,86] with an annual incidence in the United States of approximately 17.5 new cases per 1 million women.[87] The rarity of this lesion has resulted in reports on breast sarcoma typically addressing a heterogeneous group of tumors, including malignant phyllodes tumors. Mammary sarcomas should be limited to tumors arising from interlobular mesenchymal elements comprising the supporting stroma.[3] These tumors include liposarcoma, leiomyosarcoma, osteogenic sarcoma, chondrosarcoma, malignant fibrous histiocytoma, fibrosarcoma, rhabdomyosarcoma, primary angiosarcoma, and hemangiopericytoma. Also included in this category, but discussed separately in this review, are postradiotherapy angiosarcomas. Phyllodes tumors, which arise from intralobular and periductal stroma, should be excluded.

Typically, breast sarcomas present as painless, mobile, well-circumscribed breast masses.[3,15,88,89] There is commonly a history of rapid growth in a pre-existing mass.[15,89] Skin involvement and nipple changes have been reported but are infrequent.[88,90] Enlarged axillary lymph nodes may be palpable, but pathologically confirmed axillary metastases are rare. The mean age at the time of presentation in three recent reports ranged from 44 to 55 years (range 16 to 87 years).[89–91] Mammographically, these lesions typically appear as well-circumscribed, dense masses. Rarely, the presence of osseous trabeculae within an osteogenic sarcoma may be noted.[92]

Grossly, the majority of breast sarcomas are well circumscribed. The tumors usually grow as expansile masses, compressing surrounding tissue as they enlarge. The margin of a liposarcoma may be multinodular and infiltrative. The cut surface is typically yellow, gray or white in color. There may be a whorled texture as well as areas of necrosis. Gelatinous areas are frequently noted in liposarcomas. Histologically,

sarcomas of the breast are similar to their more common counterparts occurring in other areas of the body (Figure 6–7). In the breast, however, metaplastic carcinoma must be excluded prior to establishing a diagnosis of mammary sarcoma.[3] Diagnosis of this lesion requires extensive sampling to rule out the presence of in situ or invasive carcinoma. Immunohistochemical studies for epithelial markers may be useful in difficult cases. Axillary lymph node involvement is exceedingly uncommon.[3] Gutman and colleagues identified axillary nodal metastases only in the context of disseminated disease.[89]

Breast sarcomas should be treated similarly to sarcomas occurring elsewhere in the body. Surgery is the mainstay of treatment. Wide local excision with histologically negative margins is required.[15,89,93] Mastectomy may be necessary to ensure complete excision of larger tumors. Neoadjuvant chemoradiation should be considered in patients with large tumors. No staging or therapeutic role for axillary lymphadenectomy has been demonstrated.[89] Axillary lymph node dissection need be performed only if required for complete excision of the tumor.

Gutman and colleagues, reporting on 60 cases, found a median disease-free survival of 17.7 months and median overall survival of 67 months (median follow-up of 120 months).[89] Local failure was reported in 19 patients. Those suffering local failure typically did so within the first 24 months. Patients with sarcomas < 5

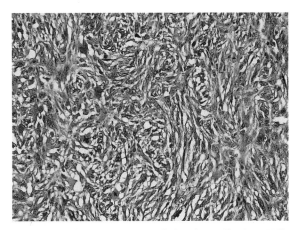

Figure 6–7. High grade sarcoma (original magnification x100).

cm in size were found to have a significantly better prognosis.[89] Pollard and colleagues identified an overall 5-year mortality of 64 percent with a local recurrence rate of 44 percent in the 25 patients in their series.[90] The role of adjuvant radiotherapy has yet to be defined.[89]

POSTRADIOTHERAPY ANGIOSARCOMA

The occurrence of sarcoma following radiotherapy has been well described.[94,95] The widespread acceptance of breast preservation in the treatment of breast cancer may have an unforeseen secondary result: an increase in the number of patients at risk for developing post irradiation sarcoma. Postradiotherapy sarcoma was defined by Cahan and colleagues in 1948 as sarcoma developing in a previously irradiated field after a latency period of several years.[96] Angiosarcoma, osteosarcoma, malignant fibrous histiocytoma, and fibrosarcoma have all been reported in the irradiated breast. Angiosarcoma has been the topic of many recent reports.[97–100] The rarity of these tumors makes the true incidence of postradiotherapy angiosarcoma of the breast difficult to determine. The estimated risk of patients treated with whole breast irradiation ranges from 0.06 to 0.4 percent.[97,100–102] Strobbe and colleagues, reporting on 21 patients with postradiotherapy angiosarcomas of the breast collected from the Netherlands cancer registry, cite a potential incidence as high as 1.59 per-

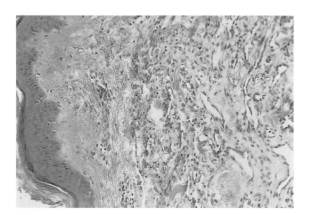

Figure 6–8. Angiosarcoma (original magnification x100).

cent when a median latency period of 74 months is considered.[97]

The median interval between breast-preserving therapy and the occurrence of angiosarcoma of the breast has been reported to be between 6 and 11 years (range 2 to 44).[95,97,98,100] Patients typically present with skin changes reminiscent of a hematoma. These changes may be present over a broad area within the radiation field. An underlying breast mass may be present. Reddish-purple skin patches as well as vesicles have also been reported.[97] Findings on mammography, ultrasound, and MRI are nonspecific.[103]

Grossly, the tumors may be friable, firm, or spongy. Areas of cystic hemorrhagic necrosis are common in high-grade lesions.[3] Histologically, the postirradiated angiosarcoma of the chest wall primarily occurs in the skin, with occasional extension to underlying subcutaneous tissue or breast. It shows a wide spectrum of degree of differentiation but is commonly high grade. Well-formed inter-anastomosing vascular channels corresponding to low-grade angiosarcoma frequently merge with high-grade solid or spindle-cell-containing regions (Figure 6–8). Distinction from postirradiation benign vascular changes including vascular or lymphatic ectasia and the so called "atypical vascular lesions" in addition to hemangiomas is mandatory.[104] Axillary lymph node involvement is uncommon. Gutman and colleagues, reporting on 17 patients with angiosarcoma, identified axillary nodal metastases only in the context of disseminated disease.[89]

Surgical treatment of postradiotherapy angiosarcoma should consist of complete resection with wide negative margins. Salvage mastectomy with en-bloc resection of involved skin and adjacent structures is often required.[97,105] Reconstruction of the resulting defect may require musculocutaneus flaps and/or skin grafts. Rarely, patients with small lesions may be adequately treated with a partial mastectomy.[105] Axillary dissection need be performed only if required for complete excision of the tumor.[105,106]

7

Prognostic and Predictive Markers in Breast Cancer

ANN D. THOR, MD
DAN H. MOORE II, PHD

OVERVIEW

Breast cancer is a highly prevalent and morbid disease, afflicting approximately 1 in 9 women in the United States. The death rate from breast cancer in the United States has recently declined for most age groups, although it remains a major killer with 45,000 deaths annually.[1] Despite the overall decline, the incidence of ductal carcinoma in situ (DCIS) and stage I disease has risen significantly. In parallel, therapeutic opportunities (both traditional and alternative) for breast cancer patients have rapidly expanded. Surgical, radiologic, and medical oncologic modalities are increasingly diverse, including both therapeutic and preventive strategies. In this era of diversity, individualization of treatment strategies to maximize response and minimize morbidity and mortality has become the goal.[2,3]

As documented in the literature of the 1930s, breast masses identified at surgery and presumed to be cancer could be immediately removed by mastectomy on the basis of physical findings.[4] The evolution of biopsy followed by histopathology as the diagnostic test preceding definitive surgery began in the second quarter of the 20th century[5–7] and became firmly established within decades. Histologic criteria became further defined with experience, resulting in subclassification of preneoplastic and malignant processes.[8] Needle biopsies (fine-needle aspiration [FNA] and core-needle biopsy) have contributed to this process, although their role in screening, diagnosis, and subclassification is variable and still in evolution.[9–13] Marker studies represent another phase in this evolution.

Randomized clinical trials (RCTs) have provided important data that allow comparison of chemotherapeutic strategies for adjuvant, neoadjuvant, palliative, or preventive treatments. Tissues acquired from patients enrolled on these randomized trials have become an important resource for correlative studies, allowing analysis of tumor markers for prognosis, prediction of therapeutic benefit, or molecular epidemiologic studies. Knowing which option to choose, in what order, and in which combination is the challenge that drives prognostic and predictive breast cancer marker studies.

This explosion in breast cancer care options has occurred nearly simultaneously with the molecular revolution that occurred in the later decades of the 20th century. The identification and characterization of deoxyribonucleic acid (DNA), the introduction of monoclonal antibodies, and molecular biologic methods have given scientists and physicians new tools to study old problems. As a result, our understanding of breast carcinogenesis and cancer biology has been greatly modified. We now appreciate the immense genetic heterogeneity of the disease, both within and between individual patients. Numerous genetic, transcriptional, and protein alterations may someday be used to diagnose and subclassify breast cancers, augmenting and perhaps replacing histopathology as the gold standard (Figure 7–1). Until the value of these new markers is determined by careful study, however, use of classic markers in breast cancer remains critical to the practice of breast cancer care. It is likely that, over the next decade, emphasis will be placed on predictive markers and quantitation of molecular targets to guide novel therapeutics (see Figure 7–1).

Clinical Use of Usual Breast Cancer Markers in the 1990s

Breast cancer markers can be broadly subdivided into (1) clinical or histologic "markers" or characteristics (such as tumor size, nodal metastases), which are useful to define or subdivide the disease; and (2) markers that are identifiable by specialized testing of the cancer, sera, nipple aspirate, or other biologic sample. Both types of markers have clinical relevance[14–22] and utility (Table 7–1).

Many physicians currently use breast cancer markers only for prognosis. Pathologists

regularly perform careful histopathologic analyses as recommended by the Association of Directors of Anatomic and Surgical Pathology.[23] The clinical application of markers, such as proliferative rate and oncogenes, has been more controversial. The American Society of Clinical Oncology (ASCO) and other specialty groups have been reviewing these issues and are expected to publish updated recommendations. Markers for therapeutic prediction, including *erb*B-2 (*HER-2/neu*), represent the new frontier.

Identification of New Markers

Potential new breast cancer markers are generally evaluated using at least one of three types of studies: (1) early exploratory studies, which generally seek associations between markers and disease characteristics; (2) studies to determine whether factors provide improved means of identifying patients at high or low risk for disease progression or death (using various statistical methods, see below); and (3) studies to determine if markers predict benefit from a given therapeutic regimen.[24] In general, analyses seek to determine if a marker is specific for the disease or tissue type, whether it relates to other disease characteristics of interest, or if it has prognostic (the ability to portend outcome independent of therapy) or predictive (the ability to portend outcome dependent on therapy) value.

Widely accepted methodologic principles have been published to guide the design, conduct, and analysis of clinical trials.[16,20,21] However, few guidelines have been published for clinical testing of prognostic or predictive markers. General guidelines, which are not marker specific, have been reported and are summarized in Table 7–2. For specific breast cancer markers, relevance and applicability may change with time. Recommendations published by governing bodies or professional organizations (such as National Cancer Institute [NCI], Food and Drug Administration [FDA], American Cancer Society [ACS], ASCO, College of American Pathologists [CAP],

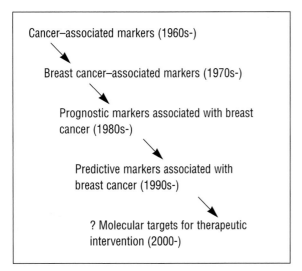

Figure 7–1. Evolution of cancer markers.

American College of Surgeons) are usually updated every few years. Referral to their recommendations on a regular basis is advisable.

To exemplify the evolving nature of the field, the NCI convened a consensus conference in 1985. Only nodal status and tumor size were recognized. In 1990, five factors were recommended by a similar group of experts: nodal metastases, tumor size, histologic grade, histologic subtype, and steroid receptor status.[3] Additional markers, including proliferation rate, ploidy, and oncogenes (such as *p53* mutation/overexpression and *erb*B-2 amplification/overexpression), were recognized as promising markers. At that time, predictive markers (associated with a treatment response) were not recognized except for steroid receptors.

Lymph Node Metastases

Nodal metastases are a well-recognized risk factor for poor outcome in breast cancer patients (discussed in detail elsewhere).[23,25,26] Nodal positivity and the number of nodes with metastases are associated with an increased risk of disease recurrence or progression.[27] Nodal metastases have often been divided into subgroups for prognostic purposes or randomized trial entry. While subclassification can be afforded using this technique, the biologic value of nodal metastases should be considered as a continuum that correlates with outcomes data on survival and recurrence.[27] Lymph node metastases are often the strongest independent variable (marker) of outcomes in breast cancer patients.

There are several important issues related to lymph node metastases that have not yet been clarified. These include the biologic significance (and definition) of microscopic nodal metastases, nodal metastases detected by only immunohistochemical assay (and the need to perform such assays), and issues related to limited axillary dissections (sentinel node procedures). There is no consensus regarding the use of frozen sections or cytology techniques on sentinel lymph nodes, the optimal protocol for

Table 7–1. UTILITY OF BREAST CANCER MARKERS

- Risk assessment
- Early detection
- Cancer subclassification
- Differential diagnosis
- Prognosis
- Therapeutic prediction
- Disease monitoring

sentinel node processing (step sections, immunohistochemistry), or the clinical relevance of micro- or single-cell metastases. Resolution of these issues will better define the role of the pathologist in this procedure. It will also determine whether microscopic cellular metastases is itself a marker of prognosis.

Tumor Size

Tumor size is an independent prognostic marker that is particularly important in node-negative breast cancer patients.[17] Most actuarial survival data have emphasized 1 cm and larger tumors, broken into subgroups, for prognostication. Given the increased incidence of tumors ≤ 1 cm, subclassification of these smaller tumors by size is important as well.[27–33] Subsetting this group into ≤ 0.5 cm versus 0.5 to 1 cm has been used by some. Further subdivisions of this group are likely as more data are available. For these small, node-negative tumors (T1a), proliferation rate appears to be a very important prognostic marker as well.[34,35]

Table 7–2. GENERAL GUIDELINES FOR CLINICAL MARKER UTILIZATION

- Markers should exhibit significant and independent predictive value, validated by clinical testing (ie, they should not be implemented solely on the basis of retrospective data analysis).[3]
- Assays used should be feasible, reproducible, widely available, and subject to quality control.[3]
- Marker analysis should provide data that are readily interpretable by the clinician, with therapeutic implications.[3]
- The measurement of a factor should not consume tumor specimen needed for other tests, particularly careful cytologic and/or histologic analysis.[20]

Tumor Grade

Several schemes have been proposed for grading breast carcinomas. These generally include architectural cellular arrangement, nuclear features, and other items such as mitotic rate. The Surveillance, Epidemiology, and End Results (SEER) data from thousands of patients have shown that breast tumor grading, irrespective of the scheme used, has prognostic significance.[36,37] The 1990 Consensus Conference recommendation—that nuclear grade be evaluated—has now been largely superseded by increasing consensus that a single classification scheme should be adopted. The Elston scheme, which includes nuclear and architectural features and mitotic count, is increasingly used.[38,39] Consensus on a preferred grading scheme is likely to be forthcoming.[40–44] Nuclear grading is also possible on cytology preparations from touch imprint or fine-needle aspiration. Athough not equivalent to the combined architectural/cytologic systems used in surgical pathology, it may provide important data on nuclear grade.[9–11] Clearly, patients with low-grade (better-differentiated) breast cancers have a better prognosis than those with high-grade (poorly differentiated) carcinoma. The reader is referred to Chapters 5 and 6 for a detailed discussion on breast pathology.

Steroid Receptor Analysis

Steroid receptors have been routinely determined on surgically resected primary breast cancers since the late 1970s.[45] Receptor-containing tumors have a better short-term prognosis, although the magnitude of this difference is relatively small (8 to 10 percent difference in recurrence rate for node-negative patients at 5 years).[17,46] Long-term relapse and survival rates between receptor-positive and receptor-negative tumor patients, however, tend to merge.[17,44,47] Despite this, steroid receptor assays are often used as a marker of probable sensitivity to tamoxifen or other agents that bind the estrogen receptor.

Determination of steroid receptors on cytologic or surgical preparations of primary breast tumors is standard and almost universally performed. Such tests should also be obtained on presurgical breast cancer samples (cytology or core biopsy) if neoadjuvant chemo- or radiotherapy will be given. Receptor determination may also be performed on tumor metastases if the steroid receptor status was not determined on the primary tumor or if there is reason to suspect biologic cancer progression (the development of an estrogen receptor–negative phenotype).

Immunochemical assays for estrogen and progesterone receptors (ER, PgR) are most often used.[17] Pathologists evaluate the receptor status of the invasive component only. Generally, immunopositivity of benign breast epithelium adjacent to the cancer is sought as an internal positive control for the assay. Many pathologists have developed their own definition of positivity, which is used in reporting. This may include evaluation of the percentage of cells staining as well as consideration of stain intensity. An effort should be made to have the local institutional scoring system defined and the methodology clearly stated in the assay report. Methods and scoring differences have been estimated to contribute to disagreements between laboratories in up to 30 percent of specimens. Data on ER from archival cases often used different methodologies for ER or PgR, and cut-off levels for positivity were generally determined by the local laboratory. Immunohistochemical methods now in use for ER and PgR can be applied to archival fixed-embedded tissue specimens that are decades old, should concern arise about old hormone receptor data.

The estrogen receptor is a good example of a marker that is both prognostic and predictive. Patients with tumors that are ER positive are more likely to have a better outcome independent of treatment. These same patients are also more likely to respond to tamoxifen therapy (a positive predictive factor).[17] Adding to the complexity of the issue, recent data suggest that optimal ER assay cut points may be different to optimize either prognostic or predictive estimations.[48] In summary, ER and PgR have both positive prognostic and predictive values associated with a more favorable patient outcome.

Cancer Subtyping

Tumor subtyping has been recognized to have independent prognostic significance in breast cancer.[22] Ten to 30 percent of invasive ductal carcinomas are of a special type, many of which can be recognized on cytology preparations. Three of these were recognized by the 1990 National Institutes of Health (NIH) Consensus Conference as having a favorable prognosis—the tubular, colloid, and papillary variants.[3] Each of these three patterns have cytologic correlates and are often classifiable on FNA (refer to Chapters 5 and 6). With the rapid expansion of molecular technologies, including the promising array-based formats (which may be used simultaneously to measure hundreds to thousands of genes or proteins from a breast cancer), subtyping based on gene expression will soon be possible.

Proliferation Rate

Cellular proliferation is an important biologic characteristic of cancer but has been less widely accepted as an independent prognostic marker. Part of the reticence to adopt it as a routinely reported marker may be due to the wide variety of tests for quantitation. The proliferation rate is based on the principle of cell replication (cell cycle states G1, S, M, G2). Cells can also be in a resting phase, known as G0. The mitotic rate, which is generally scored from routine hematoxylin and eosin–stained slides of primary tumor, has been quantitated using several systems, including mitotic figures per 10 high-powered fields, mitotic figures per 1,000 cells, or as a percentage of invasive cancer cells. The strengths and weaknesses of these visual counts have been

reviewed elsewhere.[18] Mitotic counts are now a composite of a commonly used grading system.[39,40] Separate reporting of the mitotic score, in addition to the Elston grade, is supported by a recent multivariate analysis of outcomes, which included both statistical models.[34] When other systems of mitotic quantitation are reported, the mitotic rate should be compared with the mean or median for other similar breast cancers at the same institution, using the same scoring methodology. In general, invasive lobular carcinomas have a significantly lower mitotic rate than infiltrating ductal carcinomas.[34] Scoring of in situ carcinomas has not yet been associated with prognostic or predictive value. Although mitotic counting was first reported nearly a century ago, it remains an important prognostic marker of breast cancer biology.[34,49]

Other techniques that estimate the percentage of cells in the S phase include flow cytometry and thymidine (or thymidine analogue) uptake and immunohistochemical detection of proliferation associated antigens, such as Ki-67 or proliferating cell nuclear antigen (PCNA)/cyclin.[18,49] Of these, flow cytometry or the immunohistochemical detection of proliferation associated antigens (such as Ki-67) are the most commonly used. When flow cytometry is performed on a small sample, macrodissection to increase the tumor/benign ratio is advisable, as a false diploid reading may result.

Summary of Commonly Reported Breast Cancer Markers

Clearly, no single agent or combination treatment is appropriate for all patients.[44] Improvements in outcome, with accurate forecasting of who will derive the greatest benefit, are important. "Therapeutic modeling" using markers has been evaluated in detail by a multidisciplinary panel sponsored by the ASCO. Three steps were suggested for the clinical integration of prognostic data: (1) analysis of a given patient's risk of recurrence and survival based on historic outcome and multiple prognostic factors; (2) identification of various treatment options and their potential therapeutic benefit and risk; and (3) an overall assessment of the expected benefit, risks, cost, and other personal factors that might influence treatment decisions and outcome.[19] Determination of prognostic factors in breast cancers, with subsequent use of those data to make therapeutic decisions and predict outcome, is complicated but feasible. The goal of using markers should be to "contribute to a decision in practice that results in a more favorable clinical outcome for the patient."[19] Similar guidelines should be applicable to predictive factor analysis.

Evolving Markers Based on Cancer Biology

In the early days of marker development, it was assumed that we could subset patients for counseling and treatment on the basis of marker and clinical data that predicted outcome. Unfortunately, clinical and tumor biology heterogeneity among breast cancer patients made an exact prediction of outcome for an individual patient more difficult than anticipated. While prognostic studies can provide an estimate of risk, translation to a single patient is inherently more complex. Recently reported treatment/marker interactions have made prognostic marker studies even more difficult. The use of archival tumor banks, comprising heterogeneously treated patients is no longer acceptable for verification studies of prognostic markers. Increasingly, such studies are performed on patient samples derived from cooperative group-based randomized trials. This design allows testing for treatment/marker interactions.[50,51] Marker/therapy interactions may be confounding. While the relationship may be similar (a poor prognosis and marker of poor response to outcome), it is not always so. A marker may be associated with a negative prognostic value and a positive predictive value, or vice versa. Given the complexity of such inter-

actions, rapid progression of prognostic markers from the research arena to translational (clinical) applications may be ill advised.

While centralized banking has met resistance from some local institutions and pathologists, nationally applied standards and safeguards may eventually make these a safer place than local archives for long-term storage of slides or blocks. Given the evolving technologies, banks of tumor DNA may someday be commonplace as well. The emergence of predictive factors and a new format for marker validation (the RCT) has greatly affected the laboratory development and analysis of new markers. Marker/chemotherapy interactions may also explain, to some extent, discordant marker data on distinct patient subsets, obtained using retrospective archival tumor tissues.[50,51]

Historic Overview: Identification of Novel Cancer Markers

The first widely studied cancer-associated marker was carcinoembryonic antigen (CEA). It was detectable in tumors as well as body fluids and generated great excitement as a marker for the diagnosis or monitoring of cancer. It is expressed by adenocarcinomas (including breast cancers); however, benign epithelium and inflammatory states produce CEA as well. The challenges in CEA research were making reagents and assays that were specific for CEA, quantitating the protein in human tissues and body fluids, determining the associations with clinical and disease parameters, and better definition of CEA biology and structure. We know now that CEA is a member of a large family of proteins with homology to other cross-reacting antigens.[52–55] Many of the early studies used nonspecific reagents and generated conflicting results. The CEA has shown limited usefulness in breast cancer immunodiagnostics and as a marker of disease progression. Because it is not part of a critical molecular pathway, targeting of CEA for therapeutic intent has not been useful.

In the early 1980s, scientists used breast cancer cells, cell lines, or derived cellular products (eg, membrane extracts) to generate monoclonal antibodies against breast cancer associated antigens. Numerous reagents were discovered, such as the human milk fat globule (HMFG) membranes.[56,57] Expression patterns of these antigens were variable. None have demonstrated independent value as prognostic or predictive tumor markers, although some of these reagents have been used to monitor disease progression.

The development of molecular methods, with subsequent studies of critical cell surface receptors, oncogenes, and tumor suppressor genes, has significantly altered the emphasis of breast cancer marker studies away from antigens identified by chance. In the early 1980s, gene sequence data were first used to generate monoclonal antibody probes against peptides, such as the mutant *ras* gene.[58] This allowed visualization and quantitation of *ras* gene alterations in situ in human colon and breast adenocarcinomas.[57–60] Rapid expansion of these technologies to other important breast cancer markers, including the clinical acceptance of immunohistochemical assays to analyze estrogen and progesterone receptors, firmly established this approach.

Some have suggested a "growing backlash of negative sentiment concerning breast cancer prognostic factors in the oncology community today."[61] However, with a shift in emphasis from prognosis to prediction and an increased use of targeted molecular therapeutics, the field of markers in breast cancer care has solidified. The ability of scientists to insert (transfect) genes into cells and the development of knock-in and knock-out transgenic mice now allows hypothesis testing to determine the specific biologic role(s) of specific genes or signal transduction pathways. These tools have revolutionized our understanding of cancer biology and, in the process, have identified entirely new targets (markers) for molecular therapeutics.

Promising Prognostic and Predictive Markers

A number of biology-associated markers with reported prognostic or predictive value have been reported (Table 7–3). While many of these are of biologic interest, relatively few will likely have independent prognostic value. With or without prognostic value, genes or their encoded products may be useful as therapeutic targets.

Growth Factors and Receptors

Breast epithelial cells are, by necessity, responsive to a wide range of growth factors and their receptors including hormones and their cognate receptors, ER and PgR, prolactin, insulin, and a variety of other factors. Estrogen and ER promote cancer development through an indirect process that includes the promotion of cell growth and the activation of estrogen-responsive genes. Some growth factors/receptors are considered oncogenes as well because in the aberrant state, they may cause cancer. Members of the type I growth factor receptor family (epidermal growth factor receptor [EGFR], *erb*B-2 [*HER-2/neu*], *erb*B-3, *erb*B-4) have prognostic, predictive, and therapeutic target value. For the purpose of this chapter, only the highlights of the voluminous literature will be cited.

*erb*B-2

Over a decade has passed since the *HER-2/neu* (*erb*B-2) gene was first identified in chemically

Table 7–3. IMPORTANT MARKER GROUPS IN BREAST CANCER

- Oncogenes
- Tumor suppressor genes
- Programmed cell death associated
- Angiogenesis associated
- Growth factors and their receptors
- Adhesion molecules
- Proteases/Protease inhibitors
- Metastasis associated

induced glial tumors in rats.[62,63] The human equivalent of the proto-oncogenic *neu*, known as *erb*B-2 is located on chromosome 17.[64] The *erb*B-2 gene encodes a transmembrane protein, *p185*, with structural homology to EGFR. This structural homology is one of the features linking these two genes as members of the type 1 receptor tyrosine kinase (RTK) gene superfamily, which also contains the less well studied members *erb*B-3 and *erb*B-4.[65,66] Although encoded by individual genes, these members are highly homologous. Each possesses an extracellular ligand-binding domain, and ligands that bind to all but *erb*B-2 have been identified. These four members can form homo- and heterodimers, with 10 possible dimers. The biologic differences in a prognostic or predictive sense are not yet known for these different configurations.

The *erb*B-2 overexpression/amplification is a complex process,[67–69] which occurs in approximately one-third of invasive and up to two-thirds of in situ carcinomas.[70–77] The *erb*B-2 alterations have been associated with a poor prognosis in breast cancer patients,[17,50,78–89] although it is usually less predictive of outcome than lymph node metastases. A resurgence of interest in *erb*B-2 as a breast cancer marker has recently occurred because *erb*B-2 alterations may predict chemoresponsiveness[81,83,85] and the FDA has recently approved the drug Herceptin® (Trastuzumab, Genentech, Inc.), which targets *erb*B-2.

Cancers without *erb*B-2 alterations have two copies of the gene (unless deletions have occurred) and encode low levels of protein. All normal cells and the majority of breast cancer cells bear two copies of the *erb*B-2 gene and produce low levels of the encoded protein *p185*. Assays to evaluate *erb*B-2 generally measure either gene copy number or protein expression. Abnormal *erb*B-2 can be defined as protein expression at levels above normal cells *or* gene copy number > 2. Assays, therefore, need to be precise and have the discriminatory power to separate abnormal from normal. Variance in assay procedures or reagents may increase or decrease the sensitivity or specificity of the test (no matter what procedure is used), resulting in false negatives or false positives. For this reason, calibration of *erb*B-2 assays, using controls with various levels of gene amplification, are necessary and can be purchased commercially. These should be fixed embedded pellets of cell lines, with and without gene amplification, rather than human tumors that have been positive before.

"Kits" that support *erb*B-2 testing from reagents to recommended scoring systems have just been released. It is possible that these systems will be superior to the currently used "in-house" technologies, although there is little data yet to support that conclusion.

While the pathologist may use a special scoring system (such as the 0, 1+, 2+, or 3+ system for the Dako HercepTest®), providing an estimate of the percentage of *erb*B-2–positive invasive cancer cells will allow greater comparison with other laboratories. While reagent issues are beyond the scope of this chapter, the methodology for scoring deserves brief mention. In general, (1) membranous reactivity only should be considered positive; (2) the invasive component of a tumor only (not in situ disease) should be scored; (3) *erb*B-2 staining should not be observed in adjacent stroma or inflammatory cells, nor should benign epithelium show strong membranous reactivity; (4) reporting should include an approximate estimate of the percentage of immunopositive invasive cancer cells; (5) positive and negative controls should be included in each assay; and (6) the method and primary reagent used by the laboratory should be reported with the assay result. While some recommend a reporting/ scoring of staining intensity, few have compared that data with outcome. There is little data that intensity, by itself, has prognostic or predictive value.[81] Cells with concentric membranous staining *only* are recommended for scoring by some (Dako HercepTest®). This has not been proven to be superior to focal membrane staining for prognostic or predictive purposes. However, in general, intensity and concentric staining are associated with higher levels of gene amplification. Discrete cut points used for data analysis in some studies are suboptimal; the biologic relevance of *erb*B-2 likely represents a continuum.

Two commercial fluorescence in situ hybridization (FISH) assays for *erb*B-2 have recently been approved by the FDA for prognosis (not qualification of patients for Herceptin). The majority of studies have shown comparability between immunohistochemical data and FISH,[77] although some have reported that FISH methods are superior.[84] The FISH methodology is generally similar to immunohistochemistry, although reagents are more expensive, requiring special microscopic equipment and greater pathologist time for scoring. Differences between kits include probe labeling (direct via indirect) and the use of a centromeric probe for chromosome 17 in addition to the *erb*B-2 probe. Intratumor heterogeneity of *erb*B-2 gene copy number and chromosome 17 centromeric copy number are common.[79] Scoring systems that reflect this heterogeneity have not been widely applied and, therefore, the biologic relevance is unknown.

erbB-2 as a Predictive Marker in Breast Cancers. The *erb*B-2 data from nearly 1,000 stage II breast cancers derived from a randomized three-arm trial (Cancer and Leukemia Group B, CALGB trial 8541) of cytoxan, adriamycin, and 5-fluorouracil (CAF) have suggested interactions between *erb*B-2 and chemotherapy (dose of CAF[81,83,85]). This conclusion is supported by both molecular and immunohistochemical *erb*B-2 data. Patients whose tumors had amplified or overexpressed *erb*B-2, treated with dose intensive CAF, had a significantly better survival than patients without *erb*B-2 abnormalities assigned to the same treatment arm.[81,83] In this study, stage II breast cancer patients whose tumors had alterations of both *erb*B-2 and *p53* treated with dose-intensive CAF had the most favorable outcome (90% 10-year survival).[81] Interactions between *erb*B-2 and response to

CAF have now been reported by others as well.[85,86] Data from older cooperative group trials suggest a relative resistance of *erb*B-2–altered breast cancers to methotrexate-based regimens.[50,87,88] Taxol resistance has also been associated with *erb*B-2 overexpression/amplification, although this issue remains controversial.[80] Some reports have also suggested resistance of patients with ER+ tumor to tamoxifen if *erb*B-2 and/or EGFR are overexpressed,[89–93] although the interaction has not been demonstrated by all.[94–96]

erbB-2 as a Therapeutic Target. In 1998 the FDA announced approval of Herceptin® (Trastuzumab, Genentech, Inc.) for the treatment of metastatic breast cancer. This approval occurred in five months, a nearly unparalleled "fast-track." Herceptin is thought to offer a less toxic approach for treating breast cancer, as it directly targets *erb*B-2 associated growth promotion.[97] Herceptin is a genetically engineered (humanized) monoclonal antibody which binds *erb*B-2. Early studies of breast cancer patients with advanced disease have shown that as a single agent, or in combination with other chemotherapy, Herceptin significantly improved outcome for some patients.[98,99] It is somewhat unclear how patients should be selected for treatment with this agent. Most believe that breast cancers without *erb*B-2 alterations will not be responsive to Herceptin, although there has not been a clinical trial to test this hypothesis. In completed trials, patients with the greater number of cells with concentric *erb*B-2 immunostaining had a greater response rate.

Epidermal Growth Factor Receptor

The EGFR gene is amplified with overexpression or is overexpressed in many breast cancers. This receptor allows breast cancer cells to bind a variety of autocrine or paracrine growth factors (including epidermal growth factor [EGF], transforming growth factor-alpha [TGF-α]).[100–103] The EGFR is upregulated by estrogens via direct binding to the promotor region of the gene.[104–106] It is also constitutively activated by amplified *erb*B-2.[107] Binding of ligands such as EGF to EGFR triggers rapid tyrosine phosphorylation of the *erb*B-2 protein[108] as well as other downstream substrates.[109,110]

The EGFR is overexpressed by over one-third of infiltrating ductal carcinomas, is universally expressed by medullary carcinomas, and is generally not detected in lobular or colloid carcinomas.[111] Overexpression of EGFR has been reported in male breast cancers, although infrequently.[112] Overexpression of EGFR has been associated with increased metastatic potential and a worse prognosis in both node-positive and node-negative breast cancer patients.[113–118] The EGFR may interact with *erb*B-2 to confer relative resistance to tamoxifen in ER-positive patients,[89–93,115,116] although, as stated above, this issue is somewhat controversial. Co-overexpression of *erb*B-2 and EGFR is seen in approximately one-fifth of breast cancers. In summary, EGFR should be considered prognostic and possibly predictive on the basis of the data that are currently available.

p53

Nearly one-third of breast cancers have mutations of the tumor suppressor gene *p53*. This has been associated with histologic and clinical aggressiveness.[86,119–123] Mutations often result in overexpression of the encoded protein as a result of a prolonged half-life and protein accumulation. Fortunately, this effect allows immunohistochemical detection of *p53* as a surrogate for mutational analyses.[81,120,124–128] This should be considered a screening method, as some mutations are clearly not detected. The *p53* gene as a breast cancer marker appears more prognostic in node-negative as compared with node-positive breast cancer patients. In addition to prognostic value, *p53* data may help identify patients likely to respond to chemo- or radiotherapy.[129–131]

The *p53* gene is relatively large, and mutations have been reported in both introns and exons. In breast cancers, mutations appear to cluster in exons 5 to 9. Given the molecular complexity of this large gene, studies of mutations based on genetic sequencing have been limited. Newer technologies are being developed for sequencing in high-throughput formats. Given the size of the gene and its many functions, the location and type of genetic abnormality may be important to determine its clinical value.

Patients with germline *p53* mutations (LiFraumeni syndrome) have an increased incidence of breast cancers.[132] Recent evidence suggests a relationship between *BRCA-1* and *p53* in hereditary breast cancer such that *p53* acts as a cancer cofactor in these patients.[133] Most *p53* abnormalities identified in breast cancers, however, occur as spontaneous, somatic events. The *p53* abnormalities have been reported in invasive and in situ carcinomas as well as in rare precursor lesions.

STATISTICAL ISSUES IN CANCER MARKER STUDIES

There are many statistical tools for studying the relationships between patient characteristics (such as age at diagnosis and genetic makeup), tumor parameters (eg, tumor size and grade), adjuvant therapy (primarily radiation and chemotherapy), markers, and length of survival. This subsection will highlight key issues that are important in marker analyses.

Randomized Clinical Trials

An RCT is the most rigorous way to evaluate treatment efficacy, compare different treatments, or test the predictive value of a given marker. The FDA requires proof of efficacy from one or more RCTs for approval of any new treatment for cancer. The key to an RCT is blinded randomization of patients into treatment arms. Randomization minimizes the likelihood that differences in outcome between two treatment groups are due to factors other than the difference in treatment. Formal statistical methods for ensuring that patients are assigned at random to a treatment group must be applied. The importance of this step cannot be overemphasized. Promising results from small studies without randomization are often discovered to be due to baseline differences between those who received the new treatment and those who did not, rather than the differences in treatment. Failures in randomization can result in statistical nightmares in the interpretation of marker data. The study by Thor[34] is a case in point.

An RCT usually involves patients from multiple treatment centers. Once such trials have been reviewed and approved, patients are assigned at random to treatment groups during the enrollment period. Enrollments cease when trials are closed. Patients "on protocol" are then followed up for a predetermined length of time, and their outcome is recorded. The usual outcomes of interest are disease recurrence (otherwise known as disease-free survival [DFS]), disease-specific death (DSS), and death from other causes. Recurrence or death is often referred to as "events" in statistical jargon. Depending on the eligibility criteria, many patients will not have had a recurrence and/or will still be alive at the end of the study so that the survival time for those patients is not known. These patients are generally removed from analyses of outcomes, a process called "censoring." The number of patients who are censored or have events determines the statistical power of a given study.

Kaplan-Meier Survival Curves

Survival experience is usually quantitated as the length of time patients are followed up and whether or not outcomes of interest, or events, occurred. When an event has occurred, the length of time is recorded as length of follow-up to the event time. Time after the event is disregarded. The simplest way to summarize data of this type is to plot them as Kaplan-Meier

(K-M) survival curves. A description of how to calculate points for drawing this curve can be found in many medical-statistical books.[134] Comprehensive statistical software can calculate these curves with precision. The K-M curve is nonparametric, that is, there are no parameters to be estimated to determine its shape. It is highly flexible and can be used to fit any set of survival data consisting of time and a censoring indicator. The basic idea underlying the K-M curve is that it starts with 100 percent survival at time 0 (usually the left side of the curve along the Y axis). A decrement is made at each event, and the size of the decrement is equal to the number of patients who experience that event at that time, divided by the number of patients who were still alive and being followed immediately prior to the event time. A little known but useful feature of the curve is that the number of patients at the end of the study can be estimated by examining the horizontal decrement at the last event. The number remaining is equal to the reciprocal of this decrement. For example, if the survival curve falls by 0.1 at the time of the last event, there were, with high probability, 10 patients followed up for this length of time.[134]

Comparisons of Survival

The survival experience of any number of groups can be compared visually by plotting K-M survival curves for each group. There are many statistical tests for comparing survival curves; the most widely used is the log-rank test. It summarizes the survival experience of two (or more) groups by forming a 2×2 contingency table each time an event occurs. This leads to a series of contingency tables and different weighting schemes for combining the results. The log-rank test weights the chi-square statistics from these tables equally. Harrington and Fleming proposed a weighting scheme under greater control by the user. This allows comparisons of survival curves at specific time points, such as early or late. These might be appropriate to determine if the effect of a new treatment or marker is most pronounced early on. Similarly, later events may be analyzed by changing the Harrington-Fleming parameter.[135]

Proportional Hazard Statistical Models

The K-M survival curves can be used to study the effect of a continuous variable (eg, age), but it is necessary to define one or more cut points to subdivide patients into strata. A K-M curve can be calculated for each stratum, and the strata can be compared using the log-rank or other tests. However, results of such comparisons are usually highly dependent on the cut points; therefore, a researcher who finds conflicting results may not know how to report his findings. Cut points are also commonly used to maximize the p values, a practice which should be discouraged.

The most widely used statistical tool for studying the effects of continuous variables on survival or recurrence is the proportional hazards model. This method was formulated by Cox;[136] hence, it is also known as the Cox model. It is based on an assumption that the hazard (defined as the instantaneous risk of experiencing an event at any given time) for a patient with a risk factor, say age, at level x is proportional to the hazard for another patient at level x' and that the ratio of these hazards is constant over the follow-up time. A simple equation describes the ratio of these hazards for any values of x and x':

$$\text{Ratio of hazards} = \exp[\_ (x - x')]$$

where _ is a parameter to be estimated from the data. This model is readily extended to many variables.

Comprehensive statistical software programs include routines for estimating the parameters of the Cox proportional hazards model and for testing their statistical significance. This method is widely used for studying the relation between multiple factors and survival. It is said to be semiparametric because even though the shape of the survival function is not specified, the relative hazards associated with different factors require estimation of parameters. In using this model to assess the importance of factors on survival, it is important to test the proportional hazards assumption. For example, when the number of positive nodes is used, the model assumes that the relative hazard of having 1 positive node compared with none is the same as that of having 20 nodes compared with 19. Some software programs have the capability of testing these assumptions statistically. However, it is important for the user to understand the meaning of the assumptions behind the proportional hazards model and to make adjustments when possible to make the assumptions more relevant. For example, the logarithm of the number of positive nodes (with 1 added before taking the logarithm to avoid taking the log of 0) is often a more realistic way to model the effects of positive nodes than using the actual number. A similar transformation may be appropriate for tumor size. This kind of variable transformation is often applied in marker analyses, although it is usually described in detail only in figure legends or the statistical methods section.

Univariate and Multivariate Analyses

When establishing the usefulness of a breast cancer marker, it is important to perform both univariate and multivariate analyses. Univariate analysis determines whether the factor predicts the end point. It does not consider the influence of other factors and, therefore, can be misleading. In evaluating novel markers, it is often unknown whether the marker is a cause or a result of the cancerous process. Thus, associations between the presence or absence of a marker with a better or worse survival does little to advance our understanding of the underlying biology or improve predictability of outcome. Probability values (p-values) are poor indicators of relative statistical ranking of the importance of multiple factors. For example, a factor that is "significant" at $p = .001$ may or may not be a better predictor of outcome than one with a $p = .02$. Each factor may interact with others in ways that are not assessed by the size of the p value. The only robust way to evaluate the performance of different subsets of factors is to perform randomization tests of their performance.[137]

A much better understanding of the relationship of the marker can be acquired when it is tested in the "presence" of other well-established factors (ie, multivariate analyses). For example, a factor that is highly correlated with the number of positive nodes may provide no additional independent prognostic/predictive information when the latter factor is added to the predictive equation. The only way to find this out is to perform a multivariate analysis, where all factors are considered together in a statistical model for predicting outcome. The Cox multivariate model described above is a widely used and useful tool for determining the statistical utility of a new factor in the presence of established factors. When this analysis is performed, it is important to include the most powerful usual markers in the model. Failure to do so may cause a new marker to appear important, when in reality it lacks independent value.

SUMMARY

It is important for clinicians and translational scientists to work closely with statisticians for both marker study design and analysis. Statisticians who regularly participate in breast cancer marker or outcome studies often have the greatest insights; they know which variables should be considered in the analysis and what patient populations are best suited for hypothesis testing. Survival analysis requires "expert knowledge" as many variables can affect study outcomes.[138] One of the most common errors that is made in breast marker studies is the use of diverse patients with short-term follow-up. Well-established factors associated with survival, such as tumor stage and patient age, must be considered in trial design and statistical analyses.

In deciding how many patients should be included in a study, it is important to realize that statistical power is dictated by the number of events (ie, recurrences or deaths), not the number of subjects at the start of follow-up. When multiple factors are under study, a rule of thumb is that 10 events are required for every factor studied. In node-negative disease where 5-year survival is often above 90 percent, this means that 100 patients per factor under study will be required. Prognostic marker studies should include both univariate and multivariate analyses of outcomes. Prognostic marker studies generally exclude consideration of treatment/marker interactions. If such interactions exist, they will go unrecognized when the study population is treated heterogeneously. To identify such interactions, study of tumors derived from patients entered in RCTs is necessary.

REFERENCES

1. Parker SL, Tong T, Bolden S, Wingo PA. Cancer statistics, 1996. CA Cancer J Clin 1996;46(1): 5–27.
2. Ernster VL, Barclay J, Kerlikowske K, et al. Incidence of and treatment for ductal carcinoma in situ of the breast. JAMA 1996;275(12):913–8.
3. NIH Consensus Conference. Treatment of early stage breast cancer. JAMA 1991;265:391–5.
4. Tod MC, Dawson EK. The diagnosis and treatment of doubtful mammary tumours. Lancet 1934;II:1041–5.
5. Muir R. The pathogenesis of Paget's disease of the nipple and associated lesions. Br J Surg 1934; 22:728–37.
6. Foote FW Jr, Stewart F. Lobular carcinoma in situ. A rare form of mammary cancer. Am J Pathol 1941;7:491–6.
7. Ewing J. Epithelial and other tumours of the breast. Neoplastic disease. Philadelphia: W. B. Saunders; 1940.
8. Page DL, Anderson TJ. How should we categorize breast cancer? Breast 1993;2:217–9.
9. Kreuzer G, Boquoi E. Aspiration biopsy cytology, mammography and clinical exploration: a modern set up in diagnosis of tumors of the breast. Acta Cytol 1976;20:319–23.
10. Kline TS, Joshi LP, Neal HS. Fine-needle aspiration of the breast: diagnoses and pitfalls. A review of 3545 cases. Cancer 1979;44:1458–64.

11. Dabbs DJ. Role of nuclear grading of breast carcinomas in fine needle aspiration specimens. Acta Cytol 1993;37(3):361–6.

12. Abiati A, Consensus Committee. The uniform approach to breast fine needle aspiration biopsy: a synopsis. Acta Cytol 1996;40:1120–6.

13. Bassett L, Winchester DP, Caplan RB, et al. Stereotatic core-needle biopsy of the breast: a report of the Joint Task Force of the American College of Radiology, American College of Surgeons, and College of American Pathologists. CA Cancer J Clin 1997;47(3):171–90.

14. Aziz K. Tumour markers: current status and future applications. Scand J Clin Lab Invest 1995; Suppl 221:153–5.

15. Miller WR, Ellis IO, Sainsbury JR, Dixon JM. ABC of breast diseases. Prognostic factors. BMJ 1994;309:1573–6.

16. Levine MN, Browman GP, Gent M, et al. When is a prognostic factor useful? A guide for the perplexed. J Clin Oncol 1991;9:348–56.

17. Clark GM. Prognostic and predictive factors. In: Harris JR, Hellman S, Lippman M, Morrow M, editors. Diseases of the breast. Philadelphia: J. B. Lippincott-Raven; 1996.

18. Thor AD, Edgerton SM. Cellular markers of proliferation and oncogenes. In: Colvin RB, Bhan AD, McCluskey RT, editors. Diagnostic immunopathology. 2nd ed. New York: Raven Press, Ltd; 1995.

19. Hayes DF, Bast RC, Desch CE, et al. Tumor marker utility grading system: a framework to evaluate clinical utility of tumor markers. J Natl Cancer Inst 1996;88(20):1456–66.

20. Gasparini G, Pozza F, Harris AL. Evaluating the potential usefulness of new prognostic and predictive indicators in node-negative breast cancer patients. J Natl Cancer Inst 1993;85(15): 1206–19.

21. McGuire WL. Breast cancer prognostic factors: evaluation guidelines. J Natl Cancer Inst 1991; 83(3):154–5.

22. Page DL. Prognosis and breast cancer. Recognition of lethal and favorable prognostic subtypes. Am J Surg Pathol 1991;15(4):334–49.

23. Connolly JL, Fechner RE, Kempson RL, et al. Recommendations for the reporting of breast carcinoma. Association of Directors of Anatomic and Surgical Pathology. Hum Pathol 1996;27(3):220–4.

24. Simon R, Altman DG. Statistical aspects of prognostic factor studies in oncology. Br J Cancer 1994;69(6):979–85.

25. Carter CL, Allen C, Henson DE. Relation of tumor size, lymph node status and survival in 24,740 breast cancer cases. Cancer 1989;63: 181–7.

26. Cazin JL, Gosselin P, Boniface B, et al. Comparative values of several tumour markers: example of untreated breast carcinoma. Br J Cancer 1990;62(6):1031–3.

27. Harris JR, Morrow M, Norton L. Malignant tumors of the breast. In: DeVita VT, Hellman S, Rosenberg SA, editors. Cancer: principles and practice of oncology. 5th ed. New York: Lippincott-Raven Publishers; 1997.

28. Mansour EG, Ravdin PM, Dressler L. Prognostic factors in early breast carcinoma. Cancer 1994;74:381–400.

29. Hermanek P, Sovin LH, Fleming ID. What do we need beyond TNM? Cancer 1996;77(5):815–7.

30. Goldhirsch A, Wood WC, Senn HJ, et al. International Consensus Panel on the Treatment of Primary Breast Cancer. Eur J Cancer 1995; 31A:1754–9.

31. Bast RC, Desch CE, Hayes DF, et al. Update of recommendations for the use of tumor markers in breast and colorectal cancer. J Clin Oncol 1997;16:793–5.

32. Nemoto T, Vana J, Bedwani RN, et al. Management and survival of female breast cancer: results of a national survey by the American College of Surgeons. Cancer 1980;45(12):2917–24.

33. Koscielny S, Tubiana M, Le MG, et al. Breast cancer: relationship between the size of the primary tumour and the probability of metastatic dissemination. Br J Cancer 1984;49(6):709–15.

34. Thor AD, Liu S, Moore DH, Edgerton SM. Comparison of mitotic index, in vitro bromodeoxyuridine labeling, and MIB-1 assays to quantitate proliferation in breast cancers. J Clin Oncol 1999;17(2):470–7.

35. Rosen PP, Groshen S, Saigo PE, et al. A long-term follow up study of survival in stage I (T1NoMo) and stage II (T,N, M0) breast carcinoma. J Clin Oncol 1989;7:355–66.

36. Henson DE. The histologic grading of neoplasms. Arch Pathol Lab Med 1988;112:1091–6.

37. Henson DE, Ries L, Freedman LS, Carriaga M. Relationship among outcome, stage of disease, and histologic grade for 22,616 cases of breast cancer. The basis for a prognostic index. Cancer 1991;68:2142–9.

38. Elston CW, Ellis IO. Method for grading breast cancer. J Clin Pathol 1993;46:189–90.

39. Elston CW, Ellis IO. Pathological prognostic factors in breast cancer: I. The value of histological grade in breast cancer: experience from a

large study with long-term follow-up. Histopathology 1991;19:403–10.

40. Robinson IA, McKee G, Kissin MW. Typing and grading breast carcinoma on fine-needle aspiration: is this clinically useful information? Diagn Cytopathol 1995;13(3):260–5.

41. Cajulis RS, Hessel RG, Hwang S, et al. Simplified nuclear grading of fine-needle aspirates of breast carcinoma: concordance with corresponding histologic nuclear grading and flow cytometric data. Diagn Cytopathol 1994;11(2):124–30.

42. Howell LP, Gandour-Edwards R, O'Sullivan D. Application of the Scarff-Bloom-Richardson tumor grading system to fine-needle aspirates of the breast. Am J Clin Pathol 1994;101(3):262–5.

43. Dabbs DJ, Silverman JF. Prognostic factors from the fine-needle aspirate: breast carcinoma nuclear grade. Diagn Cytopathol 1994;10(3):203–8.

44. Hirshaut Y, Pressman P. Breast cancer: the complete guide. New York: Bantam; 1996.

45. Jordan VC. Tamoxifen: a guide for clinicians and patients. Huntington NY: PRR Publishers; 1996.

46. Clark GM, McGuire WL. Steroid receptors and other prognostic factors in primary breast cancer. Semin Oncol 1988;15:20.

47. Early Breast Cancer Trialists' Collaborative Group. I. Systemic treatment of early breast cancer by hormonal, cytotoxic, or immune therapy: 133 randomized trials involving 31,000 recurrences and 24,000 deaths among 75,000 women. Lancet 1992;339:1–15, 71–85.

48. Elias JM, Masood S. Estrogen receptor assay: are we all doing it the same way? A survey. J Histotechnol 1995;18:95–6.

49. Thor AD, Yandell DW. Molecular pathology of the breast. In: Harris, JR, Hellman S, Lippman M, Morrow M, editors. Diseases of the breast. Philadelphia: J. B. Lippincott-Raven; 1996.

50. Ravdin PM, Chamness GC. The c-erbB-2 proto-oncogene as a prognostic and predictive marker in breast cancer: a paradigm for the development of other macromolecular markers—a review. Gene 1995;159(1):19–27.

51. Berry DA, Thor A, Cirrincione C, et al. Scientific inference and predictions: multiplicities and convincing stories: a case study in breast cancer therapy. In: Bernardo JM, Berger JO, Dawid AP, et al., editors. Bayesian statistics. Vol 5. Oxford University Press; 1996.

52. Nap M, Klaski A, Hoor R, Fleuren G-J. Cross-reactivity with normal antigens in commercial anti-CEA sera, used for immunohistology. The need for tissue controls and absorptions. Am J Clin Pathol 1983;79:25–31.

53. Nap M, Keuning H, Burtin P, et al. CEA and NCA in benign and malignant breast tumors. Am J Clin Pathol 1984;82:526–34.

54. Thompson J, Zimmermann W. The carcinoembryonic antigen gene family: structure, expression and evolution [review]. Tumor Biol 1988;9:63–83.

55. Thor A, Muraro R, Gorstein F, et al. Adjunct to the diagnostic distinction between adenocarcinomas of the ovary and the colon utilizing a monoclonal antibody (COL 4) with restricted carcinoembryonic antigen reactivity. Cancer Res 1987;47:505–12.

56. Foster CS, Edwards PAW, Dinsdale EA, Neville AM. Monoclonal antibodies to the human mammary gland. Virchows Arch 1982;394:279–93.

57. Burchell J, Gendler S, Taylor-Papadimitriou J, et al. Development and characterization of breast cancer reactive monoclonal antibodies directed to the core protein of the human milk mucin. Cancer Res 1987;47:5476–82.

58. Thor A, Horan Hand P, Wunderlich D, et al. Monoclonal antibodies define differential *ras* gene expression in malignant and benign colonic diseases. Nature 1984;311:562–5.

59. Horan Hand P, Thor A, Wunderlich D, et al. Monoclonal antibodies of predefined specificity detect activated *ras* gene expression in human mammary and colon carcinomas. Proc Natl Acad Sci U S A 1984;81:5227–31.

60. Thor A, Ohuchi N, Horan Hand P, et al. *ras* gene alterations and enhanced levels of *ras* p21 expression in a spectrum of benign and malignant human mammary tissues. Lab Invest 1986;55(6):603–15.

61. Osborne CK. Prognostic factors for breast cancer: have they met their promise? J Clin Oncol 1992;10(5):679–82.

62. Bargmann CI, Hung MC, Weinberg RA. Multiple independent activations of the neu oncogene by a point mutation altering the transmembrane domain of p185. Cell 1986;45(5):649–57.

63. Schecter AL, Stern DF, Vaidyanathan L, et al. The neu oncogene: an erbB related gene encoding a 185,000 Mr tumour antigen. Nature 1984;312:513–6.

64. Coussens L, Yang-Feng TL, Liao YC, et al. Tyrosine kinase receptor with extensive homology to EGF receptor shares chromosomal location with neu oncogene. Science 1985;230:1132–9.

65. Kraus MH, Issuing T, Miki N, et al. Isolation and characterization of erbB-3, a third member of

the erbB/epidermal growth factor receptor family: evidence for overexpression in a set of human mammary tumors. Proc Natl Acad Sci U S A 1989;86(23):9193–7.

66. Plowman GD, Culouscou J-M, Whitney GS, et al. Ligand-specific activation of HER4/p180 erbB-4, a fourth member of the epidermal growth factor receptor family. Proc Natl Acad Sci U S A 1993;90:1746–50.

67. Nandi S, Guzman RC, Yang J. Hormones and mammary carcinogenesis in mice, rats, and humans: a unifying hypothesis. Proc Natl Acad Sci U S A 1995;92(9):3650–7.

68. Ethier SP. Growth factor synthesis and human breast cancer progression. J Natl Cancer Inst 1995;87(13):964–73.

69. Stern DF. Biology of ErbB2/HER2/Neu. [Submitted]

70. King CR, Kraus MH, Aaronson SA. Amplification of a novel v-erb-related gene in a human mammary carcinoma. Science 1985;229:974–6.

71. Kraus MH, Popescu NC, Amsbaugh SC, King CR. Overexpression of the EGF receptor-related proto-oncogene erbB-2 in human mammary tumor cell lines by different molecular mechanisms. EMBO J 1987;6:605–10.

72. Slamon DJ, Clark GM, Wong S, et al. Human breast cancer: correlation of relapse and survival with amplification of the HER-2/neu oncogene. Science 1987;235:177–82.

73. Slamon DJ, Godolphin W, Jones LA, et al. Studies of the HER-2/neu proto-oncogene in human breast and ovarian cancer. Science 1989;244:707–12.

74. Thor AD, Schwartz LH, Koerner FC, et al. Analysis of c-erbB-2 expression in breast carcinomas with clinical follow-up. Cancer Res 1989;49:7147–52.

75. Paik S, Hazan R, Fisher ER, et al. Pathologic findings from the National Surgical Adjuvant Breast and Bowel Project: prognostic significance of erbB-2 protein overexpression in primary breast cancer. J Clin Oncol 1990;8:103–12.

76. Liu E, Thor A, He M, et al. The HER2 (c-erbB-2) oncogene is frequently amplified in in situ carcinomas of the breast. Oncogene 1992;7:1027–32.

77. Kallioniemi OP, Kallioniemi A, Kurisu W, et al. erbB-2 amplification in breast cancer analyzed by fluorescence in situ hybridization. Proc Natl Acad Sci U S A 1992;89(12):5321–5.

78. Dittadi R, Catozzi L, Gion M, et al. Comparison between Western blotting, immunohistochemical and ELISA assay for p158neu quantitation in breast cancer specimens. Anticancer Res 1993;13(5C):1821–4.

79. Szollosi J, Balazs M, Feuerstein BG, et al. erbB-2 (HER2/neu) gene copy number, p185HER-2 overexpression and intratumor heterogeneity in human breast cancer. Cancer Res 1995;55(22):5400–7.

80. Press MF, Bernstein L, Thomas PA, et al. HER-2/neu gene amplification characterized by fluorescence in situ hybridization: poor prognosis in node-negative breast carcinomas. J Clin Oncol 1997;15(8):2894–904.

81. Thor AD, Berry DA, Budman DR, et al. erbB-2, p53 and efficacy of adjuvant therapy in lymph node-positive breast cancer. J Natl Cancer Inst 1998;90:1346–60.

82. Thor AD, Budman DR, Berry DA, et al. Selecting patients for higher dose adjuvant CAF: c-erbB-2, p53, dose and dose intensity in stage II, node positive breast cancer [abstract]. Proc ASCO 1997;16:128a.

83. Muss HB, Thor AD, Berry DA, et al. C-erbB-2 expression and response to adjuvant therapy in women with node-positive early breast cancer. N Engl J Med 1994;330:1260–6.

84. Pauletti G, Godolphin W, Press MF, Slamon DJ. Detection and quantitation of HER-2/neu gene amplification in human breast cancer archival material using fluorescence in situ hybridization. Oncogene 1996;13(1):63–72.

85. Paik S, Bryant J, Park C, et al. erbB-2 and response to doxorubicin in patients with axillary lymph node-positive, hormone receptor-negative breast cancer. J Natl Cancer Inst 1998;90(18):1361–70.

86. Clark GM. Should selection of adjuvant chemotherapy for patients with breast cancer be based on erbB-2 status? J Natl Cancer Inst 1998;90(18):1320–1.

87. Gusterson BA, Gelber RD, Goldhirsch A, et al. Prognostic importance of c-erbB-2 expression in breast cancer. J Clin Oncol 1992;10(7):1049–56.

88. Allred DC, Clark GM, Tandon AK, et al. HER-2/neu in node-negative breast cancer: prognostic significance of overexpression influenced by the presence of in situ carcinoma. J Clin Oncol 1992;10(4):599–605.

89. Leitzel K, Teramoto Y, Konrad K, et al. Elevated serum c-erbB-2 antigen levels and decreased response to hormone therapy of breast cancer. J Clin Oncology 1995;13(5):1129–35.

90. Borg A, Baldetorp B, Ferno M, et al. erbB-2 amplification is associated with tamoxifen resistance in steroid-receptor positive breast cancer. Cancer Lett 1994;81:137–44.

91. Benz CC, Scott GK, Sarup JC, et al. Estrogen-dependent, tamoxifen-resistant tumorigenic growth of MCF-7 cells transfected with HER2/neu. Breast Cancer Res Treat 1993;24(2):85–95.

92. Wright C, Nicholson S, Angus B, et al. Relationship between c-erbB-2 protein product expression and response to endocrine therapy in advanced breast cancer. Br J Cancer 1992; 65(1):118–21.

93. Carlomagno C, Perrone F, Gallo C, et al. c-erbB-2 overexpression decreases the benefit of adjuvant tamoxifen in early-stage breast cancer without axillary lymph node metastases. J Clin Oncol 1996;14(10):2702–8.

94. Archer SG, Eliopoulos A, Spandidos D, et al. Expression of ras p21, p53 and c-erbB-2 in advanced breast cancer and response to first line hormonal therapy. Br J Cancer 1995; 72(5):1259–66.

95. Loaiciga K, Beckmann MW, Niederacher D, et al. p185/HER2 and pS2 protein overexpression in breast cancer specimens: improvement for prediction of response to endocrine therapy? Oncol Rep 1994;1:625–9.

96. Elledge RM, Green S, Ciocca D, et al. HER-2 expression and response to tamoxifen in estrogen receptor-positive breast cancer: a Southwest Oncology Group study. Clin Cancer Res 1998;4:7–12.

97. Diamond A, The Advisory Board Company. Herceptin® offers new treatment option for advanced breast cancer patients. The Oncology Roundtable, Oncology Watch 1998;Issue #7.

98. Park JW, Hong K, Carter P, et al. Development of anti-p185HER2 immunoliposomes for cancer therapy. Proc Natl Acad Sci U S A 1995;92: 1327–31.

99. Pegram M, Lipton A, Pietras R, et al. Phase II study of intravenous recombinant humanized anti-p185 HER-2 monoclonal antibody (rhuMAb HER-2) plus cisplatin in patients with HER-2/neu overexpressing metastatic breast cancer. Proc Am Soc Clin Oncol 1995;14:A124.

100. Davidson NE, Gelmann EP, Lippman ME, Dickson RB. Epidermal growth factor receptor gene expression in estrogen receptor-positive and negative human breast cancer cell lines. Mol Endocrinol 1987;1(3):216–23.

101. Ennis BW, Lippman ME, Dickson RB. The EGF receptor system as a target for antitumor therapy. Cancer Invest 1991;9(5):553–62.

102. Falette N, Lefebvre MF, Meggouh F, et al. Measurement of occupied and non-occupied epidermal growth factor receptor sites in 216 human breast cancer biopsies. Breast Cancer Res Treat 1992;20(3);177–83.

103. Ro J, North SM, Gallick GE, et al. Amplified and overexpressed epidermal growth factor receptor gene in uncultured primary human breast carcinoma. Cancer Res 1988;48:161–4.

104. Chrysogelos SA, Yarden RI, Lauber AH, Murphy JM. Mechanisms of EGF receptor regulation in breast cancer cells. Breast Cancer Res Treat 1994;31:227–36.

105. Ishii S, Xu Y-H, Stratton RH, et al. Characterization and sequence of the promoter region of the human epidermal growth factor receptor gene. Proc Natl Acad Sci U S A 1985;82:4920–4.

106. Koenders PG, Beex LV, Geurts-Moespot A, et al. Epidermal growth factor receptor-negative tumors are predominantly confined to the subgroup of estradiol receptor-positive human primary breast cancers. Cancer Res 1991;51(17): 4544–8.

107. Worthylake R, Opresko LK, Wiley HS. ErbB-2 amplification inhibits down-regulation and induces constitutive activation of both erbB-2 and epidermal growth factor receptors. J Biol Chem 1999;274:8865–74.

108. King CR, Borrello I, Bellot F, et al. EGF binding to its receptor triggers a rapid tyrosine phosphorylation of the erbB-2 protein in the mammary tumor cell line SK-BR-3. EMBO J 1988; 7(6):1647–51.

109. Buday L, Downward J. Epidermal growth factor regulates p21ras through the formation of a complex of receptor, Grb2 adapter protein, and Sos nucleotide exchange factor. Cell 1993; 73(3):611–20.

110. Sadowski HB, Shuai K, Darnell JE Jr, Gilman MZ. A common nuclear signal transduction pathway activated by growth factor and cytokine receptors. Science 1993;261:1739–44.

111. Skoog I, Macias A, Azavedo E, et al. Receptors for EGF and oestradiol and thymidine kinase activity in different histological subgroups of human mammary carcinomas. Br J Cancer 1986;54(2):271–6.

112. Winchester DJ, Goldschmidt RA, Kahn SH, et al. Flow cytometric and molecular prognostic markers in 91 male breast carcinoma patients [meeting abstract]. 46th Annual Cancer Symposium in Conjunction with Society of Head and Neck Surgeons; 1993 March 18–21; Los Angeles, CA: Society of Surgical Oncology; 1993.

113. Toi M, Nakamura T, Mukaida H, et al. Relation-

ship between epidermal growth factor receptor status and various prognostic factors in human breast cancer. Cancer 1990;65:1980–4.

114. Sainsbury JRC, Farndon JR, Harris AL, Sherbet GV. Epidermal growth factor receptors on human breast cancers. Br J Surg 1985;72:186–8.

115. Nicholson S, Wright C, Sainsbury JR, et al. Epidermal growth factor receptor (EGFr) as a marker for poor prognosis in node-negative breast cancer patients: neu and tamoxifen failure. J Steroid Biochem Mol Biol 1990;37(6):811–4.

116. Nicholson S, Richard J. Sainsbury C, et al. Epidermal growth factor receptor (EGFr); results of a 6 year follow-up study in operable breast cancer with emphasis on the node negative subgroup. Br J Cancer 1991;63:146–50.

117. Sainsbury JR, Farndon JR, Sherbet GV, Harris AL. Epidermal growth factor receptors and oestrogen receptors in human breast cancer. Lancet 1985;1(8425):364–6.

118. Klijn JG, Berns PM, Schmitz PI, Foekens JA. The clinical significance of epidermal growth factor receptor (EGF-R) in human breast cancer: a review on 5232 patients. Endocr Rev 1992; 13(1):3–17.

119. Stark A, Hulka BS, Conway JS, et al. Her-2/neu amplification and the risk of subsequent invasive breast cancer. [In press]

120. Thor AD, Yandell DW. Prognostic significance of p53 overexpression in node-negative breast carcinoma: preliminary studies support cautious optimism [editorial]. J Natl Cancer Inst 1993;85(3):176–7.

121. Thor AD, Moore DH II, Edgerton SM, et al. Accumulation of p53 tumor suppressor gene protein: an independent marker of prognosis in breast cancers. J Natl Cancer Inst 1992;84: 845–55.

122. Yandell DW, Thor AD. p53 analysis in diagnostic pathology: biologic implications and possible clinical applications. Diagn Mol Pathol 1993; 2(1):1–3.

123. Thor AD. Prognostic and predictive markers in breast cancer: issues related to molecular determinants of outcome. Breast J 1998;4(5): 379–82.

124. Horak EK, Smith K, Bromley L, et al. Mutant p53, EGF receptor and c-erbB-2 expression in human breast cancer. Oncogene 1991;6(12): 2277–84.

125. Nigro JM, Baker SJ, Preisinger AC, et al. Mutations in the p53 gene occur in diverse human tumour types. Nature 1989;342:705–8.

126. Davidoff AM, Humphrey PA, Iglehart JD, Marks JR. Genetic basis for p53 overexpression in human breast cancer. Proc Natl Acad Sci U S A 1991;88(11):5006–10.

127. Prosser J, Thompson AM, Cranson G, Evans HJ. Evidence that p53 behaves as a tumour suppressor gene in sporadic breast tumours. Oncogene 1990;5(10):1573–9.

128. Runnebaum IB, Nagarajan M, Bowman M, et al. Mutations in p53 as potential molecular markers for human breast cancer. Proc Natl Acad Sci U S A 1991;88(23):10657–61.

129. Bergh J, Norberg T, Sjogren S, et al. Complete sequencing of the p53 gene provides prognostic information in breast cancer patients, particularly in relation to adjuvant systemic therapy and radiotherapy. Nature Med 1995;1(10):1029–34.

130. Hawkins DS, Demers GW, Galloway DA. Inactivation of p53 enhances sensitivity to multiple chemotherapeutic agents. Cancer Res 1996;56 (4):892–8.

131. Levine AJ. p53, the cellular gatekeeper for growth and division. Cell 1997;88(3):323–31.

132. Kleihues P, Schauble B, zur Hausen A, et al. Tumors associated with p53 germline mutations: a synopsis of 91 families. Am J Pathol 1997;150(1):1–13.

133. Sobol H, Stoppa-Lyonnet D, Bressac-De Paillerets B, et al. BRCA1-p53 relationship in hereditary breast cancer. Int J Oncol 1997;10:349–53.

134. Marubini E, Valsecchi MG. Analysing survival data from clinical trials and observational studies. New York: Wiley & Sons; 1995.

135. Harrington DP, Fleming TR. A class of rank test procedures for censored survival data. Biometrika 1982;69:53–56.

136. Cox DR. Regression models and life tables (with discussion). J R Statist Soc 1972;34(B):187–220.

137. Edgington ES. Randomization tests. New York: Marcel Dekker; 1995.

138. Berry DA. When is a confirmatory randomized clinical trial needed? [editorial]. J Natl Cancer Inst 1996;88:1606–7.

8

Surgical Management of Ductal Carcinoma In Situ

STEPHEN F. SENER, MD

LAURIE H. LEE, PA-C

Although Broders first defined the pathologic entity of ductal carcinoma in situ (DCIS) in 1932, in situ disease remained a clinical curiosity until the mid-1970s because of the unusual association of a palpable mass with noninfiltrating cancer.[1] With the widespread acceptance of screening mammography for breast cancer detection came a significant increase in the number of patients with nonpalpable DCIS. Reports over the last two decades have demonstrated equivalent survival results for the treatment of DCIS with mastectomy versus breast-conservation therapy. Yet, the limitations of early studies led to ambivalence about the efficacy of breast conservation. Illustrating this sentiment was the fact that mastectomy was more commonly used than lumpectomy for patients with DCIS from 1985 through 1991, as reported by the American College of Surgeons using the National Cancer Data Base (NCDB).[2]

This chapter focuses on clinical research that has attempted to predict risk factors for ipsilateral recurrence after treatment of DCIS with breast conservation therapy.

INCIDENCE

The increased incidence of DCIS over the last two decades has resulted from a significant increase in the number of screening mammograms per year, heightened awareness by radi-

ologists of the natural evolution of calcifications related to DCIS, and technologic advances in mammography equipment.

Since 1976, the Cancer Incidence and End Results (CIER) Committee of the American Cancer Society, Illinois Division, has published incidence data on approximately 85 percent of patients treated for cancer at Illinois hospitals. A retrospective report from the CIER Committee was based on 10,974 breast cancer patients diagnosed from 1970 to 1975.[3] Only 2 percent of patients during this time period had in situ disease, reflecting the stage distribution commonly seen in the era before the availability of mammography.[4,5] The number of patients with DCIS, as a percentage of the total number of female breast cancer patients, has steadily increased to 12.9 percent in 1995, corroborating data from the NCDB.[2,6] The combined statewide registry and mammography survey data from 1985 to 1994 revealed that 2.2 patients with DCIS were identified per 1,000 mammograms. Data from Evanston Northwestern Healthcare compiled from 1994 to 1996 demonstrated that the number of patients with DCIS gradually increased until age 70 years and then remained constant thereafter (Figure 8–1).[7]

Despite the fact that most investigators regard DCIS as a preinvasive phase of malignant transformation, in some women, it is present but never becomes clinically relevant. For example, the incidence of occult multicentric DCIS in mastectomy specimens is higher than the ipsilateral breast tumor recurrence rate after lumpectomy, with or without radiation.[8] As further evidence for the heterogeneous natural history of DCIS, seven autopsy series of women without a history of breast cancer were collectively evaluated, and it was demonstrated that the median prevalence of DCIS was 8.9 percent (range 0 to 14.7 percent), depending on the level of scrutiny of the pathologic examination.[9]

TREATMENT OF PRIMARY DUCTAL CARCINOMA IN SITU

Total Mastectomy

Reports on the treatment of DCIS by mastectomy serve as historical benchmarks for comparison with breast conservation therapy, consisting primarily of patients presenting prior to the wide acceptance of mammographic screening. Patients in these series frequently had nipple discharge, Paget's disease of the nipple, or palpable DCIS, and pathologic review frequently demonstrated evidence of invasion. Locoregional recurrence and disease-related mortality rates were about 1 percent.[10–13] Chest wall recurrences were invasive and defined the

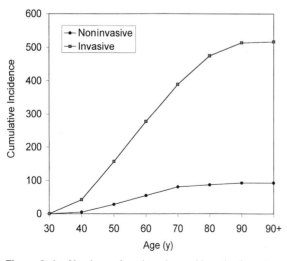

Figure 8–1. Numbers of noninvasive and invasive breast cancers by age among 609 patients treated at Evanston Northwestern Healthcare, 1994 to 1996.

cancers as biologically aggressive.[14] The risk of disease-related mortality, although low, was finite, most likely due to difficulty in identifying areas of invasion within the excised breast. Clearly distinct from these subsets are the current, more common patients with screening mammograms who present with localized, nonpalpable areas of calcification representing DCIS, in whom the incidence of multicentricity or invasion is low.

The difficulty in identifying areas of invasion continues to exist today and leads to a low but continuing risk of mortality from DCIS, especially for patients with multicentric or geographically large, comedo DCIS.[15] Treatment recommendations must take into account the risk of noninvasive and invasive recurrence as well as that of disease-related mortality. Currently, mastectomy is generally reserved for patients in whom lumpectomy results in either positive pathologic margins or unacceptable cosmesis. A small percentage of patients who might otherwise be candidates for breast conservation therapy will elect mastectomy due to a lack of interest in cosmesis, inaccessibility of radiation treatment facilities, or a history of connective tissue disease.

Lumpectomy with Radiation Therapy

The National Surgical Adjuvant Breast Project (NSABP) Protocol B-17 was initiated in 1985 to test whether radiation after lumpectomy for localized DCIS prevented recurrence of cancer in the surgically treated breast.[16–18] The updated report (1997) presented findings on 814 eligible patients through 8 years of follow-up. Of 403 patients treated by lumpectomy alone, 104 (26.8%) had an ipsilateral breast recurrence. Fifty-one (13.4%) recurrences were noninvasive and 53 (13.4%) were invasive. Of the 411 patients treated by lumpectomy and radiation, 47 (12.1%) had an ipsilateral breast recurrence. Thirty (8.2%) recurrences were noninvasive, and 17 (3.9%) were invasive. Thus, the addition of radiation to lumpectomy in the treatment of localized DCIS significantly reduced the incidence of noninvasive and invasive ipsilateral breast recurrence ($p < .000005$). Despite a better disease-free survival in those treated with lumpectomy and radiation (75% versus 62%, $p = .00003$), overall survival was equivalent (95% versus 94%).

Numerous retrospective studies have been done to determine variables associated with an increased risk of local recurrence after breast conservation therapy. The recurrence and survival results of lumpectomy and radiation for mammographically detected DCIS are shown in Table 8–1.[12,16–24] Ipsilateral breast recurrence rates ranged from 0 to 10 percent at 5 years and 8 to 23 percent at 10 years. The most comprehensive evaluations had the lowest recurrence rates and included mammographic and pathologic correlation, with microscopic margin analysis, classification of architectural pattern, determination of tumor size, and use of postlumpectomy mammography to assess the completeness of excision.

The patterns of recurrence after lumpectomy and radiation for mammographically detected DCIS are shown in Table 8–2. Most ipsilateral breast recurrences occurred in the same vicinity as the primary tumor, and approximately 50 percent were invasive cancers when detected. Solin and colleagues reported that the median time interval from diagnosis of DCIS to an invasive

recurrence was 5 years and to a noninvasive recurrence was 4 years.[24] A longer time interval to an invasive than a noninvasive recurrence has also been reported by two other groups.[20,22] In NSABP B-17, 58 percent of all recurrences were within 2 years of treatment.[17] Fowble and colleagues concluded from their data that increased attention to efforts that assure complete excision of DCIS prior to radiation (excision to negative margins > 2 mm, and negative preradiotherapy mammography) reduced the risk of noninvasive local recurrence. And, as that type of recurrence was eliminated, late invasive recurrence became the predominant type of ipsilateral breast failure.[20]

Factors Associated with Ipsilateral Breast Recurrence after Lumpectomy with Radiation Therapy

Treatment-Related Factors

Recent studies have indicated that microscopic margin status is a predictor for ipsilateral breast recurrence.[12,17,20,21,23,24] For example, in the series reported by Fowble and colleagues, the 5-year actuarial breast recurrence rate was 0 percent for patients with negative or unknown margins and 8 percent for those with positive or close margins.[20] Solin and colleagues reported a recurrence rate of 29 percent for patients with

Table 8–1. RECURRENCE AND SURVIVAL RESULTS OF LUMPECTOMY AND RADIATION FOR MAMMOGRAPHICALLY DETECTED DCIS

Authors (ref. #)	Number of Patients	Ipsilateral Recurrence (%)		Cause-Specific Survival (%)		Median Follow-Up (y)
		5 yr	10 yr	5 yr	10 yr	
NSABP B-17[16–18]	399*	10	12.1	—	75†	8.0 (mean)
Kuske, et al[19]	44	7	—	—	—	4.0
Fowble, et al[20]	110	1	15	100	100	5.3
Vicini, et al[21]	105	8.8	10.2	—	99	6.5
Hiramatsu, et al[22]	54	2	23	—	96	6.2
Sneige, et al[23]	31	0	8	—	—	7.2
Silverstein, et al[12]	133‡	7	19	—	97	7.8
Solin, et al[24]	110	7	14	100	96	9.3

*81 percent detected by mammography
†8-year disease-free survival
‡89 percent detected by mammography

Table 8–2. PATTERNS OF IPSILATERAL BREAST RECURRENCE AFTER LUMPECTOMY
AND RADIATION FOR MAMMOGRAPHICALLY DETECTED DCIS

Authors	Number of Recurrences	Local Recurrence*(%)	Invasive Recurrence(%)	Median Time (y) to Recurrence
NSABP B-17[18]	47	—	36	—
Kuske, et al[19]	3	33	100	2.6
Fowble, et al[20]	3	33	100	8.8
Vicini, et al[21]	10	70	70	2.4
Hiramatsu, et al[22]	4	75	25	6.1
Sneige, et al[23]	1	—	0	8
Silverstein, et al[12]	16	100	50	4.9
Solin, et al[24]	15	73	40	5

* recurrence within lumpectomy site

positive or close margins and 7 percent for those with negative margins.[24] The median time interval to recurrence was 3.6 years for patients with positive margins and 4.3 years for those with negative margins. From the NSABP B-17 trial, the breast recurrence rates, with a mean follow-up of 43 months, were 10 percent for patients with positive or unknown margins and 4 percent for those with negative margins.[17]

The presence of malignant-appearing calcifications on preradiation mammography has been highly predictive of recurrence. Two series have reported five such patients, all of whom had disease recurrence.[23,25] A third series reported that there were no recurrences in 37 patients with negative preradiation mammography.[20]

Pathologic Factors

Confounding the pathologist's ability to assess the adequacy of surgical margins is the growth pattern of DCIS within the duct system. Silverstein and colleagues demonstrated that even with negative margins and preradiation mammography to confirm excision of all calcifications, more than 50 percent of patients had residual DCIS in re-excision or mastectomy specimens.[15] Holland demonstrated that mammography may underestimate the extent of DCIS by 2 cm in 15 to 20 percent of patients.[26] An additional study by Faverly and colleagues demonstrated a difference in the growth patterns of well- and poorly differentiated DCIS.[27] Poorly differentiated

DCIS grew in a continuous pattern, implying that margin assessment should be accurate. However, well-differentiated DCIS grew in a discontinuous (multifocal) pattern in 70 percent of patients, making margin analysis problematic. Of specimens with multifocal DCIS, about 65 percent had gaps < 5 mm, 20 percent had gaps 5 to 10 mm, and 10 percent had gaps >10 mm.

The influence of pathologic factors on ipsilateral breast recurrence remains an area for active investigation. It was initially suggested by Solin and colleagues that high-grade DCIS or comedo necrosis was associated with a higher rate of breast recurrence.[28] However, this series with a shorter follow-up underestimated the number of recurrences in low-grade and noncomedo DCIS, and recurrences with high-grade or comedo DCIS were predominant. Longer follow-up revealed late recurrences with low-grade and noncomedo DCIS, a finding also reported by Silverstein and colleagues.[15,29]

Combination of Treatment-Related and Pathologic Factors (Van Nuys Prognostic Index)

In 1995, Silverstein and colleagues devised a scoring system, based on retrospective data, that combined three independent predictors of local recurrence after breast conservation treatment in patients with DCIS: tumor size, margin width, and pathologic classification.[30] Scores, ranging from 1 to 3, were assigned to each of the variables defined by multivariate analyses (Table 8–3). The Van Nuys Prognostic Index (VNPI) scoring system was validated using data from 394 patients treated for DCIS with breast conservation: 209 by lumpectomy alone and 185 by lumpectomy and radiation. Patients were divided into three groups with different probabilities for ipsilateral breast recurrence, on the basis of VNPI scores (3 to 4, 5 to 7, 8 to 9). The 12-year local recurrence-free survival rates were 98 percent for those with VNPI = 3 and 4; 70 percent for those with VNPI = 5 to 7; and 28 percent for those with VNPI = 8 and 9. The 12-year breast cancer-specific survival rates were 100 percent for those with VNPI = 3 and 4; 99 percent for those with VNPI = 5 to 7; and 95 percent for those with VNPI = 8 and 9.

In patients with VNPI scores of 3 and 4, there was no difference in disease-free survival in those treated with lumpectomy and radiation versus those treated by lumpectomy alone. In patients with intermediate VNPI scores (5 to 7), there was a 13 percent lower local recurrence rate in those treated with lumpectomy and radiation versus those treated with lumpectomy alone ($p = .027$). Even though there was a significantly lower local recurrence rate in patients with VNPI = 8 and 9 treated by lumpectomy and radiation versus lumpectomy alone, close to 60 percent of those treated by lumpectomy and radiation had an ipsilateral breast recurrence with an 81-month median follow-up. Although this prognostic scheme has a rational formula, it was defined using a retrospectively identified cohort. Further validation in a prospective analysis will be important to confirm its conclusions.

Clinical Factors

Solin and colleagues reported that the ipsilateral breast recurrence rate for women < 50 years of age was 25 percent compared with 2 percent for those ≥ 50 years, and the time interval to recurrence was 4.9 years for the younger women compared with 8.7 years for the single recurrence in women ≥ 50 years.[24] Van Zee and colleagues also reported an increased recurrence risk for women < 40 years of age versus those ≥ 40 years.[31] However, other investigators were unable to confirm the correlation of young age with increased risk of breast recurrence after breast conservation treatment.[20,22,23]

An increased risk of breast recurrence was associated with a family history of breast cancer by two groups of investigators.[22,25] However, this finding remains unconfirmed by others, so the impact of family history on ipsilateral breast recurrence remains uncertain at this time.[20]

Lumpectomy Alone

Lagios and colleagues proposed that lumpectomy alone was appropriate treatment for selected patients with mammographically detected DCIS.[14,32] Selection criteria included tumor size of 25 mm or less, histologically negative margins of excision, and postoperative mammography to confirm the absence of calcifications remaining in the breast. Follow-up of the original 79 patients reported in 1989 revealed a 15-year actuarial local recurrence rate of 19 percent.[33] The local recurrence rates were 33 percent for patients with high-grade DCIS, 10 percent for those with intermediate-

Table 8–3. THE VAN NUYS PROGNOSTIC INDEX (VNPI) SCORING SYSTEM

Score	1	2	3
Size (mm)	15 or less	16 to 40	41 or more
Margin width (mm)	10 or more	1 to 9	Less than 1
Pathologic class	Non–high grade	Non–high grade	High grade
	No necrosis	Necrosis	
	Nuclear grade 1 to 2	Nuclear grade 1 to 2	Nuclear grade 3

VNPI = size score + margin score + pathologic class score.

grade DCIS, and 6 percent for those with low-grade DCIS. In addition, local recurrence rates were 68 percent for patients with margins < 1 mm, 20 percent for those with margins 1 to 9 mm, and 7 percent for those with margins of 10 mm or more. Other authors have reported similar results (14 to 27% breast recurrence rates) with follow-up times of 45 to 90 months.[18,34-37] These data have led to the conclusion that there may be subsets of patients with DCIS for whom lumpectomy alone is adequate treatment.

The NSABP B-17 trial represents the only randomized comparison of lumpectomy with or without radiation therapy. Although the data from this study strongly supported the use of radiation therapy to decrease the risk of ipsilateral breast recurrence, DCIS consists of a broad spectrum of disease defined by grade and extent. Failure to scrutinize these pathologic variations has been a criticism of the study.[38] Although there may be subsets of patients that are adequately treated by lumpectomy alone, a successful outcome with this approach is dependent on careful selection of good-risk patients and demonstration of clear surgical margins after lumpectomy.

RESULTS OF TREATMENT FOR IPSILATERAL BREAST TUMOR RECURRENCE

Survival results after treatment of an ipsilateral breast recurrence following conservative surgery for DCIS are shown in Table 8–4. Patients with noninvasive recurrence were treated by complete total mastectomy and none developed distant metastases thereafter. In 707 patients treated by Silverstein and colleagues (which included 259 patients initially treated by mastectomy), the 8-year local recurrence rate was 12.5 percent.[39] There were 74 recurrences: 39 were noninvasive, and 35 were invasive. At the time of local invasive recurrence, 18 of 35 (51%) were stage I, 4 (11%) were stage IIA, 8 (23%) were stage IIB, 4 (11%) were stage IIIB,

and 1 (3%) was stage IV. However, node information was available for only 5 of the 35 patients with invasive recurrence because 30 patients initially underwent axillary dissection with the treatment of their primary tumor. Thus, some of the remaining 30 patients were probably understaged. At 8-year follow-up after treatment of the 35 patients for local invasive recurrence, the probability of developing distant metastases was 27 percent and the breast cancer–specific mortality rate was 14.4 percent. The 8-year breast cancer mortality rate for 448 patients that had breast conservation treatment for DCIS was 2.1 percent. The results indicated that, regardless of treatment choice, the overall mortality rates were low.

Re-excision of recurrent disease may be a consideration for patients treated initially with lumpectomy alone. After re-excision, radiation therapy should be included in the treatment program. For most, a recurrence occurs in the context of an irradiated breast, and a completion mastectomy is usually the treatment of choice.

RECOMMENDATIONS FOR FOLLOW-UP CARE OF PATIENTS WITH DCIS

In 1992, a collaborative effort of the American Colleges of Radiology and Surgeons, the College of American Pathologists, and the Society of Surgical Oncology led to a publication regard-

Table 8–4. RESULTS OF TREATMENT FOR IPSILATERAL BREAST RECURRENCE FOLLOWING LUMPECTOMY AND RADIATION FOR DCIS

Authors	Number Developing Metastases / Total Number	
	Noninvasive Recurrence	Invasive Recurrence
NSABP B-17[16]	0/20	1/8
Kuske, et al[19]	—	0/3
Fowble, et al[20]	—	1/3
Vicini, et al[21]	0/3	1/7
Hiramatsu, et al[22]	0/3	1/1
Sneige, et al[23]	0/1	—
Silverstein, et al[39]	0/39	5/35
Solin, et al[24]	0/9	1/6
Total	0/75	10/61 (16%)

ing standards of care for invasive and noninvasive breast cancer treated by breast conservation therapy.[40] A task force of the same four national organizations published a subsequent separate standard of care for patients with DCIS.[41]

The goals of routine follow-up include the identification of treatment sequelae and early detection of recurrent or new breast cancers. Regular clinical examinations and breast imaging are the cornerstones of effective follow-up care. Routine tests for metastatic disease are not indicated for asymptomatic patients after treatment for DCIS. Clinical examinations should be done every 6 months for at least 5 years and perhaps through 8 years, when the risk of ipsilateral breast recurrence after breast-conservation therapy approaches that of contralateral breast cancer. A preradiation therapy ipsilateral mammogram (with magnification views, as necessary) should be done to ensure that there are no residual suspicious calcifications after lumpectomy. A baseline mammogram of the treated breast should be done during the first year after breast-conservation therapy, and thereafter annually or more frequently, if warranted by clinical or radiographic findings. Mammography of the contralateral breast should be done at least annually, depending on clinical or radiographic findings.

REFERENCES

1. Broders AC. Carcinoma in situ contrasted with benign penetrating epithelium. JAMA 1932;99:1670–4.
2. Winchester DJ, Menck HR, Winchester DP. National treatment trends for ductal carcinoma in situ of the breast. Arch Surg 1997;132:660–5.
3. Cancer Incidence and End Results Committee. Cunningham MP, Chairman. Breast cancer: a report by 53 Illinois hospitals on cases diagnosed 1970–1975. Chicago: American Cancer Society, Illinois Division, Inc.; 1982.
4. Hughes KS, Lee AK, Rolfs A. Controversies in the treatment of ductal carcinoma in situ. Surg Clin North Am 1996;76(2):243–65.
5. Rosen PP, Braun DW, Kinne D. The clinical significance of pre-invasive breast carcinoma. Cancer 1980;46:919–25.
6. Cancer Incidence and End Results Committee. Cancer in Illinois: incidence reports. Chicago: American Cancer Society, Illinois Division, Inc.; 1983–1995.
7. Sener SF, Winchester DJ, Winchester DP, et al. Spectrum of mammographically detected breast cancers. Am Surg 1999;65:731–6
8. Schwartz GF, Patchefsky AS, Feig SA, et al. Multicentricity of non-palpable breast cancer. Cancer 1980;45:2913–6.
9. Welch HG, Black WC. Using autopsy series to estimate the disease "reservoir" for ductal carcinoma in situ of the breast: how much more breast cancer can we find? Ann Intern Med 1997;127:1023–8.
10. Ashikari R, Hajdu SI, Robbins GF. Intraductal carcinoma of the breast (1960–1969). Cancer 1971;28:1182–7.
11. Kinne D, Petrek JA, Osborne MP, et al. Breast carcinoma in situ. Arch Surg 1989;124:33–6.
12. Silverstein MJ, Barth A, Poller DN, et al. Ten-year results comparing mastectomy to excision and radiation therapy for ductal carcinoma of the breast. Eur J Cancer 1995;37:1425–7.
13. Rosner D, Bedwani RN, Vana J, et al. Noninvasive breast carcinoma: results of a national survey by the American College of Surgeons. Ann Surg 1980;192:139–47.
14. Lagios MD, Westdahl PR, Margolin FR, Rose MR. Duct carcinoma in situ: relationship of extent of noninvasive disease to the frequency of occult invasion, multicentricity, lymph node metastases, and short-term failures. Cancer 1982;50:1309–14.
15. Silverstein MJ, Waisman JR, Gamagami P, et al. Intraductal carcinoma of the breast (208 cases): clinical factors influencing treatment choice. Cancer 1990;66:102–7.
16. Fisher B, Constantino J, Redmond C, et al. Lumpectomy compared with lumpectomy and radiation therapy for the treatment of intraductal breast cancer. N Engl J Med 1993;328:1581–6.
17. Fisher ER, Constantino J, Fisher B, et al. Pathologic findings from the National Surgical Adjuvant Breast Project (NSABP) Protocol B-17. Intraductal carcinoma (ductal carcinoma in situ). Cancer 1995;75:1310–9.
18. Fisher B, Dignam J, Wolmark N, et al. Lumpectomy and radiation therapy for the treatment of intraductal breast cancer: findings from NSABP B-17. J Clin Oncol 1998;16(2):441–52.
19. Kuske RR, Bean JM, Garcia DM, et al. Breast conservation therapy for intraductal carcinoma of the breast. Int J Radiat Oncol Biol Phys 1993;26:391–6.

20. Fowble B, Hanlon AL, Fein DA, et al. Results of conservative surgery and radiation for mammographically detected ductal carcinoma in situ (DCIS). Int J Radiat Oncol Biol Phys 1997;38(5):949–57.

21. Vicini FA, Lacerna MD, Goldstein NS, et al. Ductal carcinoma in situ detected in the mammographic era: an analysis of clinical, pathologic, and treatment-related factors affecting outcome with breast-conserving therapy. Int J Radiat Oncol Biol Phys 1997;39(3):627–35.

22. Hiramatsu H, Bornstein BA, Recht A, et al. Local recurrence after conservative surgery and radiation therapy for ductal carcinoma in situ. Possible importance of family history. Cancer J Sci Am 1995;1:55–61.

23. Sneige N, McNeese MD, Atkinson EN, et al. Ductal carcinoma in situ treated with lumpectomy and irradiation: histopathologic analysis of 49 specimens with emphasis on risk factors and long term results. Hum Pathol 1995;26:642–9.

24. Solin LJ, McCormick B, Recht A, et al. Mammographically detected, clinically occult ductal carcinoma in situ (intraductal carcinoma) treated with breast conserving surgery and definitive breast irradiation. Cancer J Sci Am 1996;2:158–65.

25. McCormick B, Rosen PP, Kinne D, et al. Ductal carcinoma in situ of the breast: an analysis of local control after conservative surgery and radiotherapy. Int J Radiat Oncol Biol Phys 1991;21:289–92.

26. Holland R, Hendriks JHCL, Verbeek ALM, et al. Extent, distribution, and mammographic/histological correlations of breast ductal carcinoma in situ. Lancet 1990;335:519–22.

27. Faverly DRG, Burgers L, Bult P, Holland R. Three dimensional imaging of mammary ductal carcinoma in situ: clinical implication. Semin Diagn Pathol 1994;11:193–8.

28. Solin LJ, Yeh IT, Kurtz J, et al. Ductal carcinoma in situ (intraductal carcinoma) of the breast treated with breast-conserving surgery and definitive irradiation. Cancer 1993;71:2532–42.

29. Solin LJ, Kurtz J, Fourquet A, et al. Fifteen-year results of breast conserving surgery and definitive breast irradiation for the treatment of ductal carcinoma in situ of the breast. J Clin Oncol 1996;14:754–63.

30. Silverstein MJ. The Van Nuys Prognostic Index. In: Silverstein MJ, editor. Ductal carcinoma in situ of the breast. Baltimore: Williams and Wilkins; 1997. p. 491–501.

31. Van Zee P, Liberman L, McCormick B, et al. Long term follow-up of DCIS treated with breast conservation: effect of age and radiation [Abstr]. Soc Surg Oncol 1996;82:26.

32. Lagios MD, Margolin FR, Westdahl PR, Rose MR. Mammographically detected ductal carcinoma in situ. Frequency of local recurrence following tylectomy and prognostic effect of nuclear grade and local recurrence. Cancer 1989;63:618–24.

33. Lagios M. Lagios experience. In: Silverstein MJ, editor. Ductal carcinoma in situ of the breast. Baltimore: William and Wilkins; 1997. p. 361–5.

34. Shreer I. Conservation therapy of DCIS without radiation. Breast Dis 1996;9:27–36.

35. Arnesson LG, Olsen K. Linkoping experience. In: Silverstein MJ, editor. Ductal carcinoma in situ of the breast. Baltimore: Williams and Wilkins; 1997. p. 373–8.

36. Schwartz GF. Treatment of subclinical ductal carcinoma in situ by excision and local surveillance. In: Silverstein MJ, editor. Ductal carcinoma in situ of the breast. Baltimore: Williams and Wilkins; 1997. p. 353–60.

37. Silverstein MJ. Van Nuys experience by treatment. In: Silverstein MJ, editor. Ductal carcinoma in situ of the breast. Baltimore: Williams and Wilkins; 1997. p.443–8.

38. Page D, Lagios M. Pathologic analysis of the National Surgical Adjuvant Breast Project (NSABP) B-17 Trial. Unanswered questions remaining unanswered considering current concepts of ductal carcinoma in-situ [Editorial]. Cancer 1995;75:1219–22.

39. Silverstein MJ, Lagios MD, Martino S, et al. Outcome after invasive local recurrence in patients with ductal carcinoma in situ of the breast. J Clin Oncol 1998;16:1367–73.

40. Winchester DP, Cox JD. Standards for breast-conservation treatment. CA Cancer J Clin 1992; 42:134-62.

41. Winchester DP, Strom EA. Standards for diagnosis and management of ductal carcinoma in situ of the breast. CA Cancer J Clin 1998;48 (2):108–28.

9

Evaluation and Surgical Management of Stage I and II Breast Cancer

DAVID J. WINCHESTER, MD, FACS

Implementation of screening mammography and increased breast cancer awareness account for the vast majority of breast cancers presenting at an earlier stage. This combined with extensive data supporting the choice of breast preservation has lead to a dramatic change in the treatment for early stage breast cancer. Halsted firmly established radical mastectomy as the sole surgical procedure for breast cancer. Although this provided improved locoregional control of disease, the results were disfiguring (Figure 9–1, right breast). Clinical trials have led to the evolution of therapy that has lessened physical deformity (Figure 9–1, Figure 9–2) and improved survival.

DIAGNOSTIC EVALUATION

Although the surgeon is sometimes the first physician that encounters the patient with breast cancer, this diagnosis may be initially suspected by primary care physicians or other specialists. Although few of these physicians will be directly involved in the diagnostic procedures, all should be familiar with the key issues relevant to the initial evaluation of women with suspected breast cancer.

A suspicious finding or an interval change on a mammogram may require additional imaging studies. Prior to obtaining a histologic or cytologic diagnosis, a thorough breast examination and an explanation of options should be conducted by the surgeon. If a stereotactic core biopsy is performed prior to surgical evaluation, it is possible that a subtle physical finding may be overlooked, leading to a more complicated image-directed biopsy instead of an in-office needle biopsy. If complicated by a postprocedural hematoma, the therapeutic surgical procedures may also require localization. Although large postprocedural hematomas are unusual, when they do occur, the physical examination may have very little role in formulating a treatment plan.

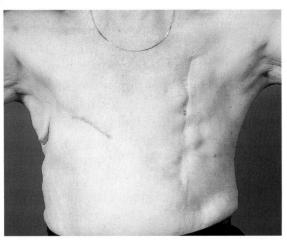

Figure 9–1. Metachronous bilateral breast cancers treated with radical mastectomy (*left*) and modified radical mastectomy (*right*).

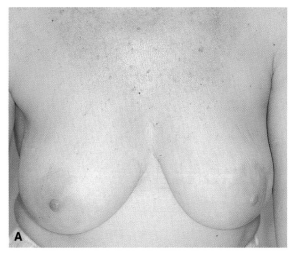
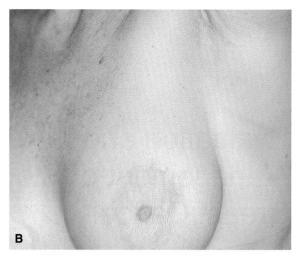

Figure 9–2. *A* and *B,* Excellent cosmetic outcome from breast preserving therapy (*left breast*).

The same concerns also apply to the radiographic evaluation. Prior to embarking on a tissue diagnosis, it is important to obtain a mammogram and additional views or a sonogram, if indicated. The usefulness of these studies is adversely affected by a breast hematoma. It is also imperative that the contralateral breast be thoroughly evaluated by physical examination, mammography, and, if indicated, sonography.

After the physical examination and radiographic studies, a cytologic or histologic diagnosis is required prior to any therapeutic procedures. If the lesion can be appreciated on physical examination, an office-based aspiration or core biopsy is simple, cost effective, and expeditious and simplifies the subsequent treatment in terms of localization of the malignancy. The diagnosis can be reliably obtained with either a cytologic aspiration or a histologic core biopsy.

Establishing a diagnosis with core biopsy provides histologic confirmation of malignancy and has the ability to distinguish between invasive and in situ carcinoma. This approach requires a local anesthetic and has a greater potential for formation of a hematoma. Compared with core biopsy, fine-needle aspiration (FNA) cytology is a simpler, less invasive technique but requires expertise in the preparation and interpretation of cytologic preparations. It has very limited capabilities in distinguishing invasive from in situ tumors, although there may be reliable signs in certain tumor types.[1] Hormone receptor assays and immunohistochemical stains for prognostic markers such as *HER-2/neu* and *p53* can be determined from both core samples and cytology preparations. The false-negative and false-positive rates of core biopsy and FNA cytology are comparable.[2,3]

THERAPY

The treatment of breast cancer continues to be refined to an individualized approach that strives to preserve the breast, chest wall muscles, and lymphatics, when possible. To achieve improved survival, multimodality therapy has also been increasingly used, but according to need and efficacy. To define the optimal local, regional, and systemic therapies of breast cancer, the patient needs to be staged according to the TNM (tumor, nodes, metastases) staging system defined by the American Joint Committee on Cancer[4] (Tables 9–1 and 9–2). For most patients with early stage breast cancer, surgical intervention serves as the first phase of treatment. This step also moves beyond clinical staging to pathologic staging to provide important prognostic information to direct adjuvant therapy decisions. In addition to the stage of the tumor, the presence of ductal carcinoma in situ

Table 9–1. TUMOR-NODE-METASTASIS (TNM) CLASSIFICATION SYSTEM FOR BREAST CANCER

Primary Tumor (T)
TX	Primary tumor cannot be assessed
T0	No evidence of primary tumor
Tis	Carcinoma in situ or Paget's disease of the nipple, with no associated tumor
T1	Tumor 2 cm in greatest dimension
	T1a 0.5 cm
	T1b > 0.5 cm and 1.0 cm
	T1c > 1.0 cm and 2.0 cm
T2	Tumor > 2 cm, and 5 cm in greatest dimension
T3	Tumor > 5 cm in greatest dimension
T4	Tumor of any size with direct extension to chest wall or skin
	T4a Extension to chest wall
	T4b Edema, ulceration, or satellite nodules
	T4c Both T4a and T4b
	T4d Inflammatory carcinoma

Regional Lymph Nodes (N)
NX	Regional lymph nodes cannot be assessed
N0	No regional lymph node metastasis
N1	Metastasis to ipsilateral axillary lymph node(s)
N2	Metastasis to ipsilateral axillary node(s) fixed to one another
N3	Metastasis to ipsilateral internal mammary lymph node(s)

Distant Metastasis (M)
MX	Presence of distant metastasis cannot be assessed
M0	No distant metastasis
M1	Distant metastasis (includes metastases to supra clavicular lymph node[s])

(DCIS) also has implications for the local management of breast cancer. Small invasive breast cancers accompanied by extensive DCIS may require total mastectomy.

Breast Preservation Therapy

Adherence to screening mammography guidelines has made most patients candidates for breast preservation therapy (BPT). Acceptance of this treatment approach has been gradual and dependent upon regional preferences and availability of radiation therapy facilities.[5] When considering treatment options for early breast cancer, good cosmesis is an important goal. Improvements in surgery and radiotherapy have minimized the incidence of poor results seen initially (Figures 9–4 and 9–5). For most patients, the best cosmetic result can be achieved with breast preservation therapy and,

along with that, the shortest recovery as compared with a mastectomy with reconstruction. Multiple prospective randomized studies have confirmed the efficacy of BPT.[6–11] No study has identified a survival disadvantage of this approach. A nonrandomized comparison[12] as well as a meta-analysis of randomized trials[13] have shown equivalent survival rates between these two approaches.

Patient Selection

Despite the extensive data to support the use of BPT, there are still patients who are not candidates for this approach. As surgery is usually the first treatment modality, the choice of therapy is guided by the surgeon's evaluation. A more effective evaluation process ideally includes the preoperative evaluation from other treating physicians to provide a cohesive and comprehensive treatment plan before therapy begins.

Most randomized clinical trials included patients with T1 and T2 tumors.[6–11] Thus, tumors up to 5 cm can be safely managed with this approach. A good cosmetic result may be difficult to achieve with large T2 tumors, and neoadjuvant chemotherapy may improve the ability to preserve breast tissue without compromising survival.[14,15] Saving the breast is important for psychological and cosmetic reasons. This requires sound surgical judgment and meticulous techniques. A large breast can more

Table 9–2. BREAST CARCINOMA STAGES

STAGE	T	N	M
0	Tis	N0	M0
I	T1	N0	M0
IIA	T0	N1	M0
	T1	N1	M0
	T2	N0	M0
IIB	T2	N1	M0
	T3	N0	M0
IIIA	T0	N2	M0
	T1	N2	M0
	T2	N2	M0
	T3	N1 or N2	M0
IIIB	T4	Any N	M0
	Any T	N3	M0
IV	Any T	Any N	M1

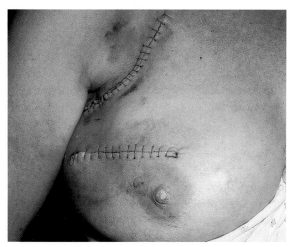

Figure 9–4. Poor cosmetic outcome resulting from poor incision placement, incision size, and hematoma formation.

readily accommodate a larger lumpectomy than a smaller breast. Resection of more than a quadrant of the breast begins to have a significant impact on the cosmetic result and leads to consideration of alternatives such as mastectomy with reconstruction.[16] With the development of microvascular techniques, reconstructive options and results have made total mastectomy a good option for many patients.

In the preoperative evaluation of the patient, the size of the primary tumor is an important discriminator in the selection of the surgical therapy. Given an acceptable ratio between the size of the tumor and the size of the breast,

patients who are interested in cosmesis and committed to radiation therapy are good candidates for BPT. Centrally located lesions including Paget's disease (Figure 9–6) were at one time considered a relative contraindication to BPT. Adequate treatment of tumors in this location may necessitate resection of a portion or all of the nipple-areolar complex (Figure 9–7). This treatment has the distinct advantage of maintaining the breast mound and a sensate breast. Nipple reconstruction may be performed, if desired.

Physical findings and mammographic dimensions may not correlate with the histologic findings after a lumpectomy is performed.[17] Thus, the choice of lumpectomy is ultimately contingent upon the ability to achieve histologically clear surgical margins. Close or involved surgical margins are important predictors of local failure and should prompt consideration of either re-excision or completion mastectomy, depending on the extent of the margin involvement.[18–20]

Placement of the incision is important to create a good cosmetic result and to allow for additional surgery in the case of microscopically involved margins. Optimal cosmesis usually places incisions within skin folds or in a curvilinear fashion around the nipple (Figure 9–8). Incisions should be placed directly over

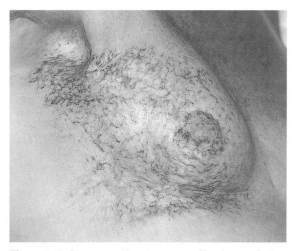

Figure 9–5. Poor cosmetic outcome resulting from radiation injury.

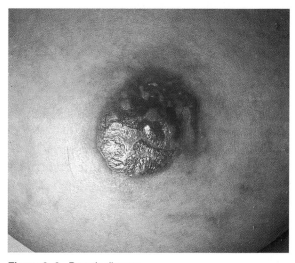

Figure 9–6. Paget's disease.

the primary to avoid tunneling and limit the deformity and extent of dissection in the breast. With the exception of superficial lesions, resection of skin or subcutaneous tissue is not required. A small ellipse of skin may be helpful for specimen orientation.

Aside from the size of the tumor, multicentric tumors or extensive intraductal cancer are also important in identifying poor candidates for BPT. Clearing the surgical margin for in situ disease is equally important for local control. Mammographically occult in situ disease may therefore have the potential to alter the surgical therapy for even small invasive tumors. Synchronous tumors located in different quadrants must be approached with the same margin criteria as those for solitary lesions, leading to a compromised cosmetic result. In addition, multicentric disease also suggests that other areas in the breast may contain unrecognized foci of cancer. Two or more ipsilateral tumors should lead to strong consideration of a mastectomy with reconstruction.

The histologic subtype of the breast primary may have an impact on the local management. In addition to DCIS, which has the propensity to extend great distances in the breast without any mammographic or physical findings, invasive lobular carcinoma may also have a pervasive presentation. In the case of in situ ductal carcinoma, preoperative magnification views may help identify extensive pleomorphic calcifications around a stellate mass. The surgical procedure should attempt to remove all suspicious calcifications.

Invasive lobular carcinomas have a more indolent presentation with a less defined mass with indistinct borders. Mammographic findings are subtle[21,22] and more likely to underestimate tumor dimensions, compared with other invasive cancers.[17] These characteristics account for the greater likelihood of requiring re-excision after lumpectomy.[17] The histologic evaluation of the lumpectomy and regional lymph nodes is more difficult because of the frequency of single malignant lobular cells that

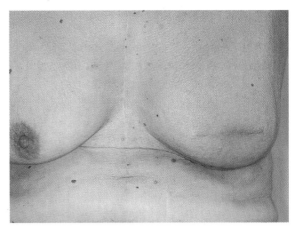

Figure 9–7. Central lumpectomy.

can extend into the breast parenchyma. Cytokeratin stains may facilitate the identification of lobular cells but have uncertain prognostic information in axillary staging.[23]

Randomized clinical trials addressing breast preservation therapy have not separated or excluded lobular carcinomas.[6–11] Several nonrandomized studies have found no difference in the local disease-free survival rates between breast preservation patients with lobular carcinoma and those with ductal carcinoma[24–26] whereas others have noted a difference.[17,27–29] Analysis of the National Cancer Data Base did not identify any significant differences in size, stage, or survival according to histology.[30] It would appear that there are not any specific histologic categories that should exclude consideration of BPT. The same principles of a careful preoperative assessment and microscopic evaluation of lumpectomy margins should lead to successful BPT for all histologic variants.

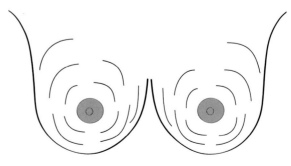

Figure 9–8. Incision placement for lumpectomy.

Risk Factors for Local Recurrence

Several important variables exist for local recurrence after lumpectomy. The only variable to predict local recurrence from analysis of National Surgical Adjuvant Breast and Bowel Project (NSABP) B-06 was age under 45 years.[31] Other variables analyzed included vascular and lymphatic invasion, tumor grade, and size.[31] Treatment-related variables include the extent of resection, margin involvement, and the implementation of radiotherapy. Thus, the risk of local recurrence can be dramatically affected by treatment decisions.

Defining the optimal margin distance is based on a subjective and individualized assessment of each patient, balancing the cosmetic outcome and pathologic characteristics. When comparing a more extensive quadrantectomy with lumpectomy, the risk of a local recurrence is reduced significantly in the former.[32] Despite a significant reduction in local recurrence with a more extensive resection,[32] radiation therapy has been shown to add to local control in these patients.[33] Margin involvement is a strong predictor of local recurrence, and identification of an involved margin should prompt consideration of re-excision or completion mastectomy.[19,20] Despite the usefulness of a microscopic margin assessment, clear surgical margins under the most stringent conditions still do not ensure local control rates that are equivalent to those achieved with the addition of radiotherapy. In the Uppsala Swedish trial, only patients with tumors < 20 mm were included. Each patient underwent a sector resection consisting of removal of a portion of the skin and pectoralis fascia. Each margin was assessed twice. Any microscopic margin involvement or lymph node involvement was an exclusion criterion. Patients were randomized to observation or radiotherapy after sector resection. Despite these favorable conditions and careful analysis of margins, local recurrence was significantly more common in the observation arm of the study.[34] Serial sectioning studies of mastectomy specimens of patients that would be lumpectomy candidates have also shown that microscopic foci of cancer are identified beyond 2 cm of the primary in 41 percent of patients.[35] Although an adequate margin is important, a more extensive resection needs to be balanced with the cosmetic result of the operation. In most instances, resection of the pectoralis fascia with the lumpectomy specimen will avoid concerns about posterior extension. Without muscle involvement, inclusion of the pectoralis fascia with the lumpectomy specimen should assist in good local control, even with a close margin.

The handling of the surgical specimen becomes critical when close or involved microscopic margins are identified on the lumpectomy specimen. Inability to accurately define specimen orientation risks having to remove too large a specimen or removing the wrong area of persistent involvement. The surgeon and the pathologist should work closely together at the time of surgery. Specimens should either be inked on six sides by the surgeon or have appropriate markers to allow the pathologist to do so. Specimens should be submitted fresh for pathologic examination so that any questions about the orientation can be addressed immediately.

Achieving good hemostasis is important for obvious reasons. Large lumpectomy cavities can be defined for the radiotherapist by placing radiopaque surgical clips at the borders of the specimen. This may help facilitate the delivery of a radiation therapy boost to the lumpectomy site.

Total Mastectomy

Total mastectomy remains an excellent choice for many patients with breast cancer. A clear advantage of mastectomy is the avoidance of radiation therapy for patients without large tumors or multiple involved lymph nodes. This has more appeal for patients that are not motivated to achieve good cosmesis. Older, less mobile patients may find this preferable to the alternative of lumpectomy and radiation therapy.

Total mastectomy is indicated for multicentric disease or tumors with extensive coexistent

DCIS, where achieving a clear surgical margin becomes difficult with a segmental mastectomy. It is also indicated for individuals who are not radiation therapy candidates, including those with active scleroderma, history of prior radiotherapy, ataxia telangectasia, and early pregnancy and for those who opt for it. Excellent cosmetic results can be achieved with a variety of reconstructive options, which can occur either simultaneously or as a delayed procedure. If a patient is contemplating reconstruction, a skin-sparing mastectomy should be performed. This operation involves the removal of the nipple-areolar complex and breast tissue but differs from a standard incision in preserving as much of the skin over the breast as possible (Figure 9–9).

Most patients with early-stage breast cancer can undergo immediate reconstruction. This has the advantages of limiting the surgical interventions to a single-stage procedure and providing the patient with the psychological benefit of an immediately reconstructed breast. Immediate reconstruction also best preserves the elasticity of the elevated flaps and helps maintain the natural contour of the breast, including the inframammary fold, which may be affected with a delayed reconstruction. Considerations for delayed reconstruction include urgency to address adjuvant systemic treatment, a patient who remains undecided regarding reconstruction options, or a patient who is likely to receive chest wall radiation therapy. Although radiation therapy can be successfully delivered after autogenous reconstruction with good cosmetic results, the incidence of capsular contraction after radiation therapy is prohibitive in those patients undergoing implant reconstruction.[36]

For patients with a strong familial history of breast cancer, a decision may be made to combine a treatment operation with a prophylactic procedure. The identification of breast cancer susceptibility genes has fostered this concept, but in practical terms, it is very difficult to assess risk *and* screen for a genetic mutation in a timely fashion before embarking on a thera-peutic operation for a diagnosis that led to the genetic evaluation. Counseling these patients can be very difficult as they have to cope with both a diagnosis of cancer and an emotional decision as to whether or not they wish to undergo a bilateral mastectomy. For those patients who might have greater difficulty in reaching a comfortable decision regarding a bilateral operation, a safe approach is to proceed with a lumpectomy and axillary staging procedure in conjunction with genetic counseling, with or without genetic testing. With this approach, the more important delivery of systemic therapy is not delayed. During chemotherapy, the time-consuming process of genetic testing can be performed, if indicated. If the patient is found not to carry a genetic mutation, radiation therapy serves as the last step of the treatment plan. For those patients with an identified mutation, a completion mastectomy and contralateral prophylactic mastectomy with reconstruction can be performed. Although a prophylactic mastectomy does not guarantee prevention of future breast cancer events, recent data suggest that it is an effective means of reducing risk.[37] As an alternative, tamoxifen can be used for both adjuvant treatment and chemoprevention. Although data are relatively early, a clear reduction in high-risk patients was identified in a randomized study of tamoxifen users.[38] If elected, compartmentalizing treatment and prophylactic issues helps to ease the sudden burden of complex decisions that a patient will face at the time of diagnosis.

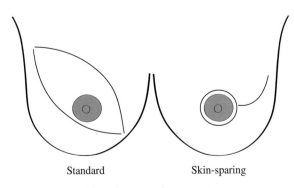

Standard   Skin-sparing

Figure 9–9. Incision placement for mastectomy.

Radical Mastectomy

In the context of early breast cancer, there is virtually no need to resect the pectoralis muscles and axillary tissue. Occasionally, tumors located posteriorly along the chest wall may focally invade the pectoralis muscle. It should be pointed out that invasion of the pectoralis muscle does not constitute chest wall invasion and is staged according to the size of the primary tumor.[4] Small breast cancers that present with muscle involvement are usually located peripherally or posteriorly, and extension, in part, reflects proximity to the muscle. This scenario can be safely managed with resection of a portion of the muscle as part of either a lumpectomy or a total mastectomy. With either surgical approach, radiation therapy should be considered.

Management of the Axilla

Just as treatment of the primary tumor of the breast has evolved from a single, radical operation for all scenarios to a more directed approach consisting of lumpectomy, the standard axillary dissection is quickly being replaced by sentinel lymphadenectomy. Introduced by Morton and colleagues in 1992 for the treatment of melanoma,[39] this technique was quickly applied to breast cancer.[40,41] Like lymphatic mapping for other disease sites, the sentinel lymph node is identified through the constant anatomic relationship between a tumor and draining lymphatics. Conceptually, each specific area in the breast drains to a sentinel lymph node which may be located anywhere within the axilla or internal mammary chain (Figure 9–10). Larger tumors may have more than one draining lymphatic (Figure 9–11). The sentinel lymph node biopsy continues to be refined and defined for patients with early breast cancer; in several studies, it has been demonstrated to yield reliable correlation to an axillary dissection.[40–46]

The axillary dissection has always been recognized as an excellent procedure for two important reasons: staging of the breast cancer and providing regional control. Lymph node involvement represents the most important variable, aside from metastatic disease, to predict outcome.[47] This information is important in defining the prognosis and in tailoring the adjuvant therapy of patients with breast cancer. Staging of the axilla represents a critical variable in defining the prognosis of patients presenting with early breast cancer. In the context of early detection and screening mammography, nodal involvement is at times the only prognosticator that leads to the clear recommendation of chemotherapy.

Aside from providing important prognostic information, axillary dissection represents the most effective means of controlling regional disease.[48] What constitutes an adequate axillary dissection? This has been well established with multiple studies analyzing the inclusion of metastatic disease based on the arbitrary division of level I, II, and III axillary lymph nodes.[49–51] On average, there is a one percent chance of metastatic disease in level III lymph nodes that would not be detected in levels I and II.[49–51] Mathiesen demonstrated that the potential for identifying micrometastases increased till 10 lymph nodes were removed from the axilla.[52] Unless extensive axillary involvement is recognized at the time of surgery, a level I/II node dissection should encompass axillary disease in 99 percent of patients.

In the presence of axillary disease, an axillary dissection is an excellent operation for regional control and prognostic information. However, for the great majority of patients with early breast cancer, an axillary dissection does not confer any therapeutic benefit. The greatest concern, particularly for younger, active patients is the risk of developing lymphedema. This risk is directly related to the extent of the axillary dissection and is further increased with the addition of radiation therapy.[53] This risk remains indefinitely for the life of the patient. Other potential side effects include paresthesias, loss of mobility, and cosmetic deformity.

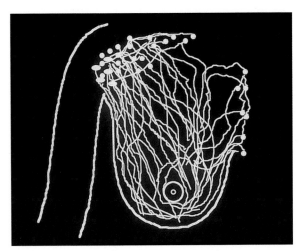

Figure 9–10. Breast lymphatic drainage patterns.

Avoiding the side effects of an axillary dissection in a substantial number of patients who do not achieve any therapeutic benefit has been a major impetus in identifying an alternative means of staging the axilla. Other methods that have been evaluated to replace axillary dissection have been imaging studies including ultrasonography, computed tomography, and scintigraphy. All these techniques have had the same major limitation of an unacceptably high false-negative rate.[54–56] Positron emission tomographic (PET) scanning has emerged as a more sensitive test that relies on the metabolic differences of tumors rather than on anatomic changes. To date, this test shows promise but is still not sensitive enough to exclude the presence of axillary disease.[57] It is unlikely that any imaging technology will compare with the sensitivity of a microscopic examination, which has the potential to identify single metastatic cells. The shortcoming of a standard axillary dissection is that pathologists are incapable of reviewing every cell of every lymph node. The ability to detect micrometastases is directly related to the intensity with which a lymph node is analyzed. Serial sectioning studies have identified a higher incidence of true nodal positivity and mortality in those with unrecognized micrometastases.[23,58] Outside of investigational studies, serial sectioning of axillary dissection specimens is impractical.

Sentinel lymphadenectomy has several conceptual advantages over standard axillary dissection. Most significant to the patient is that the risk of long term complications is virtually eliminated by avoiding an extensive axillary dissection. Recovery is much shorter, and for most, BPT, under these circumstances, can be accomplished as an outpatient procedure. Compared to a standard axillary incision, the sentinel lymph node can be removed through a smaller incision with transcutaneous localization of the node with a hand held gamma probe (Figure 9–12). In addition to the reduction in morbidity, sentinel lymphadenectomy provides the pathologist with the opportunity to perform a much more comprehensive analysis of the specimen, given the more limited material to analyze. Although diffi-

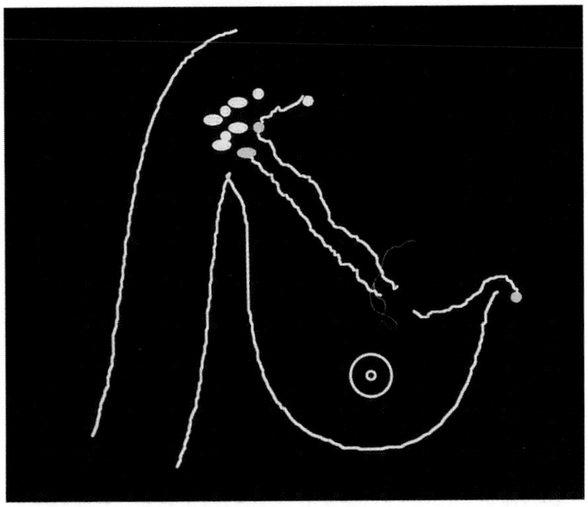

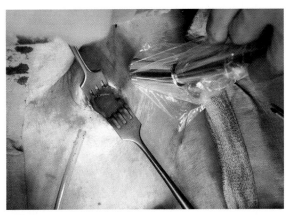

Figure 9–12. Transcutaneous localization of axillary sentinel lymph node.

Figure 9–11. Lymphatic drainage pattern of an upper breast tumor.

cult to prove, this may, in fact, provide a more sensitive means of staging the axilla, provided the sentinel node is correctly identified.

The immediate question addressed by preliminary studies has been the ability of sentinel lymphadenectomy to detect micrometastases as efficiently as an axillary dissection can. As a result, comparative studies have included both operations in the same patient. Although the end points for these studies have all been the same, the technique has varied widely. Conceptually, a visual tracer, a radiolabeled protein, or a combination of both are injected around the breast tumor. Initially, this process was performed with isosulfan blue, a vital blue dye used for lymphatic mapping for melanoma. This approach created difficulties in defining the breast lymphatics because of the three-dimensional nature of breast cancers and the potential for missing multiple sentinel nodes located within the three-dimensional axillary nodal basin. Because of the brevity of time in which isosulfan blue migrates through the sentinel node, the timely identification of multiple sentinel nodes is difficult.

The introduction of radiocolloid for this technique greatly enhanced this procedure by providing a second means of localizing a sentinel node using a hand-held gamma probe. This has simplified the procedure by obviating the lymphatic mapping required to identify the blue lymph node. Additionally, technitium-labeled sulfur colloid binds to lymphatic tissue and provides a much greater window of opportunity to localize sentinel lymph nodes. Lymphoscintigraphy done prior to the surgical procedure can assist in confirming the migration and location of radiocolloid (Figure 9–13). Another conceptual benefit of the use of radiocolloid is that it makes it possible to localize internal mammary nodes. For tumors located medially in the breast, these may be the only sentinel nodes for the tumor.

Although data are quickly emerging to support sentinel lymphadenectomy in the staging of breast cancer, it has not yet become uniformly accepted as the standard of care. A question yet to be answered is the optimization of the tech-

nique to most accurately identify the sentinel node. Variables to be defined include the location of the injection, the radiopharmaceutical compound and optimal size, the time interval between the injection and the surgical procedure, the combination of radiocolloid with isosulfan blue, size limitations of the tumor, effect of excisional biopsy on the accuracy of sentinel node localization, and the microscopic and submicroscopic evaluation of nodal tissue. The long-term regional recurrence risk after a sentinel lymph node biopsy has yet to be addressed. Until these questions have been answered, sentinel lymphadenectomy should be performed as a protocol.

Adjuvant Therapy

The surgical treatment for early breast cancer serves as a very important therapeutic step but also provides important prognostic information to define subsequent adjuvant therapy decisions. Adjuvant chemotherapy has evolved from a narrowly defined node-positive indication to more encompassing indications based on identified benefits. Nonetheless, the efficacy of combination chemotherapy is well correlated with nodal involvement, and surgical staging, particularly for early breast cancer, is important in defining optimal adjuvant therapy decisions.

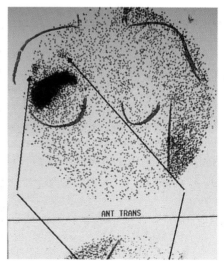

Figure 9–13. Lymphscintigram of breast primary and axillary sentinel lymph nodes.

RECURRENCE

An ipsilateral breast recurrence after BPT may be difficult to distinguish from a second primary tumor. Information important to help make this distinction includes the location of the recurrence relative to the initial primary tumor, the histologic features, and the disease-free interval. Proximity to a previous lumpectomy site increases the likelihood of the tumor being a recurrence. In the absence of any previous history of in situ carcinoma, an in situ component is suggestive of a new primary lesion. Local recurrences are most likely to occur within several years of initial treatment. A long disease-free interval is more suggestive of a second primary tumor. The distinction between a new primary tumor and recurrent breast cancer is more important in understanding the biology of the disease and the efficacy of the treatment selected. In practical terms, an ipsilateral event is managed in a similar fashion with either scenario. Without the ability to deliver additional radiotherapy in most patients, re-excision is not a safe option, and most patients are treated with a completion mastectomy. An ipsilateral event should also lead to a metastatic evaluation; recurrences are commonly the harbinger of metastatic disease.[59]

In patients previously treated with mastectomy, a chest wall recurrence can usually be managed with a local excision. The goal of excision should be a margin-free resection. In some situations, this may necessitate resection of muscle or a portion of the chest wall. In patients who have undergone previous radiation treatments, a more extensive resection may represent the only therapeutic option to achieve local control. Closure of the chest wall defect may be facilitated by a myocutaneous flap closure. Hormonal and cytotoxic chemotherapy must also be considered at the time of a local recurrence.

CONCLUSION

Local and regional surgical treatment of early breast cancer continues to evolve toward a more limited and tailored approach. Diagnostic evaluation also continues to improve in defining the extent of the disease and in providing accurate staging information to guide resection and adjuvant therapy. With these strategies, the treatment of breast cancer has become more precise and effective.

REFERENCES

1. Shin HJ, Sneige N. Is a diagnosis of infiltrating versus in situ ductal carcinoma of the breast possible in fine-needle aspiration specimens? Cancer 1998;84:186–91.
2. Shabot M, Goldberg I, Schick P, et al. Aspiration cytology is superior to Tru-Cut needle biopsy in establishing the diagnosis of clinically suspicious breast masses. Ann Surg 1982;196: 122–26.
3. Ballo SM, Sneige N. Can core needle biopsy replace fine-needle aspiration cytology in the diagnosis of palpable breast carcinoma? A comparative study of 124 women. Cancer 1996; 78:773–7.
4. American Joint Committee on Cancer. Breast. In: Fleming ID, Cooper JS, Henson DE, et al. editor. AJCC Cancer Staging Manual. 5th Edition. Philadelphia: J. B. Lippincott; 1997. pp. 171–80.
5. Winchester DJ, Menck HR, Winchester DP. National treatment trends for ductal carcinoma in situ of the breast. Arch Surg 1997;132(6): 660–5.
6. Sarrazin D, Le M, Rouesse J, et al. Conservative treatment versus mastectomy in breast cancer tumors with macroscopic diameter of 20 millimeters or less. Cancer 1984;53(5):1209–13.
7. Fisher B, Anderson S, Redmond CK, et al. Reanalysis and results after 12 years of follow-up in a randomized clinical trial comparing total mastectomy with lumpectomy with or without irradiation in the treatment of breast cancer. N Engl J Med 1995;333(22):1456–61.
8. Veronesi U, Banfi A, Del Vecchio M, et al. Comparison of Halsted mastectomy with quadrantectomy, axillary dissection, and radiotherapy in early breast cancer: long term results. Eur J Can Clin Oncol 1986;22(9):1085–9.
9. Van Dongen J, Bartelink H, Fentimen I, et al. Randomized clinical trial to assess the value of breast-conserving therapy in stage I and II breast cancer, EORTC 10801 trial. J Natl Cancer Inst Monogr 1992;11:15–8.

10. Blichert-Toft M, Rose C, Anderson JA, et al. Danish randomized trial comparing breast conservation therapy whit mastectomy: six years of life table analysis. J Natl Cancer Inst Monogr 1992;11:19–25.

11. Lichter A, Lippman M, Danforth D, et al. Mastectomy versus breast conserving therapy in the treatment of Stage I and II carcinoma of the breast: a randomized trial at the National Cancer Institute. J Clin Oncol 1992;10:976–83.

12. Winchester DJ, Menck HR, Winchester DP. The National Cancer Data Base report on the results of a large nonrandomized comparison of breast preservation and modified radical mastectomy. Cancer 1997; 80:162–7.

13. Early Breast Cancer Trialist's Collaborative Group. Effects of radiotherapy and surgery in early breast cancer. N Engl J Med 1995;333:1444–55.

14. Fisher B, Bryant J, Wolmark N, et al. Effect of preoperative chemotherapy on the outcome of women with operable breast cancer. J Clin Oncol 1998;16:2672–85.

15. Fisher B, Brown A, Mamounas E, et al. Effect of preoperative chemotherapy on local-regional disease in women with operable breast cancer: findings from NSABP B-18. J Clin Oncol 1997;15:2483–93.

16. Olivotto IA, Rose MA, Osteen RT, et al. Late cosmetic outcome after conservative surgery and radiotherapy: analysis of causes of cosmetic failure. Int J Radiat Oncol Biol Phys 1989;1: 747–53.

17. Yeatman TJ, Cantor AB, Smith TJ, et al. Tumor biology of infiltrating lobular carcinoma. Implications for management. Annals of Surg 1995;222(4):549–59.

18. Gage I, Schnitt SJ, Nixon AJ, et al. Pathologic margin involvement and the risk of recurrence in patients treated with breast conserving surgery. Cancer 1996;78:1921–8.

19. Smitt MC, Nowels KW, Zdeblick MJ, et al. The importance of the lumpectomy surgical margin status in long term results of breast conservation. Cancer 1995;76:259–67.

20. Anscher M, Jones P, Prosnitz L, et al. Local failure and margin status in early-stage breast carcinoma treated with conservative surgery and radiation therapy. Ann Surg 1993;218:22–8.

21. Krecke KN, Gisvold JJ. Invasive lobular carcinoma of the breast: mammographic findings and extent of disease at diagnosis in 184 patients. AJR Am J Roentgenol 1993;161(5):957–60.

22. Le Gal M, Ollivier L, Asselain B, et al. Mammographic features of 455 invasive lobular carcinomas. Radiology 1992;185(3):705–8.

23. Clare SE, Sener SF, Wilkens W, et al. Prognostic significance of occult lymph node metastases in node-negative breast cancer. Ann Surg Oncol 1997;4(6):447–51.

24. Weiss MC, Fowble BL, Solin LJ, et al. Outcome of conservative therapy for invasive breast cancer by histologic subtype. Int J Radiat Oncol, Biol, Phys 1992;23(5):941–7.

25. Poen JC, Tran L, Juillard G, et al. Conservation therapy for invasive lobular carcinoma of the breast. Cancer 1992;69(11):2789–95.

26. White JR, Gustafson GS, Wimbish K, et al. Conservative surgery and radiation therapy for infiltrating lobular carcinoma of the breast. The role of preoperative mammograms in guiding treatment. Cancer 1994;74(2):640–7.

27. du Toit RS, Locker AP, Ellis IO, et al. An evaluation of differences in prognosis, recurrence patterns and receptor status between invasive lobular and invasive carcinomas of the breast. Eur J Surg Oncol 1991;17(3):251–7.

28. Silverstein MJ, Lewinsky BS, Waisman JR, et al. Infiltrating lobular carcinoma. Is it different from infiltrating duct carcinoma? Cancer 1994;73(6):1673–77.

29. Mate TP, Carter D, Fischer DB, et al. A clinical and histopathologic analysis of the results of conservation surgery and radiation therapy in stage I and II breast carcinoma. Cancer 1986; 58(9):1995–2002.

30. Winchester DJ, Chang HR, Graves TA, et al. A comparative analysis of lobular carcinoma of the breast: presentation, treatment, and outcome. J Am Coll Surg 1998;186(4):416–22.

31. Fisher ER, Sass R, Fisher B, et al. Pathologic findings from the National Surgical Adjuvant Breast Project (protocol 6). II. Relation of local breast recurrence to multicentricity. Cancer 1986;57(9):1717–24.

32. Veronesi U, Volterrani F, Luini A, et al. Quadrantectomy versus lumpectomy for small size breast cancer. Eur J Cancer 1990;26:671–3.

33. Veronesi U, Luini A, Del Vecchio M, et al. Radiotherapy after breast preserving surgery in women with localized cancer of the breast. N Engl J Med 1993;328:1587–91.

34. Liljegren G, Holmberg L, Adami HO, et al. Sector resection with or without postoperative radiotherapy for stage 1 breast cancer. Five year results of a clinical trial. J Natl Cancer Inst 1994;86:717–22.

35. Holland R, Veling S, Mravunac M, et al. Histologic multifocality of Tis, T1–2 breast carcinomas: implication for clinical trials of breast conserving treatment. Cancer 1985;56:979–90.

36. Schuster RH, Kuske Rb, Young VL, Fineberg B. Breast reconstruction in women treated with radiation therapy for breast cancer: cosmesis, complications, and tumor control. Plast Reconstr Surg 1992;90:445–52.

37. Hartmann LC, Schaid DJ, Woods JE, et al. Efficacy of bilateral prophylactic mastectomy in women with a family history of breast cancer. N Engl J Med 1999;340:77–84.

38. Fisher B, Joseph P, Constantino D, et al. Tamoxifen for prevention of breast cancer: report of the National Surgical Adjuvant Breast and Bowel Project P-1 study. J Natl Cancer Inst 1998;90:1371–88.

39. Morton DL, Wen DR, Wong JH, et al. Technical details of intraoperative lymphatic mapping for early stage melanoma. Arch Surg 1992;127: 392–9.

40. Krag DN, Weaver DL, Alex JC, Fairbank JT. Surgical resection and radiolocalization of the sentinel lymph node in breast cancer using a gamma probe. Surg Oncol 1993;2:335–9.

41. Giuliano AE, Kirgan DM, Guenther JM, Morton DL. Lymphatic mapping and sentinel lymphadenectomy for breast cancer. Ann Surg 1994;3:391–8.

42. Albertini JJ, Lyman GH, Cox C, et al. Lymphatic mapping and sentinel node biopsy in the patient with breast cancer. JAMA, 1996;276: 1818–22.

43. Veronesi U, Paganelli, Galimberti V, et al. Sentinel-node biopsy to avoid axillary dissection in breast cancer with clinically negative lymphnodes. Lancet 1997;349:1864–7.

44. Krag D, Weaver D, Ashikaga T, et al. The sentinel node in breast cancer: a multicenter validation study. N Engl J Med 1998;339:941–6.

45. Guiliano AE, Jones RC, Brennan M, Statman R. Sentinel lymphadenctomy in breast cancer. J Clin Oncol 1997;15:(6):2345–50.

46. Winchester DJ, Sener SF, Winchester DP, et al. Sentinel lymphadenectomy for breast cancer: Experience with 180 consecutive patients: efficacy of filtered technetium 99m sulphur colloid with overnight migration time. J Am Coll Surg 1999;188:597–603.

47. Ciatto S, Cecchini S, Iossa A, Grazzini G. "T" category and operable breast cancer prognosis. Tumori 1989;75:18–22.

48. Fisher B, Redmond C, Fisher ER, et al. Ten-year results of a randomized clinical trial comparing radical mastectomy and total mastectomy with or without radiation. N Engl J Med 1985;312: 674–81.

49. Rosen P, Martin M, Kinne D, et al. Discontinuous or "skip": metastases in breast carcinoma: analysis of 1228 axillary dissections. Ann Surg 1983;197:276.

50. Veronesi U, Rilke F, Luini A, et al. Distribution of axillary node metastases by level of invasion. Cancer 1987;59:682–7.

51. Boova R, Bonanni R, Rosato F. Patterns of axillary nodal involvement in breast cancer. Ann Surg 1982;196:642–4.

52. Mathiesen O, Carl J, Bonderup O, Panduro J. Axillary sampling and the risk of erroneous staging of breast cancer. An analysis of 960 consecutive patients. Acta Oncol 1990;29:721–5.

53. Larson D, Weinstein M, Goldberg I, et al. Edema of the arm as a function of the extent of axillary surgery in patients with Stage 1 and 2 carcinoma of the breast treated with primary radiotherapy. Int J Radiat Oncol Biol Phys 1986;12:1575–82.

54. Tate JJ, Lewis V, Archer T, et al. Ultrasound detection of axillary lymph node metastases in breast cancer. Eur J Surg Oncol 1989;15:139–41.

55. March DE, Wechsler RJ, Kurtz AB, et al. Ct-pathologic correlation of axillary lymph nodes in breast cancer. J Comput Assist Tomogr 1991;15:440–4.

56. Kao Ch, Wang SJ, Yeh SH. Technetium-99m MIBI uptake in breast carcinoma and axillary lymph node metastases. Clin Nucl Med 1994;19: 898–900.

57. Avril N, Dose J, Janicke F, et al. Assessment of axillary lymph node involvement in breast cancer patients with positron emission tomography using radiolabeled 2–(fluorine-18)-fluoro-2–deoxy-D-glucose. J Natl Cancer Inst 1996;88:1204–9.

58. International (Ludwig) Breast Cancer Study Group. Prognostic importance of occult axillary lymph node metastases from breast cancers. Lancet 1990;335:1565–8.

59. Bedwinek J, Fineberg B, Lee J, et al. Analysis of failures following local treatment of isolated local-regional recurrence of breast cancer. Int J Radiat Oncol Biol Phys 1981;7:581–5.

10

Locally Advanced Breast Cancer

S. EVA SINGLETARY, MD, FACS

Integration of systemic chemotherapy and/or hormonal therapy with surgery and irradiation is considered the standard of care in the treatment of locally advanced breast cancer (LABC). Because the greatest risk for patients with LABC is the development of distant metastases and subsequent death, the goals of surgery are to provide maximal locoregional control with minimal disfigurement and to permit accurate staging to determine prognosis. Breast conservation surgery is sometimes possible after tumor downstaging with induction chemotherapy, but close cooperation between the medical and surgical oncologists and the radiation therapist is required to determine the feasibility of this option. Similarly, the surgeon must be familiar with the natural history of LABC to assess the advisability of major resections of either persistent advanced primary disease or locoregional recurrences. If life expectancy is very short, as is the case with patients who have bulky visceral disease or metastases nonrespondent to multiple chemotherapy regimens, the true benefit of a complex but technically feasible operation should be evaluated carefully. However, in selected patients with advanced disease, surgery may achieve quality palliation of local symptoms of pain, hemorrhage, and malodorous ulceration.

This chapter defines LABC and addresses the role of surgery after tumor downstaging with induction chemotherapy, the use of mastectomy for inflammatory breast cancer, the feasibility of immediate reconstruction in selected patients with LABC, and recent innovations in systemic therapy.

DEFINITION OF LOCALLY ADVANCED BREAST CANCER

Locally advanced breast cancer generally refers to large primary tumors (> 5 cm) associated with skin or chest-wall involvement or with fixed (matted) axillary lymph nodes (T3/T4; N2/N3).[1] In the most recent TNM staging system,[1] tumors associated with disease in the ipsilateral supraclavicular nodal basin have been eliminated from the LABC category because the supraclavicular basin lies outside the primary lymphatic drainage pathways of the axilla and internal mammary nodes; tumors associated with supraclavicular disease have been reclassified as stage IV disease. However, as patients with distant metastases confined to supraclavicular nodes have a better prognosis than patients with metastases at other distant sites and can be rendered disease free with locoregional therapy,[2] metastases limited to the ipsilateral sub- or supraclavicular fossa will be included in the definition of LABC offered here. Large primary tumors (> 5 cm) with no evidence of nodal involvement (T3;N0) have a more favorable prognosis than LABC, with a 5-year survival rate of 70 to 80 percent; thus, in the most recent TNM staging system, T3N0 lesions have been reclassified as stage IIB disease. However, as most series have classified T3N0 lesions as LABC for the purposes of treatment, these tumors will also be included in the present definition of LABC.

ROLE OF SURGERY AFTER INDUCTION CHEMOTHERAPY

Since the mid-1970s, patients with LABC treated at The University of Texas M. D. Anderson Cancer Center have received three to four cycles of doxorubicin-based combination chemotherapy prior to local therapy; local therapy is followed by the completion of systemic therapy and irradiation. Between 1974 and 1996, patients with LABC were treated in four trials addressing four major concerns about the use of induction chemotherapy: (1) whether tumor progression will occur during induction chemotherapy, rendering the tumor unresectable even with radical surgery; (2) whether operative morbidity is increased after induction chemotherapy; (3) whether the histologic staging information obtained from the surgical specimen after induction chemotherapy maintains its prognostic correlations with survival; (4) and whether breast conservation therapy with or without an axillary node dissection is feasible and safe in patients with LABC.

In the first clinical trial at M. D. Anderson Cancer Center (1974 to 1985), induction combination chemotherapy was administered to 174 evaluable patients (191 registered) with noninflammatory stage III breast cancer.[3] After three cycles of 5-fluorouracil, doxorubicin, and cyclophosphamide (FAC), patients with an excellent tumor response underwent irradiation of the chest wall and regional lymph nodes. Patients with a substantial volume of residual tumor underwent mastectomy and irradiation. After completion of locoregional therapy, FAC was reinitiated and continued until a dose of 450 mg/m^2 of doxorubicin was reached. Then treatment with cyclophosphamide, methotrexate, and 5-fluorouracil (CMF) was instituted and continued for a total treatment period of 2 years.

After the three cycles of induction chemotherapy with FAC, 17 percent of patients had a complete response (no evidence of tumor by physical or radiographic examination). Seventy-one percent had a partial response (≥ 50 percent tumor shrinkage). Only 10 percent had a minor or no significant response to induction chemotherapy. Tumor progression occurred in 2 percent of patients. This trial demonstrated that the majority of patients will have significant tumor shrinkage with induction chemotherapy and that the likelihood of tumor progression is low. As the virulence of a tumor is associated with chemoresistance, tumors that progress during aggressive chemotherapy are unlikely to be controlled with surgery, and a crossover chemotherapy regimen should be considered. This study also confirmed that induction chemotherapy is well tolerated and that surgical procedures after induction chemotherapy can be completed without an increased rate of infection or delayed wound healing.[4]

The above trial refuted the concept that histologic staging information obtained after induction chemotherapy would not have predictive power. The histologically confirmed response in the mastectomy specimen after induction chemotherapy was an excellent prognostic factor for survival and was more accurate than clinical assessment of response.[5,6] The number of positive axillary nodes after induction chemotherapy also remained prognostic for survival: actuarial 5-year survival rates were 70 percent for patients with negative lymph nodes, 62 percent for patients with one to three positive lymph nodes, 47 percent for patients with four to ten positive lymph nodes, and 21 percent for patients with more than ten positive lymph nodes.[6] The 5-year disease-free survival rates were 72, 46, 35, and 6 percent, respectively. When the subsets of patients with four or more positive lymph nodes were combined, the overall survival rate at 5 years was 38 percent, and the disease-free survival rate dropped to only 20 percent. As patients with four or more positive lymph nodes after induction chemotherapy have a survival rate similar to that obtained in historical trials of mastectomy and postoperative irradiation without systemic ther-apy,[2,7] these patients should be considered for innovative clinical trials.

The second M. D. Anderson clinical trial (1985 to 1989) was designed to determine whether the extent of residual disease in the mastectomy specimen after induction chemo-therapy can be used as a guide in planning post-operative adjuvant therapy. Three cycles of vin-cristine, doxorubicin, cyclophosphamide, and prednisone (VACP) were administered at 21-day intervals, then a modified radical mastec-tomy was performed. Patients with histologi-cally confirmed complete remission and those with < 1 cm^3 of residual tumor received five additional cycles of VACP; those with no response to induction chemotherapy were crossed over to receive five cycles of methotrex-ate, 5-fluorouracil, and vinblastine (MFVb). Patients with partial response and ≥ 1 cm^3 or more of residual tumor were randomly assigned to receive five additional cycles of either VACP or MFVb. All patients received radiation to the chest wall and regional lymph nodes. Eight patients whose tumors remained inoperable after induction chemotherapy underwent irradi-ation before mastectomy and MFVb. Irradiation had a minimal effect on wound healing provided wound tension and thin skin flaps were avoided. If mastectomy resulted in a large defect, flap coverage consisting of healthy autogenous tis-sue was preferred to the use of skin grafts.

Of 193 evaluable patients in this second trial (200 registered), 161 had a partial or greater clinical response to the three cycles of induc-tion chemotherapy. Among the patients with a partial response, no statistically significant dif-ference ($p = .64$) was detected in the 4-year sur-vival rates for the MFVb and VACP groups (75 and 58%, respectively).[8] Of the 32 patients in this study whose tumors showed a minor or no response to the induction chemotherapy, only 16 remain alive and only 8 are disease-free at the time of writing. The lack of impact on sur-vival of the crossover regimen in this study was probably due to the absence of an effective sec-ond-line therapy. Significantly, there was exten-sive downstaging in a large proportion of patients in the study: 17 mastectomy specimens had no evidence of residual tumor, and 54 mas-tectomy specimens had < 1 cm^3 of residual tumor. This finding led us to consider the pos-sibility of performing breast conservation surgery for locally advanced disease.

In a retrospective review of the mastectomy specimens in which the tumor shrank by ≥ 50 percent with induction chemotherapy, the fac-tors most commonly associated with multiple-quadrant involvement that would exclude breast conservation surgery were demonstrated to be persistent skin edema, residual tumor size > 4 cm, extensive intramammary lymphatic invasion, and known mammographic evidence of multicentric disease.[8]

The objective in the third M. D. Anderson clinical trial (1989 to 1992) was to determine prospectively what fraction of patients with LABC may be candidates for breast conserva-tion surgery after induction chemotherapy.[9] Of 203 evaluable patients with LABC who com-pleted four cycles of induction chemotherapy with (FAC), 51 (25 %) elected and underwent breast conservation surgery (Figure 10–1). The breast preservation rate for patients with ulcer-ative lesions or dermal lymphatic involvement (stage IIIB) was only 6 percent. With a median follow-up of > 60 months, only 5 (ten %) of the 51 patients who underwent breast conservation surgery had relapses in the breast.

In the fourth M. D. Anderson clinical trial (1992 to 1996), the objective was to determine if high-dose chemotherapy would increase the extent of tumor downstaging with induction chemotherapy and allow more patients the option of breast conservation surgery. One hun-dred and seventy patients with LABC were ran-domly assigned to receive either four cycles of standard FAC (1000 mg/m^2 5-fluorouracil, 50 mg/m^2 doxorubicin, and 500 mg/m^2 cyclophos-phamide) at 21-day intervals or dose-intensive FAC (1200, 60, and 1000 mg/m^2 of the three drugs, respectively) at 18-day intervals with

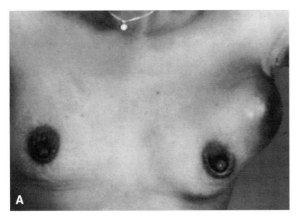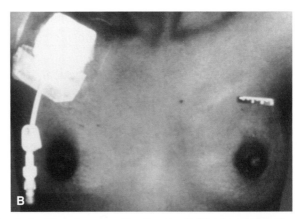

Figure 10–1. *A,* Patient with locally advanced breast cancer who desired breast conservation therapy. *B,* After four cycles of induction chemotherapy, a segmental mastectomy and axillary node dissection were performed. The patient then completed chemotherapy followed by irradiation of the breast and regional nodal basins.

prophylactic subcutaneous administration of recombinant human granulocyte colony-stimulating factor (G-CSF). After surgery, patients with < 1 cm³ of residual tumor received four additional cycles of FAC or dose-intensive FAC. Patients with a clinical partial response but with > 1 cm³ of residual tumor and those with four or more positive lymph nodes in the surgical specimen were treated postoperatively with four more cycles of FAC or dose-intensive FAC followed by four cycles of methotrexate and vinblastine. Patients with no change or progression of disease received six cycles of methotrexate and vinblastine. In all patients, locoregional radiotherapy was instituted within 6 weeks of completion of chemotherapy.

One hundred and sixty-six patients were evaluable for response. Patients who received FAC plus G-CSF were more likely to have a complete or partial clinical response compared with patients who received standard FAC (84 v 66%). However, the two regimens produced similar results in terms of histologic downstaging of the primary tumor. There was a complete histologic response (no tumor present) seen in 25 percent of patients treated with FAC plus G-CSF and in 16 percent of patients treated with FAC alone ($p = .155$). There was a near-complete histologic response (< 1 cm³ of tumor present) seen in 25 percent of patients treated with FAC plus G-CSF and in 24 percent of patients

treated with FAC alone ($p = .963$). Although a higher percentage of patients underwent breast conservation therapy in the group that received FAC plus G-CSF (42 v 29 %), this difference did not achieve statistical significance.

To determine if there may be an alternative to axillary node dissection after tumor downstaging, we analyzed 147 consecutive patients in the FAC versus high-dose FAC study who had both physical and ultrasound examinations of the axilla at diagnosis and prior to surgery[10] (Figure 10–2). Of the 133 patients with palpable axillary disease on initial examination, 43 patients (32%) were downstaged to a negative axilla as assessed by physical and ultrasound examination following induction chemotherapy. There was a pathologic complete axillary lymph node response found in 30 patients (23%). Of the 72 patients with axillary metastases that were cytologically proven by fine-needle aspiration on initial evaluation, 15 (21%) were confirmed to have histologically negative axillary lymph nodes following induction chemotherapy. Of the 28 patients in whom the axilla became clinically negative but the findings on axillary ultrasound remained positive after induction chemotherapy, 21 (75%) were found to have macroscopic axillary nodal disease upon dissection. When both the physical and ultrasound examination were negative following induction chemotherapy, 53 percent of patients (29 of 55) were found to still have axillary nodal metastases. However, 96 percent (25 of 26) had only 2 to 5 mm foci of disease.

On the basis of our analysis of the FAC versus high-dose FAC study, we are currently conducting a clinical trial to assess whether patients with a negative axilla by physical and ultrasound examination can be safely treated without axillary node dissection. In this clinical trial, patients with T2-3, N0-1 breast cancer are initially randomized to receive four cycles of either paclitaxel or standard FAC preoperatively.[11] After the completion of induction chemotherapy, patients who have become candidates for breast conservation surgery and who have clinically negative axilla are further randomly assigned to either irradiation of the axilla or a standard level I and II axillary lymph node dissection. After completion of four cycles of postoperative FAC, irradiation is delivered to the breast and, in patients with a nondissected axilla, the lower axilla and the supraclavicular

fossa. Preliminary analysis based on 78 evaluable patients (104 patients registered at the time of the analysis) who had completed the induction chemotherapy and surgery showed that paclitaxel and FAC have a similar ability to downstage both the primary tumor and the axillary nodal disease.[11] No or minimal residual disease was found in the breast in 41 percent of the 41 patients on the FAC treatment arm, compared to 32 percent of the 37 patients who received induction chemotherapy with paclitaxel ($p = .44$). Sixty-nine patients underwent an axillary node dissection. Negative or < 4 positive lymph nodes were found in 68 percent of the 41 patients who received FAC chemotherapy, compared to 77 percent of the 37 patients treated with paclitaxel ($p = .75$). In the eight patients who did not undergo an axillary node dissection, no axillary recurrences had been detected in a 24-month follow-up period.

How safe is conservative surgery for LABC in terms of long-term local control? In review

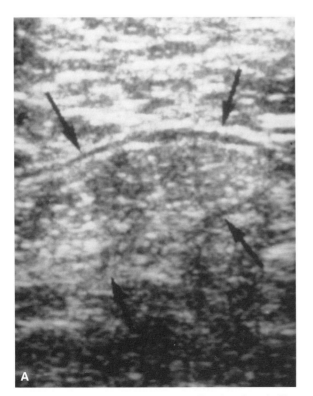 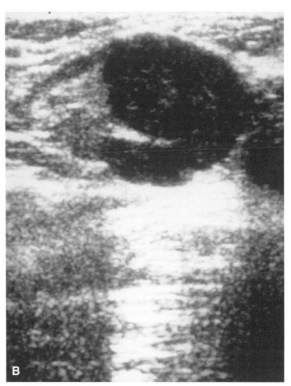

Figure 10–2. *A,* Normal fat-replaced axillary lymph node. The sonogram shows a large node completely replaced by echogenic fat with a thin hypoechoic rim outlining the periphery of the node. *B,* Hypoechoic metastatic foci in an axillary lymph node confirmed by ultrasound-guided fine needle aspiration.

of our database of all patients treated at M. D. Anderson with breast conservation therapy (patients with early-stage breast cancer and those with LABC), 949 patients were found to have been treated with breast conservation surgery at our institution between 1982 and 1994.[12] Of this group, 93 patients received induction chemotherapy prior to surgery on or off protocol. The initial stage distribution of these 93 patients was as follows: stage IIA, 22.6 percent; stage IIB, 24.7 percent; stage IIIA, 32.3 percent; stage IIIB, 16.1 percent; and stage IV (supraclavicular lymph node metastases only), 4.3 percent. In most patients (88%), induction chemotherapy consisted of FAC or high-dose FAC for three to five cycles. After segmental mastectomy and axillary node dissection, patients underwent four to eight cycles of chemotherapy followed by radiotherapy. Breast irradiation consisted of 50 Gy of external-beam radiation to the intact breast and a 10 to 15 Gy boost to the segmental mastectomy site, which had been marked intraoperatively with clips. Of the 93 patients, 86 completed postoperative therapy. Two patients refused radiotherapy after chemotherapy, four patients refused chemotherapy but did receive radiotherapy, and one patient refused all postoperative therapy.

Overall, nine patients had a local recurrence, for a local failure rate of 9.7 percent. In six patients, local recurrence was the first site of relapse; recurrence was in the breast parenchyma in three patients, in the skin of the breast in two patients, and in the breast parenchyma and an axillary node in one patient. The median time to local recurrence in these six patients was 55 months. Three patients had local recurrence after the development of distant metastases. In the nine patients with local recurrence, the surgical margin of the segmental mastectomy specimens was negative in all patients but close in three patients. The six patients with local recurrence only or local recurrence prior to distant metastases had an overall survival rate of 83 percent at a median follow-up of 88 months.

This survival rate is similar to the overall survival rate of 89 percent for the entire group of 93 patients (median follow-up of 73 months). The local recurrence rate in our selected series of breast conservation therapy for LABC was similar to the local failure rate observed for breast conservation therapy in our patients with early-stage breast cancer and was also consistent with the experience of other investigators (Table 10–1).[13,15–20] The results of our study also indicate that most patients with local recurrence can be treated without an adverse effect on overall survival.

The role of axillary node dissection after induction chemotherapy in patients with LABC has become controversial. There are four main arguments against the routine use of axillary node dissection for LABC. First, induction chemotherapy in patients with LABC and operable breast cancer has been shown to downstage positive axillary lymph nodes to negative nodes in 23 to 44 percent of patients.[6,10,14,20,21] Second, in most treatment protocols, patients with LABC routinely receive additional postoperative chemotherapy and radiotherapy regardless of the findings at axillary node dissection. Third, some LABC series have reported that axillary node dissection alone, axillary irradiation alone, or a combination of surgery and irradiation produce equivalent axillary control rates after induction chemotherapy.[22–24] The fourth argument is somewhat more complex. There has been a survival advantage suggested for high-dose chemotherapy over standard anthracycline-based chemotherapy in patients with multiple positive axillary nodes after induction chemotherapy.[25,26] However, high-dose chemotherapy off-protocol cannot be recommended in the absence of prospective randomized data demonstrating such a survival benefit. One of the lessons learned from the high-dose chemotherapy protocols for metastatic breast cancer was that patients with previously demonstrated resistance to chemotherapy usually do not benefit from this procedure.[27] In addition, proponents of axillary node dissection in patients receiving induction chemotherapy assert that the number of positive nodes detected after tumor downstaging may affect whether patients should be crossed over to a different chemotherapeutic agent or be given high-dose chemotherapy. For example, phase II trials have demonstrated high activity of taxane-based chemotherapy (paclitaxel and docetaxel) in anthracycline-resistant breast cancer.[28,29] However, if the trend in therapy is toward a sequential or combined approach using anthracycline and taxane-based regimens prior to local therapy, with no further systemic intervention planned, then the histologic assessment of the axilla becomes only a prognostic tool.

Whether chemotherapy can substitute for surgery for local control of occult axillary metastases is still unknown. Data concerning locoregional recurrences of the chest wall following mastectomy show that optimal local control is provided by using both systemic therapy and irradiation rather than chemotherapy alone.[30] The use of axillary irradiation in patients with clinically node-negative stage I or stage II breast cancer reduced the rate of axillary recurrence by 1 and 3 percent, respectively.[31-33] The Early Breast Cancer Trialists' Collaborative Group overview analysis of randomized trials comparing axillary surgical clearance versus radiotherapy found no difference in mortality between groups regardless of the type of axillary treatment.[34] Sentinel lymph node biopsy in patients with LABC has not been sufficiently studied yet and will prove accurate only if metastatic deposits within each axillary lymph node respond identically to chemotherapy.[35]

Based upon the clinical trials conducted thus far, we have learned that induction chemotherapy can be given safely without increasing the morbidity of local treatment. The histologic findings after induction chemotherapy remain important in defining prognosis. Very few patients will have progression of their disease and some will become candidates for breast conservation therapy. Most importantly, neoadjuvant chemotherapy may identify

Table 10–1. RATES OF BREAST CONSERVATION THERAPY AND SUBSEQUENT LOCAL RECURRENCE AFTER INDUCTION CHEMOTHERAPY

Author	Patients	Stage	Percent BCT	Percent Local Recurrence
Bonadonna[14]	157	II/III	81	1
Calais[15]	158	II/III	49	8
Veronesi[16]	226	II/III	90	6
Schwartz[17]	160	II/III	34	2
Touboul*[18]	97	II/IV	62	16
Merajver*[19]	89	III	28	14
Fisher[20]	747	I/II	68	8
Peoples[12]	93	II/III/IV	N/A	10

*Local therapy consisted of primary radiation therapy.
BCT = breast conservation therapy
Adapted from Hunt KK, Buzdar AU. Breast conservation after tumor downstaging with induction chemotherapy. In: Singletary SE, editor. Breast cancer—M. D. Anderson Solid Tumor Oncology Series. New York: Springer-Verlag; 1999. p. 196–207.

patients who will benefit from a cross-over chemotherapy regimen if tumor response is inadequate to the initial drugs.

INFLAMMATORY BREAST CANCER

Because today's combination chemotherapy regimens can often render inflammatory breast cancer (IBC) resectable, mastectomy now has a role in the treatment of this disease. In our review of 178 women treated for IBC in doxorubicin-based multimodality therapy protocols between 1974 and 1993, the addition of mastectomy led to significant improvement in locoregional disease control.[36] Locoregional relapse rates were 16.3 percent (16 of 98 patients) for patients who underwent chemotherapy, mastectomy, and radiotherapy, and 35.7 percent (15 of 42 patients) for patients who underwent only chemotherapy and radiotherapy ($p = .016$). However, when patients were stratified on the basis of tumor response to induction chemotherapy, only patients with a partial response to chemotherapy demonstrated significant improvement in local control with the addition of mastectomy. As only 12 percent of patients (21 of 178) had a complete clinical response, demonstration of a statistically significant improvement in local control with the use of mastectomy was not feasible in this review. The amount of residual disease found on histologic examination of the mastectomy specimen was highly predictive of long-term local control: no patient with < 1 cm^3 residual disease (n = 38) had a locoregional recurrence.

The effect of the addition of mastectomy on disease-specific and disease-free survival was also dependent on the tumor response to induction chemotherapy (Figure 10–3). Patients who had a complete or partial clinical response to induction chemotherapy and were treated with mastectomy in addition to chemotherapy and irradiation had significantly improved 5-year disease-specific survival compared with patients who had a similar response to induction chemotherapy but did not undergo mastectomy (62.0 v 43.0 %; *p* = .018). No improvement in survival (disease-specific or disease-free) with the addition of mastectomy was detected in

patients who had no significant response to induction chemotherapy.

These retrospective data suggest that optimal local control for most patients with IBC is obtained with the addition of mastectomy to chemotherapy and radiotherapy. Other benefits of mastectomy are that it allows accurate assessment of the amount of residual disease after induction chemotherapy and that lower doses of radiation can be used for subclinical disease.[37] However, mastectomy should be used only selectively in patients who have no significant response to induction chemotherapy, as these patients are at high risk for both local and distant failure regardless of surgical intervention. Although accelerated fractionation radiotherapy has been proposed to exploit the biologic characteristics of IBC, an improvement in local control rates with this technique has not been confirmed.[38,39] However, this accelerated schedule

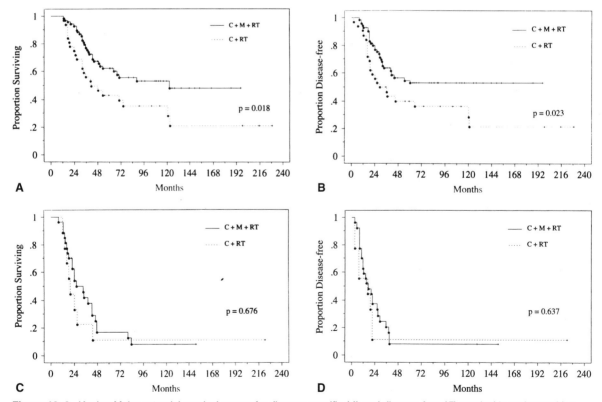

Figure 10–3. Kaplan-Meier actuarial survival curves for disease-specific (*A*) and disease-free (*B*) survival in patients with a complete or partial response to induction chemotherapy and for disease-specific (*C*) and disease-free (*D*) survival in patients with no significant response to induction chemotherapy, stratified by type of treatment received. C = chemotherapy; M = mastectomy; RT = radiotherapy. Reprinted with permission from Fleming RYD, Armar L, Buzdar AU, et al. Effectiveness of mastectomy by response to induction chemotherapy for control in inflammatory breast carcinoma. Ann Surg Oncol 1997;4:452–61.

expedites delivery of the radiotherapy, which may be especially useful if the goal of therapy is palliation. Interstitial irradiation has been studied as a possible substitute for surgery in patients who experience significant tumor reduction with chemotherapy, but early results in terms of local control do not appear promising.[40]

Attempts to improve tumor downstaging in IBC with high-dose chemotherapy have shown promise in terms of clinical response rates, but the effect on long-term survival is still unclear. In a review of five trials of either single-agent or combination chemotherapy followed by autologous bone marrow transplantation (ABMT) for IBC and other stage III breast cancers, Antman and colleagues[41] reported that 44 (79%) of 56 patients had a clinical complete response after induction chemotherapy but before ABMT, and that 89 percent had a complete response after ABMT. Disease-free status was maintained in 54 percent of patients, with follow-up ranging from 1 to 37 months.

The use of a different, crossover chemotherapy regimen prior to mastectomy in patients with IBC with less than a partial response to induction chemotherapy may also be effective, as nonanthracyline-resistant drugs such as paclitaxel and docetaxel are now available. The current trial at M. D. Anderson involves the use of paclitaxel if less than a partial response is obtained with four cycles of induction FAC. If a complete response or partial response is achieved with paclitaxel, the patient undergoes mastectomy followed by four cycles of paclitaxel and irradiation. In patients who have a complete or partial response with the initial four cycles of FAC, mastectomy is performed and an additional four cycles of FAC are given, followed by four cycles of paclitaxel and irradiation. In patients with no significant response to either FAC or paclitaxel induction chemotherapy, the radiation oncologist and surgeon plan whether to treat the breast with preoperative irradiation and then perform mastectomy or to proceed with definitive irradiation as the only local modality, with the intent of palliation.

Forty-three patients were entered in this IBC protocol between 1994 and 1998. There was a clinical complete response observed in seven percent and a clinical partial response observed in 65 percent. This overall rate of response to induction chemotherapy of 72 percent is identical to the rate of response in the 178 patients with IBC treated on FAC induction chemotherapy protocols between 1974 and 1993. However, 2-year disease-free survival and overall survival were 61 and 78 percent, respectively, in the current protocol (median follow-up, 20 months), compared to 52 and 71 percent, respectively, in our previous studies (median follow-up, 86 months). In our next protocol for IBC, patients will receive four cycles of induction chemotherapy with FAC followed by two six-week courses of paclitaxel (175 mg/m^2 as a 3-hour infusion weekly), with a two-week break between the two courses. Patients with minimal tumor response after the FAC-paclitaxel induction chemotherapy will be considered as candidates for high-dose chemotherapy with autologous peripheral blood progenitor cell support. Surgical therapy will be planned at the completion of all systemic therapy. In patients who have a complete clinical response as documented by physical examination, radiological imaging, and core needle biopsies, locoregional irradiation concomitant with weekly paclitaxel will be offered as an alternative to surgery.

RECONSTRUCTIVE SURGERY

The goal of reconstructive surgery for patients with LABC can be to (1) repair defects, or (2) repair defects and re-create a breast mound. In patients with LABC who need or elect to have standard mastectomy and who desire breast reconstruction to improve the cosmetic outcome, reconstruction is often delayed until completion of both adjuvant chemotherapy and irradiation. As most locoregional recurrences are in the skin or subcutaneous tissue of the chest wall,[42] a flat postmastectomy chest wall often makes irradiation technically easier than does a reconstructed breast mound, especially if inclusion of the internal mammary nodal basin is necessary. However, in selected patients with excellent response to induction chemotherapy or when palliative debulking surgical procedures are needed, the use of an autogenous flap to create a breast mound or provide skin coverage of the operative defect before radiotherapy is instituted if feasible.

Implant-based reconstruction in an irradiated field has been associated with a high complication rate as well as patient discomfort and dissatisfaction because of loss of skin elasticity and fibrosis of underlying tissues after irradiation.[43,44] The M. D. Anderson series of 298 patients who received submuscular implants revealed that the rates of capsular contracture (Baker III or greater), pain, implant exposure, and implant removal were significantly higher (p = .028) in 13 patients with implants within an irradiated field than in 230 patients with implants who received no radiotherapy.[45] The effects of irradiation were slightly less detrimental in patients with implants placed beneath autogenous-tissue flaps: the complication rate was 40 percent in 19 patients with implants placed in an irradiated area and 8 percent in 36 patients with implants who had not undergone radiotherapy.

The use of a myocutaneous flap for breast reconstruction, either before or after irradiation, does not interfere with the resumption of chemotherapy or the ability to detect locoregional recurrence.[46] Irradiation of the reconstructed breast-mound flap does not impair the flap's blood supply. In the M. D. Anderson series of 61 patients who required complex chest wall resections,[47] prior irradiation that included the internal mammary artery, which provides blood to the rectus abdominis flap, or the thoracodorsal artery, which provides blood to the latissimus dorsi flap, did not compromise the viability of these flaps for wound coverage. Provided that the flap has an adequate vascularization without evidence of significant fat necrosis, the irradiation itself does not alter the cosmetic result, except for the anticipated skin tanning and slight fibrosis of the reconstructed breast mound. In a series from M. D. Anderson[48] of 19 patients who received radiotherapy after reconstruction with an autogenous tissue flap, either for known local recurrence (n = 4) or as adjuvant therapy for high risk of recurrence (n = 15), the cosmetic result was dependent on the initial outcome of the reconstruction.

The two tissue flaps used most frequently for reconstruction after breast surgery are the latissimus dorsi and rectus abdominis myocutaneous flaps. The advantages of the latissimus dorsi flap include its reliable blood supply and the relative rarity of donor site morbidity. This flap is also relatively thin, so it matches the thickness of the native chest wall skin fairly closely and is excellent for providing coverage of soft-tissue defects (Figure 10–4). The chief disadvantage of the latissimus dorsi flap is its limited size; an implant is usually required if the patient desires a reconstructed breast mound. The amount of available surplus skin varies from patient to patient, but in general the latissimus dorsi flap is never > 10 cm wide or 20 cm long.

Rectus abdominis myocutaneous flaps can be quite large and are most useful for defects too large to repair with a latissimus dorsi flap. The chief disadvantage is that they tend to be bulky and thus do not closely match the thickness of the native chest wall skin. The thickness of this flap can be an advantage, however, if the defect is located directly over the central area of the chest wall; in this case, the excess flap bulk can be used to reconstruct a breast mound.

The two main types of rectus abdominis myocutaneous flaps are the transverse rectus abdominis myocutaneous (TRAM) flap and the vertical rectus abdominis myocutaneous (VRAM) flap. The TRAM flap has a greater arc of rotation and a more symmetrical and easily concealed donor site than does the VRAM flap (Figure 10–5). The VRAM flap leaves a more noticeable donor scar but is technically easier to construct and has a more reliable blood supply (Figure 10–6). The

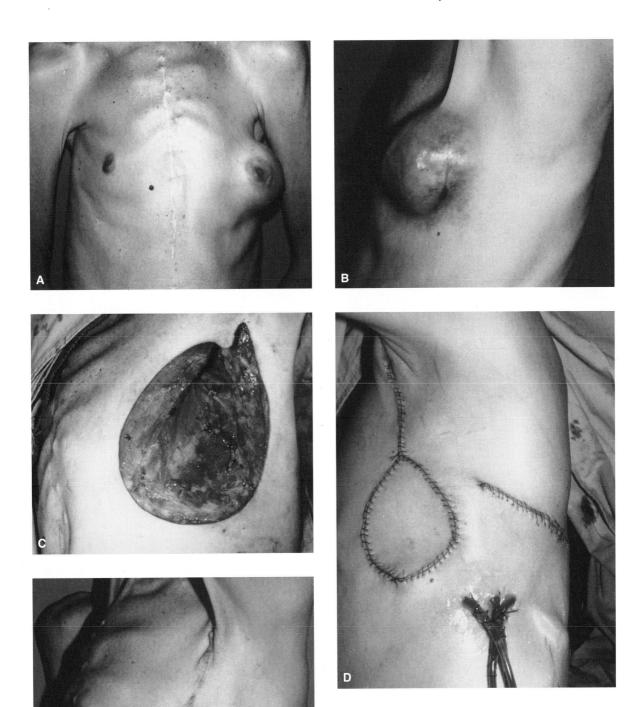

Figure 10–4. *A, B,* Patient with locally advanced cancer of the left breast who refused chemotherapy and radiation therapy. *C,* Operative defect after modified radical mastectomy. *D,* Closure of operative defect with a latissimus dorsi myocutaneous flap. *E,* Patient with excellent range of motion 10 days after surgery. (Reprinted with permission from Singletary SE. Breast surgery. In: Roh MS, Ames FC, editors. Atlas of advanced oncologic surgery. New York: Gower Medical Publishing, 1993. p. 14.1–14.9.)

TRAM flap is used most often when cosmetic considerations are important.

For major chest wall resections, the rectus abdominis flap is capable of covering a wide area from the clavicle to the costal margin and from the sternum to the midaxillary line. Because this flap is bulky, it provides sufficient chest wall stability even when up to five ribs or the entire sternum is resected, without the need for prosthetic mesh. However, if three or more ribs have been removed, the use of mesh does improve chest wall mechanics and reduces the duration of ventilator dependence. Marlex, a nonabsorbable durable mesh, can be used for flat surfaces of the chest wall. If the defect is large, a "sandwich" of Marlex mesh and methyl methacrylate can be formed to restore a more normal contour.[49] If the mesh is covered by well-vascularized tissue, the risk of infection and extrusion is usually low.

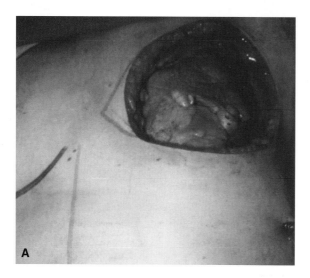

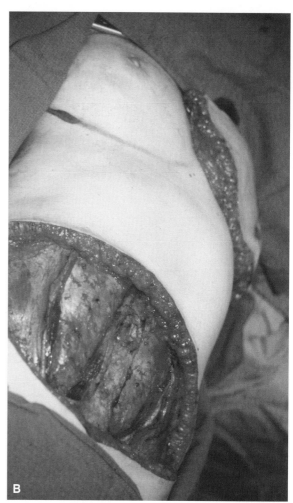

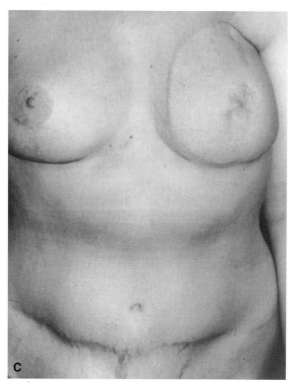

Figure 10–5. *A*, Operative defect following full-thickness chest-wall excision. *B*, Myocutaneous TRAM flap harvested from the lower abdominal wall and transferred to the chest. *C*, Postoperative result with the chest wall reconstruction shaped into a facsimile of a breast. (Reprinted with permission from Singletary SE, Hortobagyi GN, Kroll SS. Surgical and medical management of local-regional treatment failures in advanced primary breast cancer. Surg Oncol Clin N Am 1995;4(4):671–84.)

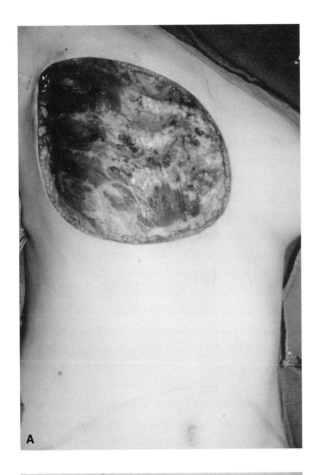

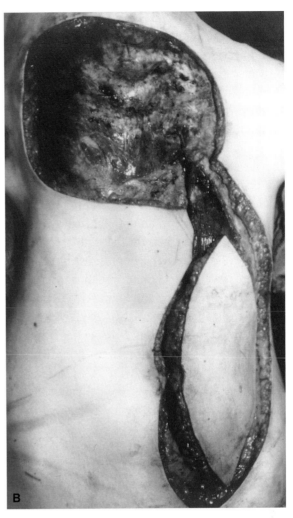

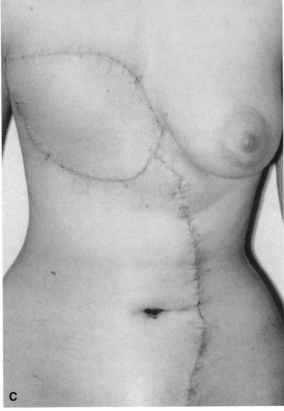

Figure 10–6. *A,* Operative defect of the chest wall after radical excision. *B,* Myocutaneous VRAM flap harvested from the lateral abdominal wall. *C,* Postoperative result. (Reprinted with permission from Singletary SE, Hortobagyi GN, Kroll SS. Surgical and medical management of local-regional treatment failures in advanced primary breast cancer. Surg Oncol Clin N Am 1995;4(4):671–84.)

STRATEGIES FOR IMPROVING SYSTEMIC THERAPY

Advances in the treatment of LABC are largely dependent on improvements in systemic chemotherapy. Two major strategies to improve systemic therapy include improved selection and individualization of chemotherapy regimens and the development of novel targeted therapies. If the chemosensitivity of a specific breast cancer could be predicted before or soon after the initiation of chemotherapy, an optimal treatment regimen could be designed for that tumor. One possible way to predict chemosensitivity is to measure levels of cellular proteins associated with drug resistance, including MDR1 (multidrug-resistance protein, or P-glycoprotein), MRP (multidrug resistance-associated protein), glutathione S-transferase, and dihydrofolate reductase.[50] Although MDR1 is often not expressed in early-stage breast cancer, it is detectable at a high frequency in patients with LABC [51] and appears to correlate with a poor response to chemotherapy. However, the other proteins associated with drug resistance are either not detectable at a sufficient frequency or have not yet been shown to be reliable enough to predict in vivo drug resistance. The earlier in vitro chemosensitivity assays were problematic because the patient's tumor cells had to be grown in culture for a prolonged period and the assays could reliably predict only chemoresistance, not chemosensitivity. Newer chemosensitivity assays that preserve the cellular spatial relationships of the tumor and do not require a prolonged culture period are currently being assessed.[52]

Another approach to predicting chemosensitivity is to measure the effects of the chemotherapy on the intact tumor in vivo. This can be done by studying sequential needle aspirates to determine changes in flow cytometric DNA profiles and nuclear morphometric features that measure alterations in DNA content and cell cycle characteristics during chemotherapy; changes in these features have been shown to correlate with subsequent tumor regression.[53,54] Alternatively,

results on positron emission tomography, which reflect the metabolic alterations in the breast cancer following chemotherapy, may hold promise as a predictor of response.[55,56] Studies are also under way to evaluate the role of magnetic resonance imaging in accurately measuring true tumor response to chemotherapy.[57] However, the optimal timing of these modalities in relation to the cycle of chemotherapy has not yet been determined.

An exciting new area is the identification of several specific targets for novel therapeutic approaches based on an understanding of the molecular genetic and biochemical features of the tumor. These therapeutic approaches may include monoclonal antibodies either alone or conjugated to a cytotoxic substance; vaccines; or gene therapy to either suppress an oncogene or replace the product of an inactivated tumor suppressor gene.[58] These strategies may be combined with current chemotherapy regimens to produce a synergistic effect. Antibodies against the *HER-2/neu* and epidermal growth factor receptor oncogene products have been demonstrated to have a synergistic effect when combined with cisplatin, doxorubicin, and cyclophosphamide.[59,60] Novel therapies may also be used to protect normal cells against the effects of chemotherapy drugs and thus lessen side effects. For example, gene therapy may allow the human multidrug-resistance gene to be transfected into human marrow progenitors to instill a preferential resistance to a chemotherapy drug such as paclitaxel.[61] Although the *BRCA1* gene is rarely mutated in sporadic breast cancer, levels of *BRCA1* mRNA and its protein are decreased in both hereditary and sporadic disease. Results of a pilot trial with an ovarian cancer nude mouse model indicate that delivery of a nonmutated *BRCA1* gene into the tumor via a retroviral vector can suppress tumor growth.[62] Encouraging observations have also been reported for an *E1B* gene-attenuated adenovirus, ONYX-015, that targets the *p53* gene of tumors but not of normal cells.[63] The tumor-specific cytolysis produced by this adenovirus appears to augment the efficacy of concomitant chemotherapy. Other therapeutic possibilities include inhibitors of angiogenesis[64–66] and matrix metalloproteinases[67]; retinoids to induce differentiation[68]; and vaccines directed against tumor antigens such as muc-1.[69]

Translational research that brings new treatment concepts from the laboratory to the clinical arena is essential for continued progress in the management of LABC. Clinicians must be prepared to consider the feasibility of molecular control of the underlying process of mammary carcinogenesis as part of their treatment armamentarium for both early-stage breast cancer and LABC.

REFERENCES

1. Anonymous. Breast. In: Fleming ID, Cooper JS, Henson DE, et al, editors. AJCC cancer staging manual. 5th ed. Philadelphia: Lippincott-Raven; 1997. p.171–80.
2. Strom EA, McNeese MD, Fletcher GH, et al. Results of mastectomy and postoperative irradiation in the management of locoregionally advanced carcinoma of the breast. Int J Radiat Oncol Biol Phys 1991;21:319–23.
3. Hortobagyi GN, Ames FC, Buzdar AU, et al. Management of stage III primary breast cancer with primary chemotherapy, surgery, and radiation therapy. Cancer 1988;62:2507–16.
4. Broadwater JR, Edwards MJ, Kuglen C. Mastectomy following preoperative chemotherapy. Ann Surg 1991;213:126–9.
5. Feldman LD, Hortobagyi GN, Buzdar AU, et al. Pathological assessment of response to induction chemotherapy in breast cancer. Cancer Res 1986;46:2578–81.
6. McCready DR, Hortobagyi GN, Kau SW, et al. The prognostic significance of lymph node metastases after preoperative chemotherapy for locally advanced breast cancer. Arch Surg 1989;124:21–5.
7. Hortobagyi GN, Singletary SE, Buzdar AU, et al. Primary chemotherapy for breast cancer: M. D. Anderson experience. In: Banzet P, editor. Proceedings of the 3rd International Congress on Neoadjuvant Chemotherapy. New York: Springer-Verlag; 1991. p. 145–8.
8. Singletary SE, McNeese MD, Hortobagyi GN. Feasibility of breast conservation surgery after induction chemotherapy for locally advanced carcinoma. Cancer 1992;69:2849–52.
9. Booser D, Frye D, Singletary S, et al. Response to induction chemotherapy for breast cancer: a prospective multimodality treatment program. [abstract] Proc Am Soc Clin Oncol 1992;11:82.
10. Kuerer HM, Newman LA, Fornage BD, et al. Role of axillary lymph node dissection after tumor downstaging with induction chemotherapy for locally advanced breast cancer. Ann Surg Oncol 1998;5(8):673–80.
11. Buzdar AU, Hortobagyi GN, Asmar L, et al. Prospective randomized trial of paclitaxel alone versus 5-fluorouracil/doxorubicin/cyclophosphamide as induction therapy in patients with operable breast cancer. Semin Oncol 1997;24:1–4.
12. Peoples GE, Regan Q, Heaton KM, et al. Breast conservation therapy for large primary and locally advanced breast cancers after induction chemotherapy. Ann Surg Oncol. In press.
13. Hunt KK, Buzdar AU. Breast conservation after tumor downstaging with induction chemotherapy. In: Singletary SE, editor. Breast Cancer-M. D. Anderson Solid Tumor Oncology Series. New York: Springer-Verlag; 1999. p.196–207.
14. Bonadonna G, Veronesi U, Brambilla C, et al. Primary chemotherapy to avoid mastectomy in tumors with diameters of three centimeters or more. J Natl Cancer Inst 1990;82:1539–45.
15. Calais G, Berger C, Descamps P, et al. Conservative treatment feasibility with induction chemotherapy, surgery, and radiotherapy for patients with breast carcinoma larger than 3 cm. Cancer 1994;74:1283–8.
16. Veronesi U, Bonadonna G, Zurrida S, et al. Conservation surgery after primary chemotherapy in large carcinomas of the breast. Ann Surg 1995;222:612–8.
17. Schwartz GF. Breast conservation following induction chemotherapy for locally advanced breast cancer: a personal experience. The Breast Journal 1996;2:78–82.
18. Touboul E, Buffat L, Lefranc J, et al. Possibility of conservative local treatment after combined chemotherapy and preoperative irradiation for locally advanced noninflammatory breast cancer. Int J Radiat Oncol Biol Phys 1996;34:1019–28.
19. Merajver SD, Weber BL, Cody R, et al. Breast conservation and prolonged chemotherapy for locally advanced breast cancer: the University of Michigan experience. J Clin Oncol 1997;15:2873–81.
20. Fisher B, Bryant J, Wolmark N, et al. Effect of preoperative chemotherapy on the outcome of

women with operable breast cancer. J Clin Oncol 1998;16:2672–85.

21. Schwartz GF, Birchansky CA, Komarnicky LT, et al. Induction chemotherapy followed by breast conservation for locally advanced carcinoma of the breast. Cancer 1994;73:362–9.

22. Scholl SM, Fourquet A, Asselain B, et al. Neoadjuvant versus adjuvant chemotherapy in premenopausal patients with tumors considered too large for breast conserving surgery: preliminary results of a randomised trial: S6. Eur J Cancer 1994;5:645–52.

23. Delena M, Varini M, Zucali R, et al. Multimodal treatment for locally advanced breast cancer. Cancer Clinical Trials 1981;4:229–36.

24. Perloff M, Lesnick GJ, Korzun A, et al. Combination chemotherapy with mastectomy or radiotherapy for stage III breast carcinoma: Cancer and Leukemia Group B study. J Clin Oncol 1988;6:261–9.

25. Rahman ZU, Frye DK, Buzdar AU, et al. Impact of selection process on response rate and long-term survival of potential high-dose chemotherapy candidates treated with standard-dose doxorubicin-containing chemotherapy in patients with metastatic breast cancer. J Clin Oncol 1997;15:3171–7.

26. Hortobagyi GN, Buzdar AU, Champlin R, et al. Lack of efficacy of adjuvant high-dose (HD) tandem combination chemotherapy (CT) for high-risk primary breast cancer (HRPBC)—a randomized trial. [abstract] Proc Am Soc Clin Oncol 1998;17: 123a.

27. Dunphy FR, Spitzer G, Buzdar AU, et al. Treatment of estrogen receptor negative or hormonally refractory breast cancer with double high-dose chemotherapy intensification and bone marrow support. J Clin Oncol 1990;8:1207–16.

28. Holmes FA, Walters RS, Theriault RL, et al. Phase II trial of Taxol, an active drug in the treatment of metastatic breast cancer. J Natl Cancer Inst 1991;83:1797–1805.

29. Valero V, Holmes FA, Walters RS, et al. Phase II trial of docetaxel, a new highly effective antineoplastic agent in the management of patients with anthracycline-resistant breast cancer. J Clin Oncol 1995;13:2886–94.

30. Buzdar AU, McNeese MD, Hortobagyi GN, et al. Is chemotherapy effective in reducing the local failure rate in patients with operable breast cancer? Cancer 1990;65:394–9.

31. Osborne MP, Ormiston N, Harmer OL, et al. Breast conservation in the treatment of early breast cancer: a 20-year follow-up. Cancer 1984;53:349–55.

32. Delouche G, Bachelot F, Premont M, Kurts JM. Conservation treatment of early breast cancer: long-term results and complications. Int J Radiat Oncol Biol Phys 1987;13:29–34.

33. Wazer DE, Erban JK, Robert NJ, et al. Breast conservation in elderly women for clinically negative axillary lymph nodes without axillary dissection. Cancer 1994;74:878–83.

34. Early Breast Cancer Trialists' Collaborative Group. Effects of radiotherapy and surgery in early breast cancer. N Engl J Med 1995;333: 1444–55.

35. Singletary SE. Management of the axilla in early stage breast cancer. In: Perry MC, editor. American Society of Clinical Oncology Educational Book. Alexandria (VA): American Society of Clinical Oncology; 1998. p.132–41.

36. Fleming RYD, Asmar L, Buzdar AU, et al. Effectiveness of mastectomy by response to induction chemotherapy for control in inflammatory breast carcinoma. Ann Surg Oncol 1997;4:452–61.

37. Singletary SE, Ames FC, Buzdar AU. Management of inflammatory breast cancer. World J Surg 1994;18:87–92.

38. Barker JL, Montague ED, Peters LJ. Clinical experience with irradiation of inflammatory carcinoma of the breast with and without elective chemotherapy. Cancer 1981;45:625–29.

39. Thoms WW, McNeese MD, Fletcher GH, et al. Multimodal treatment for inflammatory breast cancer. Int J Radiat Oncol Biol Phys 1989;17: 739–45.

40. Brun B, Ottmezguine Y, Feuilhade F, et al. Treatment of inflammatory breast cancer with combination chemotherapy and mastectomy versus breast conservation. Cancer 1988;61:1096–103.

41. Antman K, Bearman SI, Davidson N, et al. Dose intensive therapy in breast cancer: current status. In: Gale RP, Champlin RE, editors. New strategies in bone marrow transplantation. New York: Alan R Liss; 1990. p. 423–6.

42. Newman LA, Kuerer HM, Hunt KK, et al. Presentation, treatment and outcome of local recurrence after skin-sparing mastectomy and immediate breast reconstruction. Ann Surg Oncol 1998;5(7):620–6.

43. Halpern J, McNeese MD, Kroll SS, Ellerbrock N. Irradiation of prosthetically augmented breasts: a retrospective study on toxicity and cosmetic results. Int J Radiat Oncol Biol Phys 1990;18: 189–91.

44. Forman DL, Chiu J, Restifo RJ, et al. Breast reconstruction in previously irradiated patients using tissue expanders and implants: a poten-

tially unfavorable result. Ann Plast Surg 1998;
40:360–4.

45. Evans GRD, Schusterman MA, Kroll SS, et al. Reconstruction and the radiated breast: is there a role for implants? Plast Reconstr Surg 1995; 96:1111–8.

46. Schusterman MA, Kroll SS, Miller MJ, et al. The free transverse rectus abdominis musculocutaneous flap for breast reconstruction: one center's experience with 211 consecutive cases. Ann Plast Surg 1994;32:234–42.

47. McKenna RJ, Moutain CF, McMurtrey MJ, et al. Current techniques for chest wall reconstruction: expanded possibilities for treatment. Ann Thorac Surg 1988;46:508–12.

48. Hunt KK, Baldwin BJ, Strom EA, et al. Feasibility of postmastectomy radiation therapy after TRAM flap breast reconstruction. Ann Surg Oncol 1997;4:377–84.

49. Kroll SS, Walsh G, Ryan B, King RC. Risks and benefits of using Marlex mesh in chest wall reconstruction. Ann Plast Surg 1993;31:303–6.

50. Verrele P, Meissonnier F, Fonck Y, et al. Clinical relevance of immunohistochemical detection of multidrug resistance. P-glycoprotein in breast carcinoma. J Natl Cancer Inst 1991;83:111–6.

51. Ro J, Sahin A, Ro JY, et al. Immunohistochemical analysis of P-glycoprotein expression correlated with chemotherapy resistance in locally advanced breast cancer. Hum Pathol 1990;21: 787–91.

52. Blackman KE, Fingert HJ, Fuller AF, Meitner PA. The fluorescent cytoprint assay in gynecological malignancies and breast cancer. Methodology and results. Contrib Gynecol Obstet 1994; 19:53–63.

53. Brifford M, Spyratos F, Hacene K, et al. Evaluation of breast carcinoma chemosensitivity by flow cytometric DNA analysis and computer assisted image analysis. Cytometry 1991;13:250–8.

54. O'Reilly SM, Camplejohn RS, Rubens RD. DNA flow cytometry and response to preoperative chemotherapy for primary breast cancer. Eur J Cancer 1992;28:681–3.

55. Jansson T, Westlin JE, Ahlstrom H, et al. Positron emission tomography studies in patients with locally advanced and/or metastatic breast cancer: a method for early therapy evaluation. J Clin Oncol 1995;13:1470–7.

56. Nieweg OE, Wong W-H, Singletary SE, et al. Positron emission tomography of glucose metabolism in breast cancer: potential for tumor detection, staging, and evaluation of chemother-

apy. Ann NY Acad Sci 1993;698:423–8.

57. Orel SG, Schnall MD, Powell CM, et al. Staging of suspected breast cancer: effect of MR imaging and MR-guided biopsy. Radiology 1995; 196:115–22.

58. Dhingra K, Hittelman WN, Hortobagyi GN. Genetic changes in breast cancer—consequences for therapy? Gene 1995;159:59–63.

59. Baselga J, Norton L, Masui H, et al. Antitumor effects of doxorubicin in combination with anti-epidermal growth factor receptor monoclonal antibody. J Natl Cancer Inst 1993;85: 1327–33.

60. Hancock MC, Langton BC, Chan T, et al. A monoclonal antibody against the c-erbB-2 protein enhances the cytotoxicity of cisdiammine dichloroplatinum against human breast and ovarian tumor cell lines. Cancer Res 1991;51:4575–80.

61. Ward M, Richardson C, Pioli P, et al. Transfer and expression of the human multiple drug resistance gene in human CD34+ cells. Blood 1994; 84:1408–14.

62. Holt JT, Thompson ME, Szabo C, et al. Growth retardation and tumor inhibition by BRCA1. Nat Genet 1996;12:298–302.

63. Heise C, Sampson-Johannes A, Williams A, et al. ONYX-015, an E1B gene-attenuated adenovirus, causes tumor-specific cytolysis and antitumoral efficacy that can be augmented by standard chemotherapeutic agents. Nature 1997;3:639–45.

64. Thorpe PE, Burrows FJ. Antibody-directed targeting of the vasculature of solid tumors. Breast Cancer Res Treat 1995;36:237–51

65. O'Reilly MS, Holmgren L, Chen C, Folkman J. Angiostatin induces and sustains dormancy of human primary tumors in mice. Nat Med 1996; 2:689–92.

66. Folkman J. Clinical implications of angiogenesis research. N Engl J Med 1995;333:1757–63.

67. Sledge GW Jr, Qulali M, Goulet R, et al. Effect of matrix metalloproteinase inhibitor batimastat on breast cancer regrowth and metastasis in athymic mice. J Natl Cancer Inst 1995;87:1546–50.

68. Lotan R. Retinoids in cancer chemoprevention. FASEB J 1996;10:1031–9.

69. Gilewski T, Adluri R, Zhang S, et al. Preliminary results: vaccination of breast cancer patients lacking identifiable disease with muc-1-keyhole limpet hemocyanin (klh) conjugate and qs21. [abstract] Proc Am Soc Clin Oncol 1996; 15:555.

11

Breast Reconstruction

GEOFFREY C. FENNER, MD
THOMAS A. MUSTOE, MD

In contrast to the 1960s when silicone implants were the mainstay of breast reconstruction, patients in the 1990s may choose from an impressive spectrum of reconstructive options. Techniques, instruments, and materials have evolved that provide all patients, regardless of age, stage, previous treatment, or laterality, choices that may optimally represent their desires and expectations. Breast cancer awareness has increased the sophistication of patients, however, it remains the plastic surgeon's responsibility to educate patients and coordinate expectations and outcome.

Increased detection of breast cancer has paralleled improved techniques and availability of screening mammography, an increased female population, and the impact of changes in the age of childbearing, menarche, and menopause. Today, ductal carcinoma in situ (DCIS) represents 15 to 20 percent of all breast cancer cases;[1] it is treated by either localized resection or total mastectomy. Genetic testing and better elucidation of risk factors has identified additional patients as potential candidates for prophylactic mastectomy. As many as 15 percent of patients undergoing breast conservation, and who require a proportionately large lumpectomy, attain poor esthetic outcome and may be better served in the longterm, by preoperative consideration of completion mastectomy and autologous reconstruction.[2] Included in this group are patients with small breasts, proportionately large lesions, and centrally located lesions. These women, often having been diagnosed at an earlier age and stage, have excellent prognoses, and represent an increasing percentage of patients seeking consultation and alternatives for breast restoration.

The female breast is intimately associated with a woman's selfesteem, sexuality, and interpersonal relations. The response to the impact and presumed implications of breast cancer varies widely among women. Breast cancer represents a therapeutic myriad with emotional and physical implications, both for the present and future. Although breast reconstruction may be viewed as a positive alternative to breast loss, it represents only one facet newly diagnosed cancer patients must face. Each patient upholds an individual, often rigid, esthetic standard, emotional drive, and physiology which guides them towards a specific reconstructive technique. It remains the plastic surgeon's responsibility to inform, educate, and perform with this in mind.

The first breast reconstruction was performed by Czerny, in 1895, when he successfully transplanted a lipoma from a patient's flank to a submammary position.[3] Multiple developments over the past 100 years have improved reconstructive options as well as ultimate outcomes for women faced with mastectomy.

IMMEDIATE RECONSTRUCTION

Immediate reconstruction provides significant advantages for the newly diagnosed breast cancer patient (Table 11–1). Greater understanding of tumor biology and technical advances in reconstructive surgery have led to greater acceptance of immediate postmastectomy reconstruction. The first large series reported in 1982, conveyed excellent outcome, less expense than delayed reconstruction, and no apparent effect on the natural course of the malignancy.[4] Initial options for immediate reconstruction through the mid-1990s included various expanders and implants, yet now include various flaps and even free-flap reconstruction. Satisfactory outcome is dependent upon patient selection as well as communication between the ablative and reconstructive surgeons.

The advantages of immediate reconstruction include diminished psychosocial trauma, superior esthetic results, decreased surgical morbidity, and lower cost than delayed reconstruction. Historically, delayed reconstructions were more often performed due to heightened fear of recurrence, concerns that immediate reconstruction would mask subsequent detection of a recurrence, and the possibility that immediate reconstruction would be compromised by and hinder the initiation of adjuvant therapy. It was also felt that patients would be more appreciative of reconstruction if required to live for a time with the postmastectomy defect. These ideas have since been rendered obsolete by the need to consider the emotional impact of mastectomy and by the technical and therapeutic advances of the past 15 years.

Patients undergoing immediate reconstruction tend to incorporate the new breast into their body image, thereby maintaining greater selfesteem, personal sexuality, and confidence in interpersonal relationships.[5] They tend to have less "cancer anxiety," less recall, and greater freedom in choosing clothing.[6] Patients undergoing mastectomy and immediate reconstruction demonstrate a similar psychosocial outcome to that of breast conservation patients, having had lumpectomy with or without radiation.[7] Body image may be adversely affected due to greater breast and donor site scarring compared to patients having undergone breast conservation. Overall, psychologic morbidity is similar, and clearly favorable compared to that of patients having had delayed reconstruction.[8]

The opportunity to attain optimal esthetic results is enhanced with immediate reconstruction. The newly raised mastectomy skin flaps tend to preserve the shape of the natural breast, providing a structural template that determines the shape of the underlying volume, whether an implant or flap reconstruction. Skin flap fibrosis associated with delayed reconstruction represents inherent tissue loss and requires either greater tissue expansion or greater skin replacement at the time of autologous reconstruction. Fibrosis of the mastectomy skin flaps are an impediment in achieving a natural breast shape. Skin-sparing mastectomy in immediate reconstruction further increases the ability to attain a symmetric result, limits scarring to the periareolar region, and minimizes the need for contralateral procedures such as reductions and mastopexies.[9–13]

Administration of adjuvant therapy is not delayed in patients undergoing immediate breast reconstruction, nor is the rate of complications higher after immediate reconstruction.[14–15] The usual 3 to 4 week interval prior to the initiation of adjuvant chemotherapy is ample time for uncomplicated, postreconstructive wound healing and patient recovery. Only 1 to 2 percent of patients have their chemotherapy delayed beyond 3 to 4 weeks due to complications from immediate reconstruction, such as delayed healing.[16]

Although neoadjuvant and adjuvant chemotherapy have no relative impact upon immediate reconstruction, adjuvant radiation is known to unequivocally detract from the esthetic result and increase the local complication rate. This is influenced by many factors, including reconstructive technique and the type and dose of radiation. Historically, radiation exaggerated the extent of fibrous capsular contracture present, to some extent, in all expander/implant reconstructions.[17–19] Poor outcome paralleled the need for substantial expansion and the use of large, smooth, silicone implants. The rate of poor cosmetic results in early series ranged from 18 to 40 percent, with a failure rate up to 40 percent.[20] Evans and colleagues reported a 43 percent complication rate among radiated implant reconstruction patients, compared to a 12 percent rate in nonradiated patients.[18] Schuster reported a 55 percent complication rate and unacceptable cosmesis in 24 percent of postreconstructive patients requiring adjuvant radiation.[17] Of patients who had undergone a composite autogeneous/implant reconstruction, 40 percent of the radiated and 8.3 percent of the nonradiated patients had major complications.[18] Dickson reported an overall complication rate of 70 percent for patients having immediate prosthetic reconstruction with radiation, and rates of 30 percent for skin necrosis and 67 percent for capsule contracture.[21] Although the general consensus is to avoid prosthetic reconstruction in patients, an anticipated need for adjuvant radiation, the regiment is most often recommended postoperatively. Use of textured saline prosthesis as well as improved radiation techniques have demonstrated improved overall tolerance and diminished complications in some early reports, but there is no consensus.[22–24]

In contrast, tolerance of autologous tissue to radiation is generally good. Zimmerman reported the effect of postoperative radiation on immediate free transverse rectus abdominis myocutaneous (TRAM) reconstruction. He reported no total or partial losses. Cosmesis, as rated by patients, was excellent in 60 percent of cases, good in 30 percent, and fair in 10 percent.[25] Although some variable degree of cutaneous fibrous contracture may occur, this can usually be compensated for through surgical and design modifications. It is interesting that the rate of fat necrosis and volume loss in TRAM flaps, postradiation, was higher in pedicled (33%) than in free TRAMs (6%) reconstructions.[26]

Immediate postmastectomy reconstruction for locally advanced disease has been reported as encouraging. Sultan reported on 22 patients with stage IIB or III disease who had undergone neoadjuvant chemotherapy and completion of chemotherapy 3 weeks subsequent to surgery. Perioperative morbidity was 14 percent. Delay in resumption of chemotherapy occurred in no instances, and patients expressed appreciation for having been offered this option.[27] Styblo reported on 21 patients with stage III disease who had undergone immediate TRAM reconstruction. There were no delays in reinstitution of adjuvant treatment and no increase in local relapse.[28] It has been shown that breast reconstruction may facilitate resection, without an increase in local complications or relapse.

Immediate reconstruction also has economic advantages. Ablation and reconstruction are combined in one procedure, thereby limiting anesthetic risk and the time committed to postoperative recovery. Patients welcome the opportunity for a single procedure with less impact on occupational and domestic responsibilities. Avoidance of a staged second surgery and hospitalization in delayed reconstruction have obvious cost advantages.

SKIN-SPARING MASTECTOMY

Toth and Lappert first described skin-sparing mastectomy (SSM) in 1991.[9] The technique is indicated for patients with early stage (I and II) breast cancer, patients managed with prophylactic mastectomy, and in attempts to facilitate a highly esthetic outcome through maximal skin preservation (Figure 11–1). Incisions are planned that will remove the breast, nipple-areolar complex, adjacent biopsy scars, and the skin over more superficial tumors. Kroll and colleagues in

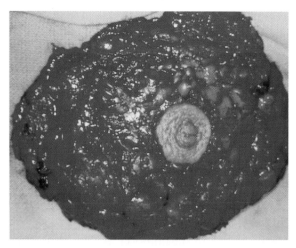

Figure 11–1. Skin-sparing mastectomy.

1991 reported only one local recurrence in 100 cases with a follow-up of 23 months.[10]

Local recurrence is dependent upon tumor size and locoregional nodal involvement. Despite variation in mastectomy technique, including SSM, the rate of local recurrence has remained stable. Skin-sparing mastectomy is more challenging for the oncologic surgeon, more time consuming, and requires delicate handling of the skin flaps to avoid ischemic complications. These efforts to preserve the skin envelope and inframammary fold are greatly appreciated by the patient and result in greater symmetry, often diminishing the need for a contralateral procedure. Subsequent areolar tatooing may completely camouflage the central incisions.

Newman reported a 6.2 percent local recurrence rate in 372 patients who underwent SSM for TI/II lesions. Ninety-six percent of these recurrences presented as palpable skin flap masses.[11] Hidalgo reported on 28 patients who underwent immediate reconstruction (92% receiving TRAM flaps) after SSM, with a mean follow-up of 27 months. Complications at the reconstructive site were limited to cellulitis and marginal periareolar skin loss. Esthetic results were judged as excellent in 75 percent of patients.[12] Carlson compared 327 patients given SSM to 188 non-SSM patients. After a mean follow-up of 41 months, the local recurrence rate was 4.8 percent in the former group and 9.5 percent in the latter; native skin flap necrosis occurred in 10.7 percent of the SSM patients and in 11.2 percent of the non-SSM patients.[13] Because local recurrence after SSM is low and the likelihood of local control and survival are high, SSM with immediate reconstruction is an acceptable treatment for breast cancer.

BREAST IMPLANTS

The number of women with breast implants ranges between 1.5 and 2 million. The modern silicone implant has been available since 1963 and has undergone a multitude of subsequent mechanical and material improvements. All implants consist of a silicone elastomer shell that may be single or double lumen, with a smooth or textured surface. Contents of single chamber implants consist of either silicone gel, which is factory sealed and nonadjustable, or saline, which may be adjusted intra- and/or perioperatively. Dual chamber implants were devised to provide the benefits and camouflage of silicone texture (outer lumen), along with postoperative saline adjustability (inner lumen). Various natural oils, triglycerides, and water soluble hydrogels are currently under investigation but are not currently available in the United States.

Silicone is ubiquitous in our environment. Individual exposure occurs through contact with needles, syringes, medications (insulin, simethicone), lipstick, creams, cosmetics, and implantable devices, such as pacemakers, joint replacements, defibrillators, shunts, stents, and implants.[29] Extensive research undertaken since the FDA-directed silicone breast implant moratorium in 1992 has confirmed that implantable medical grade silicone is among the least bioreactive, most inert substances available for implantation.[30–32] Studies have failed to show linkage between connective tissue disease and silicone gel implants. The silicone elastomer shell and gel of breast implants, however, like all implanted devices, will trigger a foreign body inflammatory cell response, with giant cell formation and eventual scarring. The extent and impact of this fibrotic capsular response upon the fluid, and physical characteristics of breast implants is dependent upon capsular density, implant–tissue incorporation, the presence of myofibroblasts, and/or the presence of intracapsular silicone or sepsis.

Capsular contracture represents the most common complication of breast implants. It consists of progressive fibrous constriction around breast implants and is unpredictable and variable. It is graded according to a scale developed by Baker (Table 11–2) and ranges from visually imperceptible (class I), to stone hard and painful (class IV). It may occur immediately or years after implantation. There is a greater incidence associated with smooth silicone implants and with subglandular placement in cosmetic augmentation. Some theories suggest local contamination with *Staphylococcus epidermidis* as one inciting cause. The powder from gloves and inflammation from even limited hematomas may play a role in some cases.

Capsular contracture may cause implant deformation, migration, and rupture (Figure 11–2) and may, on occasion, become calcified and detour from effective mammography. Individual perception is dependent upon severity and on the esthetic standard of the patient. Capsular contracture is not in itself a health risk. Twenty to 50 percent of reconstruction patients who develop contractures require operative intervention.

Contractures, historically, were released through aggressive manual compression. The goal was to "pop" the surrounding constricting capsule, leading to a softer breast. This technique of closed capsulotomy resulted in occasional implant rupture, extracapsular silicone extravasation, and surgeon injury (gamekeeper's thumb). In addition to long-term failure, the technique could potentiate liability risk if future rupture was detected. Contractures today are more commonly corrected through a limited, outpatient, open capsulotomy, whereby

Table 11–2. BAKER'S CLASSIFICATION OF CAPSULE CONTRACTURE

Class I	Augmented breast feels as soft as an unoperated-upon breast
Class II	Minimal; less soft, the implant can be palpated but is not visible
Class III	Moderate; more firm, the implant can be easily palpated and is visible
Class IV	Severe; the breast is hard, tender, painful, cold, and distorted

Reproduced with permission from Little G, Baker JL. Results of closed compression capsulotomy for treatment of contracted breast implant capsules. Plast Reconstr Surg 1980;65:30.

the fibrous capsule is surgically released and or excised (capsulectomy) (Figure 11–3).

Silicone gel is composed of an amorphous matrix consisting of silicone oils of various sizes and weights. Smaller caliber oils are known to diffuse through the elastomer shell (silicone gel "bleed") and become incorporated into the fibrous capsule. Microscopic amounts may percolate through lymphatic channels following macrophage ingestion and migrate to the regional lymph nodes. As with exposure to other medial grade silicones, there is no evidence to suggest that the minute quantities transgressing the elastomer shell have any metabolic or long-term impact.

Silicone gel implant rupture occurs in up to 63 percent of patients after 12 years, documented during surgery in patients having their implants removed.[33–36] Among asymptomatic patients, the incidence of implant rupture is unknown but is believed to be significant.

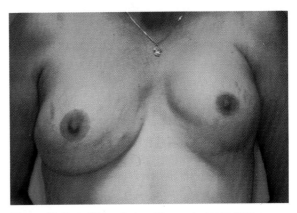

Figure 11–2. Left breast class III capsule contracture.

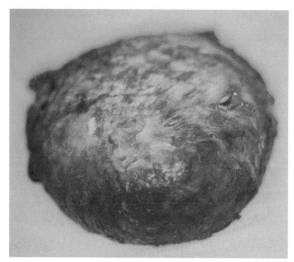

Figure 11–3. Excised implant and enveloping capsule contracture.

Gradual attenuation of the elastomer shell, with imperceptible rupture, is well documented. Abrupt or premature rupture may be prompted by capsular contracture, implant shell infolding leading to accelerated stress fractures, and trauma. Once a gel implant shell ruptures, from longevity or trauma, the contents are usually contained within the surrounding fibrous capsule. This is likely to remain undetected and has demonstrated no systemic effects.

Post-traumatic change in the form of herniation, deflation, malposition, or deformation may manifest extracapsular extravasation. When this occurs, free gel may infiltrate breast parenchyma and tissue planes, and/or elicit a granulomatous foreign body reaction. This may lead to regional silicone migration, silicone mastitis, and formation of irregular nodules that may, on physical examination and mammography, simulate a malignancy.[37] Suspected implant rupture warrants evaluation. Magnetic resonance imaging has a greater sensitivity than do either mammography or ultrasound and is the test of choice for detecting implant rupture.[38] Early removal of the free silicone and implant, with or without implant replacement, will help to avoid these sequellae and minimize subsequent confusion in mammographic screening.

Silicone and saline implants are radioopaque on mammography and have led to concerns regarding potential delay in breast cancer detection.[39–40] Implant characteristics, which may affect the sensitivity of standard mammography, include implant size, the proportion of overlying breast tissue, implant placement (subglandular versus submuscular) and the presence and immobility of capsular contracture.[41–42] As recommended by the American Cancer Society and the American Society of Plastic and Reconstructive Surgeons, women with breast implants should maintain the same schedule of mammography as all other women. They should secure a certified facility that has sufficient experience with breast implants and confirm the availability of displacement mammography (Eklund) and ultrasound. Patients with postmastectomy implant reconstruction are typically followed by physical examination only. One major epidemiologic study has confirmed that the stage at breast cancer detection in women with implants is identical or better than it is in the general population;[43] a second major study from the National Cancer Institute will be addressing this question as well. In addition, there is no evidence that silicone is carcinogenic in humans. In fact, in two large studies women with implants exhibit 10 to 30 percent less breast cancer than would be statistically expected when matched with the general population; the results, however, did not show statistical significance.[44–47] This issue needs further study with larger numbers of patients. The most recent large study, sponsored by the NCI (in press), shows an incidence no different than for the matched control group.

In 1992, a series of poorly documented case reports and the subsequent intense media scrutiny, combined with a temporary suspension of silicone gel implant usage by the FDA, led to lawsuits and an eventual multibillion dollar settlement with the major implant manufacturers. Only one implant company (Mentor) was allowed to provide gel implants for reconstruction patients, with specific and rigid criteria on a highly monitored, investigational basis. There were a plethora of syndromes, autoimmune diseases, and symptoms associated with silicone breast implants, and intense litigation followed. Many of these proposed associations, such as rheumatoid arthritis, were, in fact, shown in subsequent, large retrospective studies to occur in a lesser percentage of augmented patients than in the general population. Scleroderma-like syndromes were not shown to be associated with breast implants. The American College of Rheumatology issued on October 22, 1995, the following statement, based on accumulated data: "Studies provide compelling evidence that silicone implants expose patients to no demonstrable additional risk for connective tissue or rheumatologic disease." None of the postulated syndromes have withstood the scrutiny of prospective epidemiologic testing.[48–50] Results from a large National Cancer Institute study are still pending.

The FDA has recently submitted its requirements for submission of a "premarket approval" which will, once again, enable marketing of gel implants. The protocol requires patient monitoring during an 18-month follow-up, and submission of a limited questionnaire.

PRIMARY IMPLANT RECONSTRUCTION

One-stage primary implant reconstruction, the workhorse of breast reconstruction in the 1980s, has become less frequently used due to improved outcome with expander or autologous reconstruction. Certain patients with A- to B-sized breasts, having limited to no ptosis, sufficient soft-tissue coverage, and who desire an expeditious and simplistic approach to breast restoration, may remain candidates for either immediate or delayed single-staged implant reconstruction. Even in this group, however, a more natural shape can be achieved by an expander with a removable valve, that may also serve as a permanent implant.

Inherent to mastectomy are resection of the nipple-areolar complex, inclusion of adjacent biopsy incisions, and a resultant, variable, ipsilateral skin deficiency. Immediate reconstruction requires an initial assessment of skin flap vascularity, trauma, and tension. Only the healthiest skin flaps should signify proceeding with immediate implant reconstruction. Questionable vascularity, or marginal necrosis, warrants reappraisal and the choice of an alternative option, such as an immediate expander or autologous flap reconstruction, or delayed reconstruction. Compromised flaps, and/or insertion of a large implant under tension, risks dehiscence and implant exposure. Avoidance of tight compressive dressings and constricting bras, prompt drainage of hematomas or seromas, and early revision of marginal necrosis will minimize complications.

Implant position is determined by the dimension and esthetics of the contralateral breast. The position of the inframammary fold, breast base width, volume, and overlying skin redundancy, or ptosis, are critical in attaining optimal symmetry with the native breast. The IMF may be lowered up to 2 cm when attempting to simulate limited contralateral ptosis. Alternatively, a concurrent, or delayed contralateral reduction or mastopexy may maximize esthetic outcome and symmetry.

Delayed implant reconstruction is a safer and more popular option. The well-healed skin flaps are elevated in the subpectoral plane and may be stretched, thinned, and scored to provide improved projection without regard to vascular compromise. The final outcome may be similarly improved by a symmetry procedure.

One-stage implant reconstruction is an option ideally suited to the rare patient with small to moderate sized nonptotic breast who possesses sufficient soft tissue coverage and who desires the simplest reconstructive option. Despite an initial desire to avoid a secondary procedure, many patients require future implant adjustments or symmetry procedures. This technique has been largely supplanted by adjustable and permanent expanders/implants and the popular, time-tested, two-stage expander technique.

ADJUSTABLE IMPLANT RECONSTRUCTION

Adjustable implants or permanent expanders/implants represent an option intermediate to the single-stage implant reconstruction and the more conventional two-stage technique (Figure 11–4). Postoperatively, adjustable implants enable precision in symmetry and the ability to attain a softer, often larger reconstruction with greater ptosis. The technique offers protection against tension-related wound complications and is generally considered preferable to primary implant reconstruction. It offers an excellent alternative to patients with limited skin deficits, A- to B-sized contralateral breasts, and/or those patients who require only limited expansion. In addition, a second-stage implant exchange is often avoided.

Indications for use of an adjustable implant include patients with an immediate or delayed soft tissue deficit, with mild to moderate ptosis, or who require salvage after failed primary implant reconstruction. Patients with asymmetric deformities from hypoplasia, trauma, burns, or congenital deformities (including pectus excavatum and Poland's syndrome) are also ideal candidates. Adjustability is beneficial in augmentation candidates with inherent parenchymal asymmetries or tuberous breasts, or in patients with an unpredictable or poorly communicated esthetic standard.

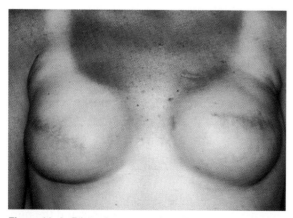

Figure 11–4. Bilateral reconstruction with adjustable expander/prosthesis.

Poor candidates for implant reconstruction are those with large, pendulous breasts. These women, often obese, represent a challenge with any technique and are unlikely to achieve satisfactory symmetry without a contralateral reduction or mastopexy. Prior radiation treatment is a strong relative contraindication. The fibrotic and relatively ischemic nature of radiated skin flaps resists expansion and tolerates an underlying implant poorly, with a tendency towards cutaneous erosion and exposure. These patients are better served with either an autologous or composite reconstruction.

There are two types of adjustable prostheses currently available. One is a round and anatomic, textured or smooth, postoperatively adjustable, saline implant. The implants are successively expanded, with saline, by percutaneous injection through a remotely positioned subcutaneous injection port. Alternatively, Becker expander/prostheses are composed of a dual chamber system. The inner lumen, like the Mentor implant, is filled and expanded with saline through a self-sealing, removable injection port. The outer lumen is factory sealed with silicone gel. It provides patients with the tangible advantages and surface camouflage of silicone and the postoperative adjustability of a saline implant.

Once optimal size and shape have been attained, as confirmed by patient and surgeon, and sufficient time for capsule maturation has been allowed (4 to 6 months), the ports may be removed under local anesthesia, usually through a short segment of the lateral mastectomy incision. Vigorous retraction of the connecting tube engages a self-sealing valve and prevents leakage of intrinsic saline. Removal of a small volume of saline prior to port removal may optimize implant softness and simulate ptosis.

Preoperative considerations include accurate assessment of size and base diameter. These determinations may be aided by the use of templates, sizers, and by the weight of the mastectomy specimen. Preoperative markings should detail breast margins in the immediate reconstruction setting or, in delayed reconstruction, mirror the contralateral breast.

Total muscular coverage, in the immediate reconstruction setting, will reduce the incidence of implant exposure, infection, and cutaneous complications. Sufficient coverage and implant camouflage is provided by a submuscular pocket composed of the pectoralis, serratus, and rectus muscles. The deflated implant is placed, precisely, within the muscular pocket and cleared of redundant folds. The injection port is connected, drawn through the lateral serratus fibers, and fixed to the lateral chest wall. Patency of the filling system should be confirmed. Skin flap viability must be assessed prior to closure and all questionable skin resected. The implants may be expanded to obliterate dead space but should not further stress the muscular or cutaneous closure.

Expansion is usually initiated 7 to 14 days postoperatively, following confirmation of skin flap viability. The frequency and extent of each expansion is dependent upon wound healing, skin sufficiency, and the patient's tolerance and comfort level. Typically, saline is injected to the point of tolerable skin tension, without blanching, on a weekly basis. Maintenance of the implant at maximum volume for a minimum of 3 months allows for capsule maturation. The implant may then be adjusted, within a narrow range, prior to port removal, to optimize consistency and ptosis.

IMMEDIATE TWO-STAGE BREAST RECONSTRUCTION

Tissue expansion in breast reconstruction was pioneered through the efforts of Chadomer Radovan and initially reported in 1976.[51] The postmastectomy defect lacks both skin for coverage and the underlying breast mound. To be reconstructed, the skin envelope must have a adequate laxity to allow the breast mound to project sufficiently, achieve symmetric ptosis, and remain soft in consistency. These goals often require the recruitment of substantial adjacent skin through temporary overexpansion. Expanders, presently available for immediate breast reconstruction, enable focused expansion and simulation of a realistic inframammary fold, without the physiologic, donor site, and rehabilitative demands of autologous reconstruction. Second-stage exchange with either saline or silicone implants is a simple, outpatient procedure. Tissue expanders remain the most popular method of immediate breast reconstruction.

The advent of textured surfaces has somewhat lessened the incidence of capsule contracture, has limited the incidence of perioperative migration, and has resulted in more predictable, successful results. The introduction of anatomic expanders and implants has enabled preferential expansion of the lower pole, to better simulate natural ptosis. Over longer follow-up, however, there are still significant limitations in the ability to consistently achieve a natural shape and soft breast.

Although all patients who undergo a mastectomy may be considered candidates for expander reconstruction, preferred patients are those with smaller, minimally ptotic breasts. Some of these patients may exhibit sufficiently vigorous skin flaps to accommodate a primary implant reconstruction. Those with limited deficits, and particularly those who increasingly undergo skin-sparing mastectomies, are candidates for the use of newer adjustable implants. The two-staged approach is a reliable, predictable reconstruction and has the ability to incorporate maximal adjacent skin, achieve greater volumes and ptosis, and enable patient-directed modifications. Final refinements, including fold adjustments and capsulotomy, are facilitated at the time of implant exchange, optimizing the esthetic result. Conversely, patients with large or pendulous breasts require greater, more prolonged expansion and often a contralateral symmetry procedure to achieve an acceptable result.

Prior or anticipated chest-wall radiation after breast conservation or mastectomy remains a strong relative contraindication to immediate expander reconstruction. Cutaneous radiation fibrosis resists effective expansion, limits ultimate projection, and increases the risk of capsule contracture, skin flap necrosis, implant exposure, and infection. Patients with compromised wound healing ability, such as those with scleroderma and lupus, may also benefit from alternative methods.

Textured, anatomic expanders with integrated ports are preferable. Smooth-surfaced expanders have been shown to result in an unacceptable rate of capsule contracture, compromising effective expansion.[52] Anatomic expanders enable preferential expansion of the lower pole, a more realistic shape, and greater projection. Use of an integrated port affords greater patient comfort, in that the overlying mastectomy skin flaps are usually anesthetic. The integrated ports, when compared to remote ports, also incur a lower rate of malfunction.

Simulating contralateral base width and the height of maximal projection are the key elements in attaining optimal cosmetic outcome. The goal is to accomplish the major surgical steps at the first procedure, which requires careful analysis of the contralateral breast. Simulation of ptosis can be accomplished through overexpansion of the skin envelope and subsequent deflation or secondary replacement with an implant of lower vertical profile. Moderate ptosis can be simulated through the use of overexpansion and anatomic expanders, and by lowering of the inframammary fold. Moderate to severe ptosis can not be accurately matched and usually necessitates either a contralateral reduction or mastopexy or composite reconstruction using the latissimus dorsi myocutaneous flap. Contralateral procedures are usually more precise when based upon the quality and extent of expansion achieved and are therefore preferentially performed during the second stage. The end point of the expansion process occurs when adequate projection is achieved in relation to the contralateral breast, rather than the ultimate volume being attained.

Patients and their reconstructions are not adversely affected if concurrent expansion adjuvant chemotherapy is imposed, pending wound stability at initiation. When implemented, completion of a chemotherapeutic regimen and granulocyte recovery is usually required prior to the second stage.

If adjuvant radiation is deemed necessary subsequent to expander placement, full, preradiation expansion, with preferably a 15 to 20 percent overcompensation, helps resist the fibrotic contracture associated with radiation. All patients undergoing postreconstruction radiation, however, risk radiation-induced implant complications. Radiation-induced capsule contracture affects the quality of the expansion, often leads to local chest wall discomfort, and potentiates the risk of expander extrusion or exposure. Patients should be monitored throughout their course and the expander incrementally deflated if skin flap compromise is noted. Treatment options for patients with radiation-induced complications include expander removal and delayed reconstruction, salvage by autologous replacement (TRAM or latissimus), and, occasionally, delayed capsulotomy. Patients with large, smooth implants seem to show the worst response.

Complications of expander reconstruction parallel those of primary and adjustable implant reconstruction[53–57] (Table 11–3). Advantages and their ranges are illustrated in Table 11–1. Capsular contracture remains the single most troublesome complication and is reported in 10 to 25 percent of patients.[58–59] Progressive contracture may lead to asymmetry, deformation, and pain, and require intervention, such as capsulotomy, in 20 percent of cases.

The advantages of prosthetic breast reconstruction include the ability to attain a reasonably good esthetic result without a complex, prolonged operation and hospital stay. Compromising a donor site, with its potential complicating morbidity, is also avoided. Prosthetic reconstruction remains appealing for bilateral cases in which symmetry is less of a problem and where bilateral autologous reconstruction would impose substantial demands on the patient and surgeon. Similarly, in patients with smaller breasts, in older patients, and in those less motivated, expander or implant reconstruction remains a desirable option.

ADVANTAGES OF AUTOLOGOUS RECONSTRUCTION

Breast reconstruction with a silicone- or saline-based implant is technically the simplest option available to mastectomy patients. Recent advances enhancing the potential esthetic outcome include permanent expander prosthesis and postoperatively adjustable implants. Most competent surgeons can insert a prosthesis, postmastectomy, in a wide range of patients. Consequently, prosthetic reconstruction is the most common mode of breast reconstruction available today.

Prosthetic reconstruction is safe and expeditious, with a limited recovery period. It is suited to the patient desiring a simple approach toward breast restoration. Candidates include those who wish to avoid an external prosthesis, those with limited expectations, those with smaller breasts and limited-to-no ptosis, those with existing medical risk factors and anxious patients who have difficulty comprehending more technical procedures, and those desiring an expeditious initiation of adjuvant treatment. Expander/implant reconstruction may also pacify younger patients who wish to ultimately convert to autologous reconstruction following anticipated pregnancies.

Implant-based breast reconstruction, however, has many disadvantages. The implant, which is clad only by a thin layer of skin and muscle, is often poorly camouflaged and leads to a round, "mechanical," unnaturally aptotic and asymmetric replacement. Peri-implant capsule contractures may impose further distortion, migration, asymmetry, and discomfort. Capsular fibrosis limits the fluidity of both saline and silicone implants. It is noticeable upon palpation and in its inability to react naturally to positional changes. This is especially

Table 11–3. IMPLANT COMPLICATIONS

	No XRT (%)	XRT (%)
Implant loss/extrusion	3.4–18	4–10
Deflation	3–4	
Infection	1.2–8	10
Capsule contracture	2.9–31	20
Skin necrosis	10–24	3–7
Satisfaction	80–98	49–55

XRT = external radiation beam therapy

apparent when lying supine, when the reconstructed breast remains fixed and projecting while the native breast falls naturally to the side. This represents the most common adverse postoperative development, occurring in 20 to 40 percent of all mastectomy patients and requiring operative intervention in up to 20 percent of cases.[58–59] Implant-based reconstruction may, therefore, be a less strategic option for younger patients. Kroll reported on 325 postmastectomy patients who had undergone either expander or autologous reconstruction. Complications occurred in 23 percent of expander patients, compared to 9 and 3 percent in latissimus and TRAM flap reconstructions, respectively.[60]

Implants are devices and are susceptible to device failure. It has been well demonstrated that the silicone elastomer shell of both silicone and saline implants fatigue over time. This may manifest itself as either a silicone or saline bleed and/or leak. An intracapsular silicone implant rupture is likely to remain undetected until some adverse event occurs. Most commonly, this may involve an increased tendency toward progressive capsular contracture. Blunt trauma resulting from a car, bicycle, or rollerblade incident, or even an overzealous mammogram, may convert a contained rupture into an extracapsular rupture. Patients typically notice a change in the shape and/or volume of the implant. This scenario warrants either mammographic, ultrasonic, or MRI imaging to rule out rupture.[38] Conversely, rupture of saline implants leads to implant deflation and a flat breast. In either case, implant replacement is warranted.

In contrast, autologous tissue has the warmth, consistency, feel, and reactive mobility of one's own tissues. It is a malleable, conformable, permanent medium that does not elicit a foreign body fibrotic response and is more tolerant of adjuvant therapy, trauma, and infection (Table 11–4). In contrast to the greater contracture and rupture rates of implants, autologous tissue softens and ages commensurate with adjacent structures and is therefore an ideal option for younger patients. An autologous flap may be contoured to match a contralateral breast of almost any size and shape. Although the initial overall cost of the flap reconstruction is greater, the long-term costs of autologous reconstruction have been shown to be less than those of prosthetic reconstruction due to subsequent secondary capsulotomies, revisions, and implant exchanges required with the latter procedure.

Autologous reconstruction is inherently more complex from both a technical and an artistic standpoint. The functional and esthetic outcome of the initial procedure, which lasts from 4 to 5 hours, largely depends upon the surgeon's experience and/or microsurgical expertise. Although the initial procedure requires a longer hospitalization (3 to 4 days) and postoperative recovery, the result is permanent and rarely requires a secondary adjunctive procedure. The TRAM flap is overwhelmingly the flap of choice when available. Alternatives include the latissimus dorsi, Ruben's or peri-iliac, lateral thigh, and gluteal flaps.

Table 11–4. ADVANTAGES OF AUTOLOGOUS RECONSTRUCTION

Soft
Warm
Pliable
Permanent
Enables wide resection
No foreign body response
Natural consistency and appearance
Tolerates adjuvant therapy well
Decreases need for symmetry procedure
More economic in the longterm

CONVENTIONAL TRANSVERSE RECTUS ABDOMINIS MYOCUTANEOUS FLAP

The transverse rectus abdominis myocutaneous flap, one of the most ingenious techniques in plastic surgery, has established itself over time as the flap of choice for autogenous breast reconstruction. It presents the reconstructive surgeon with the opportunity to a create a breast of unsurpassed esthetic beauty, is unparalleled in its ability to simulate the opposite breast, and secondarily improves the contour of the lower abdomen. Attaining consistently good results requires careful planning and technical proficiency. The lower abdomen consistently provides exceptional and sufficient tissue for unilateral and, in the majority of patients, bilateral breast reconstruction. The procedure is versatile and reliable when performed within its recognized vascular and volumetric constraints. Hartrampf's landmark introduction of the TRAM flap in 1982, still the gold standard for autologous breast reconstruction, provided the foundation for the modern era of breast reconstruction.[61]

The conventional, unipedicled TRAM flap, as originally described, consists of a transverse ellipse of skin and fat based on one rectus abdominis muscle and its intrinsic musculocutaneous perforators from the superior deep epigastric pedicle. The pedicle branches as it transgresses through the substance of the ipsilateral rectus through a network of "choke" vessels, which reconstitute in the midabdomen.[61–65] This inflow communicates with the periumbilical, myocutaneous perforators that supply the suprafacial and subcutaneous plexuses. Bostwick has determined that blood flow in the conventional TRAM is based upon pedicle caliber, number of perforators, integrity of the suprafascial plexus across the midline, and venous outflow.[64–65] Perfusion has been graded and is depicted as a sequence of zones, with zone VI, the most distal tissue, representing strictly random perfusion (Figure 11–5). Flow in the conventional TRAM is, therefore, secondary and unpredictable beyond the midline. Patient selection is critical and is limited, among experienced surgeons, to those patients who have tissue requirements met by the ipsilateral "hemi-TRAM."

In the uncomplicated case, the flap extends from the umbilicus to a point superior to the pubis. The incisions are beveled, after isolation of the umbilicus, to incorporate additional periumbilical perforators and subcutaneous fat. The flap is elevated at the suprafascial level toward the medial and lateral row of ipsilateral musculocutaneous perforators. The fascia is incised, immediately adjacent to the perforators, facilitating subsequence closure, and the underlying rectus is mobilized.

Most commonly, a full width muscle harvest with a thin strip of fascia is performed. The rectus muscle is elevated beneath the superior abdominal skin flap to the costal margin. The superior epigastric pedicle is easily identified, enabling transection of the lateral rectus fibers as well as of the intercostal nerves. This facilitates muscle atrophy and, thereby, minimizes the central xiphoid bulge, common initially after this procedure. The flap is transposed through a subcutaneous tunnel, which undermines the medial IMF, and is inset into the breast defect. Zones IV and II may be discarded prior to transposition to facilitate passage.

In an effort to preserve abdominal wall integrity, an alternative "split-muscle" harvest has been advocated.[66–68] Pedicle (muscle) width is based upon the laterality of the medial and lateral row of perforators. It is usually possible to preserve a substantial (one-third) width of the lateral rectus and often a slip of infraumbilical medial rectus. Although the muscle is, in most cases, denervated, it is thought to uphold the muscular interface of the semilunar line and adds fibrous stability in the perioperative period.

It is common practice to include a segment of skeletonized inferior epigastric pedicle in the event additional perfusion is necessary to sustain the flap.[69–70] This "lifeboat" enables sup-

plementary perfusion through a microvascular anastomosis, if intrinsic vascular insufficiency is noted. The flap is "supercharged" through an anastomosis, most commonly to an axillary recipient pedicle.

Fascial donor site closure is achieved with either interrupted figure-of-eight sutures or a running, heavy, braided, synthetic. The patient is then flexed to 45° to facilitate abdominal closure and ascertain breast symmetry. Typically, two drains are placed, both at the breast and abdominal sites. Postoperative flap monitoring is institution-specific and may encompass temperature probes, ultrasound or laser doppler, and clinical surveillance.

Optimal perioperative conditions are paramount to early and late flap success. Patient core temperature, intravascular fluid status, anxiety and pain level, and position may all have an impact on final outcome. If the start time is late in the day or there is minimal urine

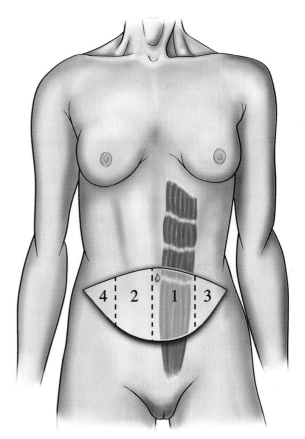

Figure 11–5. TRAM flap zones.

upon foley placement, an initial fluid bolus may be required. An intraoperative hourly urine output of 50 cc should be maintained to ensure adequate flap perfusion. In addition, maintenance of normothermia may minimize vascular vasoconstriction, spasm, and shivering, all of which may have an adverse impact on immediate postoperative flap perfusion. The use of heating blankets and fluid warmers is routine.

Use of the superiorly based unipedicle TRAM flap requires strict adherence to patient selection criteria. Obtaining consistent results demands an assessment of potential risk factors. It has been clearly demonstrated that patients who smoke, are obese, have significant abdominal scarring, or have had previous radiation have an increased risk of complications, including fat necrosis, partial flap failure, and donor site complications.[71–75] These risk factors should not eliminate patients from the procedure so much as indicate modification to enhance blood supply to the transferred tissue. For instance, nicotine from cigarette smoking has been recognized as a potent vasoconstrictor of the microcirculation. Patients who smoke or are unable to abstain 4 to 6 weeks prior to surgery are at extremely high risk for partial flap and donor site necrosis.[76] These patients, likely to fail conventional reconstruction, often succeed under the preface of a delay, bipedicle, or free technique.

Alternatively, the midabdominal TRAM was devised in response to a 20 to 60 percent of partial flap loss or fat necrosis and a high rate of hernia and abdominal wall weakness in high-risk patients.[77–78] This flap is based on the perforator-rich periumbilical region, and extends inferiorly to a tangent parallel to the anterior superior iliac spine (ASIS). Because muscle integrity is preserved below the arcuate lines, a lower incidence of hernia may be anticipated. Slavin's review of 236 midabdominal flaps showed a 2 percent rate of partial flap necrosis and a 1 percent incidence of fat necrosis.[77] The primary disadvantage is an occasionally displeasing high- or midabdominal scar and the lack of the abdominoplasty effect inherent in conventional TRAM.

Although largely supplanted by microsurgical advances, preoperative surgical delay of a conventional TRAM is another technique for augmenting reliable flap dimensions.[79–82] In 1995, Codner demonstrated improved inflow and diminished congestion after surgical delay.[82] Zones II and III proved more vigorous and reliable, especially in the high-risk patient, and lessened the need for a bipedicled approach. In 1997, Restifo documented greater pedicle caliber (1.3 versus 1.8 mm) and flow rates (7.5 versus 18.2 mL/min) compared to controls after surgical delay.[83] Staged interruption of the inferior epigastric pedicle, on a physiologic basis, is highly effective in augmenting vascularity and is beneficial in the high-risk patient.

Scars within the confines of the harvested flap, such as appendectomy, hernia, and midline scars, represent an ischemic boundary and will diminish the volume tissue available, due to variable vascular disruption. Regional incisions, such as paramedian, cholecystectomy, or extended Pfannenstiel's incisions may directly disrupt the pedicle and potentiate donor site complications. Shaw and colleagues assessed complications among TRAM patients with preexisting scars.[75] In 43 percent of the patients, abdominal wall weakness, partial flap loss, fat necrosis, and donor site morbidity developed. Paramedian scars precluded use of the free TRAM in three of three patients. Cholecystectomy scars and multiple scars showed the highest propensity toward skin-related complications. Conservatism, and often an alternative flap design, are warranted in patients with preexisting scars.

Operative assessment of the contralateral breast helps in formulating a reconstructive strategy and optimizing symmetry. The location and breadth of the IMF is a critical landmark and serves as the basis for building a symmetric breast. Attention to the condition and volume of retained skin (mastectomy skin flap), the size, shape, base width, and ptosis of the contralateral breast and how it relates to the IMF is necessary if symmetry is to be optimized. Patients with pre-existing macromastia may elect to undergo concurrent or delayed contralateral breast reduction, both to alleviate objective symptoms (shoulder pain and grooving, intertrigo, lower back pain) and improve the ultimate esthetic outcome. Patients with substantial glandular ptosis may elect to undergo mastopexy for similar reasons. It is the current authors' preference to perform these contralateral procedures as a second stage. Improved accuracy of a symmetry procedure may be attained after resolution of flap edema, muscle atrophy, and skin retraction. Staging also enables concurrent refinements (SAL, IMF revision) on the recently restored breast.

The goal of reconstructive surgeons using the TRAM flap for breast reconstruction is to increase the total efficiency, reduce operative morbidity, and to be able to offer patients an absolute minimum complication rate and hospital stay. Experience has demonstrated the vascular and volumetric constraints of the pedicled TRAM flap and led to technical refinements that are dependent upon individual patient risk factors.

FREE TRANSVERSE RECTUS ABDOMINIS MYOCUTANEOUS FLAP

The free TRAM flap, based on the dominant inferior epigastric blood supply and requiring a microvascular anastomosis, represents a reliable, versatile, highly esthetic option for both immediate and delayed reconstruction. The rationale for employing this option stems from its benefits in immediate reconstruction, where the ultimate goal of the reconstructive surgeon is to provide a highly desirable restoration, minimal complications, and an expeditious recovery that will remain invisible to the adjuvant therapeutic sequence (see Figure 11–5). Complications associated with conventional TRAM reconstruction, occurring in up to 25 percent of reported cases, are partial flap loss

and fat necrosis, and are inherent to the procedure's secondary blood supply and volume constraints.[57,66,73–76,84–86] These complications may impose prolonged wound healing and considerable delay in the therapeutic sequence. Although the free TRAM procedure requires greater technical proficiency and a slightly longer operating time, the flap has unparalleled vascular reliability and versatility, and is the flap of choice in high-risk patients. These include obese patients, smokers, and those patients with prohibitive scars or who have had prior radiation treatment.[73–76]

Suprafascial elevation is identical to that employed in the pedicled TRAM procedure. Widely dispersed perforators may be omitted due to the dominant inflow, thereby limiting the fascial harvest. The lateral edge of the rectus muscle is elevated to discern the path of the epigastric pedicle. This determines whether a medial and/or lateral muscular strip may be preserved. The pedicle is ligated at the external iliac origin. Axillary recipient vessels are normally reliable, even if prior radiation therapy has been implemented. Preference, in decreasing order, include the thoracodorsal, the circumflex scapular, lateral thoracic, and internal mammary vessels. This last option requires a peristernal costochondrectomy at the third rib interface for adequate exposure. An interrupted or running arterial microvascular anastomosis is typically performed with 9.0 nylon suture. Venous anastomosis may be similarly performed, or one may use an anastomotic coupling device (3M) for added speed. The occluding clamps are removed, and the quality of flap perfusion is confirmed both clinically and with the use of an intraoperative doppler.

Advantages of the free TRAM flap (Figures 11–6A, 11–6B) include a more limited abdominal harvest site, which corresponds to a more expeditious, often less uncomfortable postoperative recovery. The volume of rectus muscle harvested may be limited to a small cuff of fibers surrounding the perforators transgressing through the rectus muscles to supply the suprafascial and subcutaneous plexuses. Thus, a medial and/or lateral strip of rectus muscle may be preserved, which benefits young, active patients or those desiring future pregnancies. Use of the free TRAM enables preservation of an inframammary fold, does not compromise the marginal perfusion of the freshly elevated mastectomy skin flaps, optimizing the esthetic outcome. Freedom upon insetting, due to the absence of the conventional muscular "leash," facilitates a quick, easy, and highly cosmetic and symmetric reconstruction (Figures 11–7A, 11–7B). The improved blood supply may expedite wound healing and initiation of adjuvant therapy, which may also be better tolerated than in the conventional TRAM flap procedure.

The only absolute contraindications to free TRAM reconstruction include prohibitive scarring, violation of the inferior epigastric blood supply from previous abdominoplasty, suction lipectomy, extended Pfannenstiel's incision, or previous TRAM procedure. Pre-existing medical conditions may limit the patient's ability to tolerate 4 to 6 hours combined anesthesia time. This should be addressed preoperatively.

In a series of 211 free TRAM flaps, Schusterman reported a flap thrombosis rate of 3.3 percent and a flap loss rate of 1.4 percent.[87] One study compared outcome among conventional and free TRAM reconstruction. It was demonstrated that despite a higher percentage of high-risk patients (63 versus 28%), the free TRAM group had fever complications (9 versus 28%) than the conventional TRAM group. The advantages of the free TRAM procedure are outlined in Table 11–5.

The main disadvantage of TRAM flap reconstruction is the potential for weakening the abdominal wall. Questions remain as to the best technique of abdominal closure and the impact of free versus pedicled flap reconstruction on the abdominal wall. Despite all the advantages of the TRAM, it is a major surgical procedure and carries the risk of abdominal weakness, bulging, and hernia formation. True hernias resulting from the procedure are extremely rare (< 3% of cases). Abdominal wall bulges, indicating a separation and attenuation of the internal and external oblique muscles, occur more frequently (3 to 12% of cases).

Several studies have obtained objective measures of abdominal muscle strength. Trunk muscle strength as measured by an isoknetic dynamometer demonstrated postoperative recovery of 92, 96, and 98 percent at 3, 6, and 12 months, respectively, for unilateral free TRAM flap patients. Although the ability of one-half of the group to perform situps was not affected, the other half demonstrated mild impairment.[88] Kind and colleagues compared the recovery after pedicled and free TRAM reconstruction. Flexion torque as measured by dynamometer

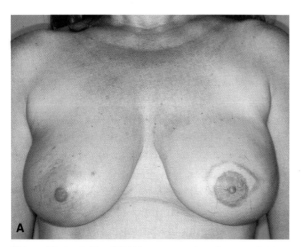 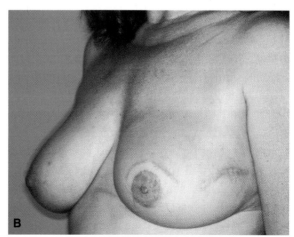

Figure 11–6. *A,* Free TRAM reconstruction; *B,* 9 months postoperative.

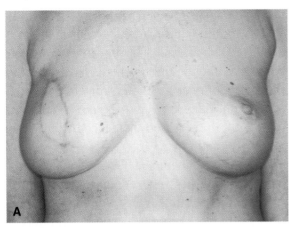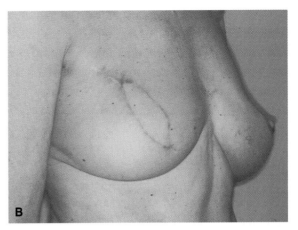

Figure 11–7. *A* and *B*, Right free TRAM reconstruction prior to nipple/areolar reconstruction.

was 58 and 89 percent at 6 weeks and 6 months, respectively, for conventional TRAMs. In contrast, the free TRAM showed 89 and 93 percent of preoperative flexion recovery at 6 weeks and 6 months respectively. The investigators concluded that the pedicled TRAM caused a significantly greater insult to the abdominal wall in the early postoperative period but that the two techniques equilibrated to over 90 percent of preoperative levels at 12 months. It was also determined that muscle splitting techniques appeared to offer no functional advantage.[89]

The ability of patients to perform situps after various modes of TRAM reconstruction has been studied. Percentages of patients able to perform a situp were 63.0, 57.1, 46, and 27 percent for the single free TRAM, conventional TRAM, bilateral free flap, and conventional flap, respectively.[90] Fitoussi reported that 47 percent of single pedicle TRAM and 0 percent of bipedicle TRAM patients could perform situps postoperatively and concluded that although the hernia rate did not vary between the two groups, functional sequellae were statistically significant.[91]

Hernias occur in 5 to 6 percent of TRAM patients, regardless of whether the procedure was conventional or free, uni- or bipedicled. The incidence appears more closely associated with the technique and detail of abdominal closure rather than with the number or extent of muscles harvested. Various modifications, outlined below, appear to have a positive impact.

Approximation of the medial and lateral remnants of the tendinous inscriptions appears to "restore the ribs" of abdominal support and relieve tension on the anterior rectus sheath.[92] Primary repair of the fascial defect should include approximation of the underlying muscular support. Kroll advocates approximation of the anterior remnant of the internal oblique to the linea alba and a reinforcing two-layer closure. Fascial sheath closure is strengthened with sutures through the semilunar line.[93]

Abdominal wall complications are probably best avoided through recognizing excessive tension during closure or undue attenuation of weakened fascia. The threshold for mesh reinforcement should correlate positively with these findings. Mesh enables reinforcement without excess tension and may facilitate postoperative mobility, diminish pain, and expedite recovery. The infection rate after using mesh is reported to be < 2 percent and is usually a result of other miscalculations that result in exposure through marginal dehiscence or necrosis.

Table 11–5. ADVANTAGES OF FREE TRAM

Primary and dominant blood supply
Greater available volume
Less muscle harvest/abdominal dissection
More comfortable recovery
More reliable in high-risk patients
Greater freedom in insetting
Good tolerance to adjuvant therapy

The other complication that has led to considerable investigation and comparison between TRAM techniques is the incidence of fat necrosis. Kroll and colleagues reported in 1998 on the incidence of fat necrosis among patients who had had conventional versus free TRAM reconstruction. Of the 49 free TRAM patients, 8.2 percent exhibited clinical fat necrosis, with one patient showing mammographic evidence. Of the 67 pedicled TRAM patients, 27 percent demonstrated fat necrosis on examination and nine patients on mammogram.[94]

BIPEDICLED TRANSVERSE RECTUS ABDOMINIS MYOCUTANEOUS FLAP

A unipedicled conventional TRAM will reliably perfuse all of zone I, 20 percent of zone II, and 80 percent of zone III.[95] An alternative technique or flap choice is warranted if tissue requirements exceed these specifications. Indications for a bipedicled TRAM include those patients who insist on autogenous reconstruction, who require additional volume, and for whom microsurgical reconstruction is not possible due to an absence of reasonable recipient axillary vessels. The indications parallel those for surgical vascular delay.

The lower abdominal pannus is isolated on the medial and lateral row of perforators, bilaterally. Once the upper abdominal apron is elevated, each superior epigastric pedicle is isolated with the assistance of doppler mapping, and a split bipedicle muscle harvest is performed. The flap is transposed and inset in much the same way as for an unipedicled TRAM flap.

Multiple reports have investigated the long- and short-term impact of bilateral rectus harvest. Hartrampf reported that 64 percent of patients could not perform a single situp after bipedicled reconstruction, compared to 17 percent in the unipedicled group. Petit reported a 20 percent incidence of subsequent severe back pain in bipedicled patients.[96]

The bipedicled flap has reduced the incidence of partial flap loss and fat necrosis in much the same manner as the free technique. The use of mesh has markedly reduced the incidence of abdominal hernia formation and bulging. Although these patients have objective loss of abdominal function, subjective interference with daily activity is rare. There are reports of an increased incidence of long-term lower back pain.

Use of the bipedicled TRAM for unilateral reconstruction has invoked substantial controversy in the plastic surgery literature. Antagonists claim the morbidity from bilateral muscle harvest, including abdominal wall weakness and the propensity toward future back pain, "can no longer be defended" in the current realm of reliable microsurgical capability and surgical delay.[97] Conversely, proponents claim that the split muscle technique and addition of mesh reinforcement limit functional morbidity and that the resultant abdominal wall integrity is dependent upon the closure technique used.[98] They adhere to its use as a reliable alternative in high-risk patients.

LATISSIMUS DORSI

The latissimus dorsi myocutaneous flap was originally described by Tansini in 1906 and used to cover radical mastectomy defects.[99] It has since demonstrated remarkable versatility and is useful in providing purely autogenous, composite implant, and partial mastectomy reconstruction (Figure 11–8). The straightforward anatomy, easy elevation, relative lack of donor morbidity, and ability to provide an additional "curtain" of conforming tissue have made it a reasonable adjunct to breast reconstruction, most commonly in healthy patients considering expander reconstruction.

The indications for latissimus reconstruction vary widely and depend upon the preferences and capabilities of the surgeon. Several subsets exist, all governed by the assumption that a TRAM flap has been ruled out for either medical, anatomic, or personal reasons. The first set includes those patients who are otherwise appropriate candidates for expander reconstruction but for whom less than optimal coverage is predicted. This may include patients who have had a prior radical mastectomy and lack a pectoralis, those who have thin mastectomy skin flaps, or those who require a large skin resection due to inclusive resection of a remote biopsy site or to prior radiation.

The second set includes those patients amenable to expander reconstruction who have sufficient coverage and high esthetic expectations. The challenge in unilateral postmastectomy expander reconstruction is to provide a breast form which simulates the contralateral side. Prosthetic reconstruction provides a round, firm, relatively immobile breast form which is ideally suited for patients with small to intermediate sized breast and limited to no ptosis. Patients who are moderate or large in size and develop some degree of ptosis with age and childbirth will demonstrate variable asymmetry with unilateral prosthetic reconstruction. These non-TRAM candidates may elect to undergo either contralateral mastopexy or composite latissimus-expander reconstruction for improved symmetry. The flap provides supplemental muscle and fat, which helps camouflage the underlying prosthesis and replaces the resected skin, leading to a more natural ptotic breast form.

The third category includes those patients who prefer an autogenous restoration but lack flap alternatives due to medical or surgical reasons. Most patients have a breast volume in excess of their available flank tissue and require supplemental volume in the form of an implant. The resultant satisfaction in esthetic outcome and greater projection and natural ptosis allay most patient's preoperative reluctance toward a supplemental implant.

The fourth and fifth sets involve autogenous latissimus reconstruction without supplemental prosthesis and apply to two patient extremes where the available flank tissue volume simulates breast volume. Solely autogenous latissimus reconstruction is routinely possible in heavier patients having substantial upper flank tissue. These patients typically have redundant flank skin and additional subcutaneous bulk that may be incorporated into the flap to provide necessary volume and ptosis. Conversely, patients with marked breast hypoplasia may also attain sufficient volume, contour, and symmetry from a purely autogenous latissimus myocutaneous flap.

The flap has an extremely reliable blood supply and is versatile even in smokers and diabetics. Partial flap necrosis has been reported in up to 7 percent of patients.[100] The most common nuisance is the persistence of seromas, which often requires prolonged drainage or aspiration. Implant-related complications include implant slippage and capsule contracture. Use of textured, saline expanders and implants has reduced these complications.

The latissimus dorsi flap represents a popular, extremely reliable option for the mastectomy patient. The results are outstanding, when used in conjunction with the newer textured, anatomic saline expanders and implants, typically better than those achieved with expanders alone.

RUBENS FLAP

Peter Paul Rubens was known for his portraits of females with particular fullness in the suprailiac region. The skin and subcutaneous tissue in this region may be sustained by the deep circumflex iliac artery, as originally

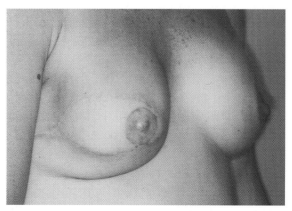

Figure 11–8. Latissimus dorsi myocutaneous flap reconstruction.

described by Taylor.[101] Hartrampf coined this peri-iliac fat pad the "Rubens flap."[102]

The TRAM is the flap of choice in autologous breast reconstruction. One of the benefits of the TRAM flap is the performance of a concurrent abdominoplasty, with resection of often large volumes of infraumbilical tissue. It is with some bewilderment that patients complain of a greater lower abdominal circumference, not a reduction, and have greater difficulty wearing their previously well-fitted clothing. Closing the anterior TRAM donor site leads to accentuation of the peri-iliac tissue and can cause an actual increase in the peri-iliac circumference. This redundancy represents the tissue available for free tissue transfer after a previous TRAM flap. The predominant indication for use of the Rubens flap is therefore a prior TRAM harvest or abdominoplasty. Other indications for use of the Rubens flap include thin patients and prohibitive anterior abdominal scars.

Flap dissection requires a precise knowledge and familiarity with the intrinsic support of the abdominal wall. The primary disadvantage of the flap is the occurrence of an occasional flank hernia. Compulsive closure of the donor site is paramount to the success of this procedure and requires a dedicated surgeon to do so. Other potential morbidity includes longstanding seromas that require prolonged drainage and compression garments. Patients with this problem also have a higher incidence of prolonged discomfort and often require monitored physical therapy.

The flap is oriented parallel to the iliac crest, with two-thirds of the skin paddle above and one-third below the crest (Figure 11–9A). An inguinal incision lateral to the femoral pulse will expose the external oblique. Once this is incised, the round ligament is identified and retracted superiorly to expose the inguinal floor. An incision through the internal oblique, transversalis, and transversalis fascia will expose the underlying deep circumflex iliac vessels. This helps guide the remainder of the flap dissection. Once the skin and fat are cut,

the muscle layers are cut immediately adjacent to the pedicle. The inferior skin flap is elevated above the tensor of fascia lata to the iliac crest. Subperiosteal dissection will ensure the integrity of both the deep circumflex iliac artery (DCIA) pedicle and perforators. The lateral femoral cutaneous nerve runs inferiorly, within 1 cm of the anterior superior iliac spine, and may lie either above or below the DCIA. This nerve should be preserved.

Donor site closure is initiated by approximation of the transversalis fascia to the iliopsoas fascia. The remaining flank muscles are secured to the iliac crest through drill holes and heavy suture or wire.

Deep circumflex iliac artery pedicle length facilitates anastomosis to the preferred thoracodorsal vessels in the majority of cases. This flap tends to be less robust than the TRAM and may exhibit a weak doppler signal, at best. The flap provides excellent projection (Figure 11–9B) and is an ideal option for bilateral reconstruction, which may be performed simultaneously, concurrent with mastectomy.

SUPERIOR GLUTEAL FLAP

The superior gluteal flap was the first free flap described for breast reconstruction.[103] Microsurgical expertise is essential for success due to a tedious flap dissection, an inherently short vascular pedicle, and because the microanastomoses are most commonly performed to the delicate and variable internal mammary vessels.[104]

Candidates include patients who fail qualification for implants due to prior chest-wall irradiation or "implant anxiety" or who have abdominal scars precluding TRAM reconstruction. Such scars may have resulted from laparotomies, enterotomies, previous abdominoplasties, liposuction, or TRAM harvests. This flap may represent the only autogenous option in thin patients who lack sufficient abdominal or lateral thigh tissue for unilateral or bilateral reconstruction.

Like the TRAM, the gluteal flap offers a permanent, soft, warm, and natural reconstruction. It has a more dense fat–septal network, providing an intermediate size reconstruction with excellent projection. It may be the flap of choice for patients who have had a previous TRAM and require a staged contralateral mastectomy. It also offers an inconspicuous donor site.

Flap dimensions typically extend from the lateral midsacrum to within 5 cm of the ASIS. The verticle height of the flap depends on the tissue needed but may vary from 10 to 15 cm. Flap dissection necessitates identification of the fragile superior gluteal vessels deep to the gluteus muscle. This pedicle emerges from the greater sciatic foramen amidst numerous branches and provides 1.5 to 2.0 cm of pedicle length. The internal mammary vessels are exposed and mobilized through a third peristernal rib resection. The external jugular vein, rotated down from the mandibular angle, may serve as a venous alternative if internal mammary vein integrity is lacking.

Like its counterpart, the inferior gluteal flap is indicated in rare patients who refuse prosthetic reconstruction and who are not candidates for either TRAM, lateral thigh, or latissimus flaps. Although the length of the donor inferior gluteal vessels enable anastomosis to the more forgiving thoracodorsal pedicle and the donor site scar is the least conspicuous of any autogenous option, harvest necessitates sacrifice of the gluteal motor nerve, occasional sacrifice of the posterior cutaneous nerve, and close dissection to the sciatic nerve, all of which may lead to transient pain syndromes and weakness with ambulation; prolonged rehabilitation may be required. For these reasons, the gluteal flap is generally the least favored flap in the breast reconstruction algorithm.

LATERAL THIGH FLAPS

The lateral transverse thigh flap and tensor of fascia lata flap are two reconstructive variants that are based upon the lateral femoral circumflex vessels and make use of the lateral "riding breeches" or "saddle bags."[105] The pedicle transgresses through and requires the sacrifice of the modest tensor muscle. Preservation of adjacent fascia lata helps to ensure lateral knee stability without functional compromise. More imposing, and representing the primary disadvantage, are the often disfiguring lateral thigh scars, which are long and remain poorly camouflaged.

Preoperative design requires experience and precision. An excessive subcutaneous harvest will result in objectionable lateral thigh contour deficits. These are difficult to correct but do

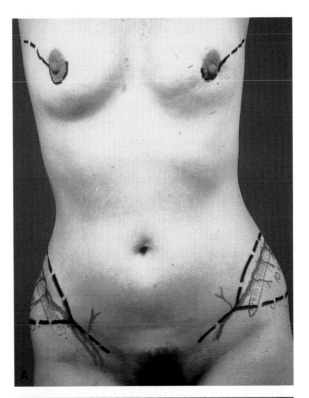

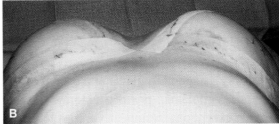

Figure 11–9. Ruben's flap *A,* Bilateral flap design; *B,* Immediate postoperative projection demonstrated. Reproduced with permission from William W. Shaw, MD, Division of Plastic Surgery, UCLA.

benefit from delayed suction lipectomy. Patients may require prolonged drainage and garment compression to limit the tendency toward seroma formation. Advantages include a 7 to 8 cm vascular pedicle, excellent flap projection, and the ability to perform concurrent bilateral simultaneous harvests and reconstruction.

BILATERAL BREAST RECONSTRUCTION

Indications for contralateral prophylactic mastectomy include a strong family history of breast cancer, positive genetic testing, lobular carcinoma in situ (LCIS), cancer anxiety, and equivocal or progressively difficult clinical and/or radiographic examinations.

With improvements in breast cancer screening, a greater number of early breast cancers are being detected in young, premenopausal patients, many of whom have some degree of familial cancer history. Patients with young families present with the intent to absolve breast cancer risk for the benefit of their young ones and represent a new indication for either prophylactic or bilateral mastectomy. Breast cancer awareness has elevated the level of sophistication of all patients. Prosthetic and autologous reconstruction is a known entity that continues to become more reliable, safe, and esthetically satisfying. As this awareness becomes more apparent and outcomes improve, it is not surprising that an increasing number of susceptible women are at least questioning the option of bilateral ablation and immediate reconstruction.

Esthetic outcome is often better in bilateral reconstruction than in unilateral reconstruction due to the symmetry achieved. Macromastia and pseudoptosis are not compounding factors since skin redundancy may be addressed symmetrically. Bilateral implants and/or permanent expander implants, postmastectomy, usually provide exceptional results, in contrast to unilateral procedures, which exaggerate implant characteristics. Postoperative adjustability ensures a symmetric result. This is ideal for the older patient or the patient with marginal reserve who desires to avoid an external prosthesis and could not tolerate a long, grueling procedure.

The TRAM flap, once again, is the flap of choice, providing reliability and minimal morbidity in bilateral autologous reconstruction (Figure 11–10). Sufficient tissue is present for bilateral reconstruction in 75 to 80 percent of patients. The majority of patients when advised of the ability to perform an immediate, single-stage, highly esthetic and symmetric, permanent, bilateral autogenous reconstruction, and simultaneously rid themselves of an often pervasive lower abdominal pannus, are, most often, highly grateful and not overly concerned about the possibility of having slightly smaller breasts if less than profound amounts of tissue are available. Advantages of bilateral TRAM reconstruction include the ability to perform a simultaneous harvest in the supine position.

Either bilateral conventional or free TRAMS may be performed. The vascular reliability of bilateral "hemi-TRAM" flaps is normally adequate, because cross perfusion across the midline is not necessary, depending on an absence of excessive scarring, obesity, prior radiation, and history of smoking. Use of the conventional flaps is usually faster and technically simpler than free TRAM reconstruction but requires inherent sacrifice of both rectus muscles, which may lead to objective and subjective abdominal wall weakness in the majority of more active patients. Extensive superior abdominal dissection and tunneling is required and may prolong postoperative discomfort and recovery. Transposition of bilateral flaps may lead to an upper abdominal bulge and violate some aspect of both inframammary folds, compromising final cosmesis.

The advantages of bilateral free TRAM reconstruction include limited muscle harvest, limited upper abdominal dissection (which minimizes discomfort and expedites recovery), unparalleled esthetic outcome, and a greater tolerance to adjuvant radiation if deemed necessary. Lateral extension of these free "hemi-flaps" may be incorporated to boost tissue volume in thin patients and is made possible by the exceptional blood supply. Assuming the presence of suitable recipient vessels and sufficient experience of the reconstructive team, free TRAM reconstruction for bilateral restoration is usually preferred for the ultimate benefit of the patient. The incidence of abdominal wall bulging and hernia formation is similar for free and conventional bilateral reconstruction and is dependent upon the security and detail of the abdominal closure. Some surgeons perform a mild bowel prep preoperatively to facilitate closure in bilateral cases. The potential to exclude medial, diminutive, or outlying perforators in bilateral free reconstruction facilitates fascial closure without the use of mesh. Although it is reported that mesh may be avoided in 60 to 80 percent of patients having bilateral TRAM reconstruction, the use of a more relaxed closure using mesh may facilitate postoperative comfort, recovery, and return of bowel motility. Prolene mesh is currently the authors' preferred choice for reinforcement. Closure may be facilitated by a preoperative bowel prep, the appropriate use of relaxing agents, avoidance of nitrous oxide (which can lead to bowel dilitation) and the use of lateral external oblique relaxing incisions. The incidence of true hernias is rare. Lower abdominal attenuation or abdominal wall bulging occurs in 4.4 to 20 percent of cases.

RECONSTRUCTION OF THE PARTIAL MASTECTOMY DEFECT

Breast conserving surgery combined with adjuvant radiation has been accepted as a regime equivalent to modified radical mastectomy for early stage (I and II) breast cancer. The technique is popular due to its ability to eradicate breast cancer while preserving a maximal volume of breast tissue.

Skin incisions are designed directly over the lesion, and skin and subcutaneous tissues are preserved unless involved in the lesion. Closure involves subcuticular closure only and the

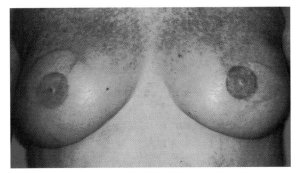

Figure 11–10. Bilateral free TRAM reconstruction.

avoidance of drains. The resulting deformity after lumpectomy or quadrantectomy depends on initial breast size, tumor size and location, radiation dose, surgical technique, and adjuvant chemotherapy. The relative excision, in proportion to breast size, is perhaps the most important factor. Patients with large, pendulous breasts may easily accommodate a 4 cm lumpectomy. The same resection in a smaller-breasted woman may lead to an unacceptable cosmetic result. Radiation therapy exaggerates the tissue deficit in the form of ischemic fibrous contracture.

The treated breast is subject to edema, retraction, fibrosis, calcification, hyperpigmentation, depigmentation, telangiectasia formation, and atrophy. It is not until 24 to 36 months postradiation that radiation-induced changes stabilize. Initial edema camouflages the initial deficit and is replaced with fibrosis and contracture that tends to worsen with time. Deficits within the lower pole tend to retract upward. Deficits along the superomedial aspect of the breast are difficult to camouflage due to the paucity of available adjacent tissue and are, unfortunately, socially conspicuous. Centrally located lesions are more forgiving unless resection involves some aspect of the nipple-areolar complex.

An assessment of the patient's overall oncologic risk for recurrence should be considered prior to any attempt at partial mastectomy reconstruction. Breast cancer history, the nature of the inciting lesion, and the patient's family history should be reviewed prior to an additional procedure that may further affect subsequent screening examinations. In any event, stabilization of the breast appearance is a prerequisite and occurs 1 to 3 years postradiation.

Investigators have attempted to classify the spectrum of partial mastectomy deficits and relate them to specific treatment options. Classification is based upon the localized deficit of skin and glandular tissue, malposition and/or distortion of the areola, and the extent of fibrous contracture of the breast.[106] Local flap transposition is recommended for mild deformities, whereas myocutaneous flaps are reserved for more extensive defects.

Approximately 15 percent of patients treated with BCT are not content with the esthetic outcome.[107] These patients often seek consultation to improve selfesteem and body image. Careful assessment of the actual and apparent tissue deficits are crucial in the selection of the appropriate reconstructive strategy. Contour deficits signify substantial parenchymal loss, whereas radiation contracture represents extensive cutaneous deficits. Nipple-areolar distortion necessitates a substantial increase in cutaneous replacement, as central areolar support requires dermal rather than subcutaneous support.

The majority of patients are poor candidates for implant reconstruction. Cutaneous fibrosis responds poorly to implant displacement, and implant radio-opacity impairs an already complex screening examination. Autologous tissues, conversely, are reliable, versatile, and provide all the components necessary for partial restoration. The inherent vascularity may actually improve the quality of the relatively ischemic and radiated recipient tissue.

Large central excisions involving the nipple-areolar complex and primary closure take on a flat, attenuated appearance, lacking projection. These defects may be reconstructed in one of two ways. It may be possible to mobilize a skin glandular flap based on inferolateral perforators from the underlying pectoral fascia, which is then mobilized into the defect. The curvilinear incision extends from the inferomedial aspect of the previous areola to the central inframammary fold. All but a central skin paddle, rotated into

the areolar defect, is de-epithelialized. Primary skin closure is facilitated by undermining at the parenchymal interface. The second technique parallels conventional mastopexy and enables superior advancement of an inferior dermoglandular pedicle. It is performed through a Wise or keyhole pattern incision.[106,108–109]

Upper outer quadrant excisions are the most frequent and, fortunately, the most forgiving.[106,108–109] The great majority of these excisions do not require reconstruction. Occasionally, delayed augmentation, scar lengthening via Z-plasty, and areolar transposition are indicated. If a discrepancy between the medial and lateral breast quadrant is recognized due to a substantial superolateral resection, immediate centralization of the nipple-areolar complex over the point of maximal projection is warranted. This involves simple areolar transposition after release of the dermal attachments. Wide excisions may require transfer of regional or distant tissue. The latissimus dorsi myocutaneous flap represents the ideal choice for these defects (Figure 11–11).

Partial inferior defects may be corrected on an immediate or delayed basis. The occasional patient, lacking significant radiation change, may benefit from delayed insertion of a small round or custom (one-third) implant for volume replacement. Most defects, however, benefit from a procedure that parallels a standard superior pedicle reduction mammoplasty.[108–109] The resection and reconstruction are facilitated through a standard keyhole pattern. Medial and

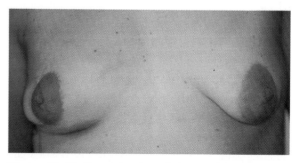

Figure 11–11. Reconstruction of the partial mastectomy defect. Superolateral reconstruction with latissimus dorsi myocutaneous flap.

lateral parenchymal flaps are mobilized from the pectoralis fascia and inframammary fold and mobilized into the inferior defect, whether it be lateral, central, or medial.

Supra-areolar defects are socially conspicuous and necessitate local reconstruction due to the paucity of available adjacent tissue and the tendency to develop a visible and depressed scar. These defects are corrected by superior advancement of the areolar complex, based on an inferior pedicle, in a procedure similar to an inferior pedicle reduction mammoplasty.[106,108–109]

The latissimus dorsi myocutaneous flap represents the flap of choice for the majority of partial mastectomy defects. Its regional location, malleability, ease of dissection, and lack of donor site morbidity are ideally suited for this indication. All breast conservation defects should be reconstructed by overcorrecting the skin and soft tissue deficits. In general, *twice* the apparent tissue loss should be inset to compensate for normal wound contracture, continued retraction of the postradiation fibrosis, and anticipated muscle atrophy inherent in raising muscle flaps. The muscle may be folded and contoured to accommodate the most irregular defects. Although small skin paddles may be harvested to precisely accommodate the apparent skin deficit, a typical 4 × 6 cm skin paddle facilitates flap harvest and replacement of compromised or contracted radiated skin.

Although partial latissimus harvests are possible, the majority of partial mastectomy defects warrant total flap elevation. Preservation of the thoracodorsal nerve will maintain greater muscle bulk but lead to early postoperative contractions. Compulsive fixation at the recipient site is necessary to avoid disruption. Transection or resection of the muscular insertion will help avoid the typical bulge within the anterior axilla. Finally, supporting the radiated native breast skin with a de-epithelialized portion of the transposed skin paddle will improve ultimate wound contour.

The TRAM flap represents a flap of substantial bulk, typically incurring greater donor site morbidity and a longer recovery. It would appear less economic in restoration of limited tissue defects. It is indicated for the reconstruction of large inferior pole deficits in large-breasted women.

Continued surveillance for recurrent cancer after partial reconstruction should proceed unimpeded. Studies comparing pre- and postoperative mammograms after partial reconstruction have confirmed the radiolucency of these flaps. The development of new microcalcifications, fat necrosis, and new lesions are easily discernible. Some reports, interestingly, have noted improved mammographic visualization and resolution of breast density and fibrosis as a result of improved local vascularity.

Immediate reconstruction of partial mastectomy defects is gaining popularity. The demand for these techniques has evolved due to a tendency toward more aggressive resection in BCT and accumulated experience with unfavorable tumors. Petit and colleagues reported that immediate reconstruction of the partial mastectomy defect was performed in 25 percent of cases. They advocated close preoperative collaboration to optimize cosmetic results and enable "improved radicality" of the surgical breast conservation.[110] Thus, the potential for immediate partial mastectomy reconstruction facilitates a more aggressive resection or marginal clearance in BCT and may lessen the need and/or frequency of re-excision. Also, it may lessen the need for staged reconstruction following radiation-induced exaggeration of the defect.

NIPPLE-AREOLAR RECONSTRUCTION

Nipple-areolar reconstruction is a critical stage in breast reconstruction and may add remarkable realism to the new breast mound (Figure 11–12). Areolar tattooing facilitates symmetry in color, may camouflage minor discrepancies and scars, and lacks the morbidity associated with skin grafts. Nipple reconstruction is typically performed at a second stage, at the time of port removal, or breast mound revision.

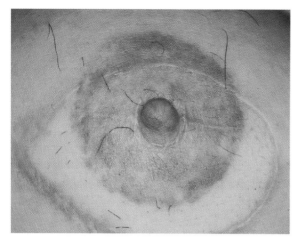

Figure 11–12. Completed nipple-areolar reconstruction.

Although single-stage reconstruction may be performed, attaining symmetry of nipple-areolar position is crucial to esthetic outcome and is most accurately attained at a second stage, when dermal edema and skin elasticity have normalized.

The insensate, adynamic nipple remains static in size, contour, and projection and will likely be visualized through undergarments, swimsuits, and clothing. The patient's final assessment and perception may closely parallel the quality and symmetry of the newly constructed nipple. Consideration of a symmetry procedure should, therefore, be entertained prior to final nipple reconstruction and should encompass whether the patient prefers support (bra) and to what extent. Simulation in a bra or sheer blouse preoperatively may help the patient's understanding of these issues.

Various techniques of nipple reconstruction are available and provide a range of caliber potential projection. Modification, reduction, or composite grafting of the contralateral nipple may be considered as an option in the patient with redundant nipples. Although this represents the most realistic reconstruction, it necessitates a procedure on the remaining intact nipple and is sensitive perioperatively.

Local flaps are the technique of choice for nipple reconstruction, most of which are variants of the original skate flap. The skate flap has proven to be a reliable workhorse, with the potential for a long projectile nipple if needed.[109] The donor site does require a skin graft, most commonly harvested from the groin, inner thigh, or axilla. Precise demarcation of the central nipple complex is critical and serves as a basis for dermal flap elevation. The lateral dermal wings are elevated, preserving the central nipple core and an inferior extension of fat. These components are elevated, preserving the subcutaneous perforators, and then surfaced by the lateral wings. The circular de-epithelialized harvest site is then covered with a full thickness skin graft.

The Star flap,[111] C-V flap,[112] fishtail flap (McCraw), and double opposing tab flap (Kroll) are additional flap options, most of which are modifications of the skate flap. Although they provide less nipple projection than does the skate flap, they avoid the need for a skin graft. These are excellent alternatives for the majority of patients with small to moderate sized contralateral nipples.

Intradermal areolar tattoo has greatly simplified the final phase of restoration and adds abrupt and striking realism to the physical breast form. It remains an artistic challenge among surgeons to simulate contralateral areolar pigment. This final phase enables the surgeon one additional opportunity to optimize symmetry. Nipple-areolar reconstruction may enhance the focus of the reconstructed breast and improve overall patient incorporation of the reconstructed breast, both physically and psychologically.

REFERENCES

1. Ernster VL, Barclay J, Kerlikowske K, et al. Incidence of and treatment for ductal carcinoma in situ of the breast. JAMA 1996;275:913–8.
2. Grisotti A. Conservative treatment of breast cancer. In: Spear S, editor. The breast: principles and art. Philadelphia: Lippincott-Raven; 1998. p. 137.
3. Goldwyn RM. Vincenz Czerny and the beginnings of breast reconstruction. Plast Reconstr Surg 1978;61:673–81.

4. Georgiade G, Georgiade N, McKarty KS Jr, et al. Rationale for immediate reconstruction of the breast following modified radical mastectomy. Ann Plast Surg 1982;8:20–28.

5. Rosenqvist S, Sandelin K, Wickman M. Patients' psychological and cosmetic experience after immediate breast reconstruction. Eur J Surg Oncol 1996;22:262–6.

6. Wellisch DK, Schain WS, Noone RB, et al. Psychosocial correlates of immediate versus delayed reconstruction of the breast. Plast Reconstr Surg 1985;76:713–8.

7. Shover LR, Yetman RJ, Tuason LJ, et al. Partial mastectomy and breast reconstruction. A comparison of their effects on psychosocial adjustment, body image, and sexuality. Cancer 1995;75:54–64.

8. Noguchi M, Kitagawa H, Kinoshita K, et al. Psychologic and self-assessments of breast conserving therapy compared with mastectomy and immediate breast reconstruction. J Surg Oncol 1993;54:260–6.

9. Toth BA, Lappert P. Modified skin incisions for mastectomy: the need for plastic surgery input in pre-operative planning. Plast Reconstr Surg 1991;87:1048–53.

10. Kroll SS, Ames F, Singletary SE, et al. The oncologic risks of skin preservation at mastectomy when combined with immediate reconstruction of the breast. Surg Gynecol Obstet 1991; 172:17–20.

11. Newman LA, Keurer HM, Hunt KK, et al. Presentation, treatment, and outcome of local recurrence after skin sparing mastectomy and immediate breast reconstruction. Ann Surg Oncol 1998;5:620–6.

12. Hidalgo DA. Aesthetic refinement in breast reconstruction: complete skin sparing mastectomy with autogenous tissue transfer. Plast Reconstr Surg 1998;102:63–70.

13. Carlson GW, Bostwick J, Styblo TM, et al. Skin sparing mastectomy: oncologic and reconstructive considerations. Ann Surg 1997;225:570–75.

14. Yule GJ, Concannon MJ, Croll G, et al. Is there liability with chemotherapy following immediate breast reconstruction? Plast Reconstr Surg 1996;97:969–73.

15. Grotting JC, Urist MM, Maddox WA, Vasconez LO. Conventional TRAM flap versus free microsurgical TRAM flap for immediate reconstruction. Plast Reconstr Surg 1989;84(6):1005–6.

16. Elliott LF, Eskenazi L, Beegle PH Jr, et al. Immediate TRAM flap breast reconstruction: 128 consecutive cases. Plast Reconstr Surg 1993; 92:217–27.

17. Schuster RH, Kuske RB, Young VL, Fineberg B. Breast reconstruction in women treated with radiation therapy for breast cancer: cosmesis, complications, and tumor control. Plast Reconstr Surg 1992;90:445–52.

18. Evans GR, Schusterman MA, Kroll SS, et al. Reconstruction and the radiated breast: is there a role for implants? Plast Reconstr Surg 1995; 96:1111–5.

19. Spear S, Majidian A. Immediate breast reconstruction in 2 stages using textured integrated-valve tissue expanders and breast implants: a retrospective review of 171 consecutive breast reconstructions from 1989–1996. Plast Reconstr Surg 1998;101:53–63.

20. Jackson WB, Goldson AL, Staud C. Post-operative irradiation following immediate breast reconstruction using a temporary tissue expander. J Natl Med Assoc 1994;86:538–42.

21. Dickson MG, Sharpe BT. The complications of tissue expansion in breast reconstruction: a review of 75 cases. Br J Plast Surg 1987;40:629–35.

22. Jacobson GM, Sause WT, Thompson JW, Plenk HP. Breast irradiation following silicone gel implants. Int J Radiat Oncol Biol Phys 1986; 12:835–8.

23. Chu FC, Kaufman TP, Dawson GA, et al. Radiation therapy of cancer in prosthetically augmented or reconstructed breasts. Radiology 1992;185:429–33.

24. Spear S. Prosthetic reconstruction in the radiated breast. In: Spear S, editor. The breast: principles and art. Philadelphia: Lippincott-Raven; 1998. p. 399–406.

25. Zimmerman RP, Mark RJ, Kim AL, et al. Radiation tolerance of transverse rectus myocutaneous free flaps used in immediate breast reconstruction. Am J Clin Oncol 1998;21:381–5.

26. Hunt KK, Baldwin BJ, Strom EA, et al. Feasibility of post-mastectomy radiation therapy after TRAM flap breast reconstruction. Ann Surg Oncol 1997;4:377–84.

27. Sultan MR, Smith ML, Estabrook A, et al. Immediate breast reconstruction in patients with locally advanced disease. Ann Plast Surg 1997;38:345–9.

28. Styblo TM, Lewis MM, Carlson GW, et al. Immediate breast reconstruction for stage III breast cancer using transverse rectus myocutaneous flaps. Ann Surg Oncol 1998;3:375–80.

29. Brody GS. Safety and effectiveness of breast

implants. In: Spear S, editor. The breast: principles and art. Philadelphia: Lippincott-Raven; 1998. p. 336–46.

30. Peters W, Keystone E, Snow K, et al. Is there a relationship between autoantibodies and silicone gel implants? Ann Plast Surg 1994;32:1–5.

31. Kossovsky N, Heggers JP, Robson MC. Experimental demonstration of the immunogenicity of silicone protein complexes. J Biomed Mater Res 1987;21:1125–33.

32. Heggers JP, Kossovsky N, Parsons RW, et al. Biocompatibility of silicone implants. Ann Plast Surg 1983;11:38–45.

33. DeCamara DI, Sheridam SM, Kammer BA. Rupture and aging of silicone breast implants. Plast Reconstr Surg 1993;91:828–34.

34. Greenwald WB, Randolph M, May JW. Mechanical analysis of explanted silicone breast implants. Plast Reconstr Surg 1996;98:269–72.

35. Phillips JW, Decamara DL, Lockwood MD, et al. Strength of silicone breast implants. Plast Reconstr Surg 1996;97:1215–25.

36. Robinson OG, Bradley EL, Wilson DS. Analysis of explanted silicone implants: a report of 300 patients. Ann Plast Surg 1995;34:1–6.

37. Ahn CY, Shaw WW. Regional silicone gel migration in patients with ruptured implants. Ann Plast Surg 1994;33:201–8.

38. Ahn CY, DeBruhl ND, Gorczyca DP, et al. Comparative silicone breast implant evaluation using mammography, sonography, and magnetic resonance imaging: experience with 59 implants. Plast Reconstr Surg 1994;94:620–7.

39. Leibman AL, Kruse BD. Imaging of breast cancer after augmentation mammoplasty. Ann Plast Surg 1993;30:111–5.

40. Silverstein MJ, Gamagami P, Handel N. Missed breast cancer in an augmented woman using implant displacement mammography. Ann Plast Surg 1990;25:210–3.

41. Carlson GW, Curley SA, Martin FE, et al. The detection of breast cancer after augmentation mammoplasty. Plast Reconstr Surg 1993;91: 837–40.

42. Gumico CA, Pin P, Young VL, et al. The effect of breast implants on the radiographic detection of microcalcifications and soft tissue masses. Plast Reconstr Surg 1989;84:772–8.

43. Birdsell DC, Jenkins H, Berkel H. Breast cancer diagnosis and survival in women with and without breast implants. Plast Reconstr Surg 1993;92:795–800.

44. Deapon DM, Bernstein L, Brody GS. Are breast implants anti-carcinogenic? A 14 years follow-up of the Los Angeles study. Plast Reconstr Surg 1997;99:1346–53.

45. Deapon DM, Pike MC, Casagrande JT, Brody GS. The relationship between breast cancer and augmentation mammoplasty: an epidemiologic study. Plast Reconstr Surg 1986;77:361–7.

46. Engel A, Lamm SH. Risk of sarcomas of the breast among women with breast augmentation. Plast Reconstr Surg 1992;89:571–2.

47. Su CW, Dreyfuss DA, Krizek TJ, et al. Silicone implants and the inhibition of cancer. Plast Reconstr Surg 1995;96:513–8.

48. Brody GS, Conway DP, Deapon DM, et al. Consensus statement on the relationship of breast implants to connective tissue disorders. Plast Reconstr Surg 1992;90:1102–5.

49. Gabriel SE, O'Faflon WM, Kurland LT, et al. Risk of connective tissue diseases and other disorders after breast implantation. N Engl J Med 1994;330:1697–702.

50. Giltay EJ, Moens HJB, Riley AH, et al. Silicone breast prostheses and rheumatic symptoms: a retrospective follow-up study. Ann Rheum Dis 1994;53:194–6.

51. Radovan C. Breast reconstruction after mastectomy using the temporary expander. Plast Reconstr Surg 1982;69:195–208.

52. Colen SR. Immediate two stage breast reconstruction utilizing a tissue expander and implant. In: Spear S, editor. The breast: principles and art. Philadelphia: Lippincott-Raven; 1998. p. 375–86.

53. Forman DL, Chiu J, Restifo RJ, et al. Breast reconstruction in previously irradiated patients using tissue expanders and implants: a potentially unfavorable result. Ann Plast Surg 1998; 40:360–3.

54. Mandrekas AD, Zambacos GJ, Katsantoni PN. Immediate and delayed breast reconstruction with permanent tissue expanders. Br J Plast Surg 1995;48:572–8.

55. Francel TJ, Ryan JJ, Manson PM. Breast reconstruction utilizing implants: a local experience and comparison of three techniques. Plast Reconstr Surg 1993;92:786–94.

56. Yeh KA, Lyle G, Wei JP, et al. Immediate breast reconstruction in breast cancer: morbidity and outcome. Am J Surg 64:1195–9.

57. Wickman M, Jurell G, Sandelin K. Technical aspects of immediate breast reconstruction: 2 year follow-up of 100 patients treated conservatively. Scand J Plast Reconstr Surg 1998;32: 265–73.

58. Caffee HH. Textured silicone and capsule contracture. Ann Plast Surg 1990;24:197–9.

59. Pakium AI, Young CS. Submuscular breast reconstruction: a one stage method of tissue expansion. Ann Plast Surg 1987;19:312–7.

60. Kroll SS, Baldwin B. A comparison of outcome using three different methods of breast reconstruction. Plast Reconstr Surg 1992;90:455–62.

61. Hartrampf CR Jr, Scheflan M, Black PW. Breast reconstruction with a transverse abdominal island flap. Plast Reconstr Surg 1982;69:216–9.

62. Boyd JB, Taylor GI, Corlett R. The vascular territories of the superior and deep inferior epigastric systems. Plast Reconstr Surg 1984;73:1–16.

63. Moon HK, Taylor GI. The vascular anatomy of the transverse rectus myocutaneous flaps based on the deep superior epigastric system. Plast Reconstr Surg 1988;82:815–32.

64. Bostwick J. Plastic and reconstructive breast surgery. St Louis: Quality Medical Publishing; 1990.

65. Watterson PA, Bostwick J, Hester TR, et al. TRAM flap anatomy correlated with a ten year clinical experience with 556 patients. Plast Reconstr Surg 1995;95:1185–94.

66. Hartrampf CR, Bennett GK. Autogenous tissue reconstruction in the mastectomy patient: a critical review of 300 patients. Ann Surg 1987;205:508–19.

67. Hartrampf CR, Michelow BJ. Breast reconstruction with living tissue. Norfolk (VA): Hampton Press; 1991.

68. Little JW. Breast reconstruction by the unipedicle TRAM operation: muscle splitting technique. In: Spear S, editor. The breast: principles and art. Philadelphia: Lippincott-Raven; 1998. p. 521–34.

69. Takayanagi S. Extended transverse rectus abdominus myocutaneous flap. Plast Reconstr Surg 1993;92:757–8.

70. Yamamota Y, Nohira K, Sugihara T, et al. Superiority of the microvascularly augmented flap: analysis of 50 transverse rectus abdominus myocutaneous flaps for breast reconstruction. Plast Reconstr Surg 1996;97:79–83.

71. Paige KT, Bostwick J, Bried JT, Jones G. A comparison of morbidity from bilateral, unipedicled and unilateral, unipedicled TRAM flap breast reconstructions. Plast Reconstr Surg 1998;101:1819–27.

72. Williams JK, Bostwick J III, Bried JY, et al. TRAM flap breast reconstruction after radiation treatment. Ann Surg 1995;221:756–64.

73. Jacobson WM, Meland NB, Woods JE. Autologous breast reconstruction with use of transverse rectus myocutaneous flap: Mayo clinic experience with 147 cases. Mayo Clin Proc 1994;69:635–40.

74. Berrino P, Campora E, Leone S, et al. The transverse rectus myocutaneous flap for breast reconstruction in obese patients. Ann Plast Surg 1991;27:221–31.

75. Takeishi M, Shaw WW, Ahn CY, et al. TRAM flaps in patients with abdominal scars. Plast Reconstr Surg 1997;99:713–22.

76. Kroll SS, Gheradini G, Martin JE, et al. Fat necrosis in free and pedicled TRAM flaps. Plast Reconstr Surg 1998;102:1502–7.

77. Slavin SA, Goldwyn RM. The midabdominal rectus abdominus myocutaneous flap: review of 236 flaps. Plast Reconstr Surg 1988;81:189–97.

78. Slavin SA, Hein KD. The mid-abdominal transverse rectus abdominus myocutaneous flap. In: Spear S, editor. The breast: principles and art. Philadelphia: Lippincott-Raven; 1998. p. 565–76.

79. Callegari PR, Taylor GI, Caddy CM, et al. An anatomic review of the delay phenomenon. I. Experimental studies. Plast Reconstr Surg 1992;89:397–407.

80. Morris SF, Taylor GI. The time sequence of the delay phenomenon: when is a surgical delay effective? An experimental study. Plast Reconstr Surg 1995;95:526–33.

81. Taylor GI. The surgically delayed unipedicled TRAM flap for breast reconstruction. Ann Plast Surg 1996;36:242–5.

82. Codner MA, Bostwick J, Nahai F, et al. TRAM flap vascular delay for high risk breast reconstruction. Plast Reconstr Surg 1995;96:1615–22.

83. Restifo RJ, Ahmed SS, Isenburg JS, et al. Timing, magnitude and utility of surgical delay in the TRAM flap. I. Animal studies. Plast Reconstr Surg 1997;99:12–16.

84. Serletti JM, Moran SL. Free versus the pedicled TRAM flap: a cost comparison and outcome analysis. Plast Reconstr Surg 1997;100:1418–24.

85. Schusterman MA, Kroll SS, Weldon ME. Immediate breast reconstruction: why the free TRAM over the conventional TRAM flap. Plast Reconstr Surg 1992;90:255–61.

86. Kroll SS, Netscher DT. Complications of the TRAM flap breast reconstruction in obese patients. Plast Reconstr Surg 1989;84:866.

87. Schusterman MA, Kroll SS, Miller MJ, et al. The free transverse rectus myocutaneous flap for breast reconstruction: one center's experience with 211 consecutive cases. Ann Plast Surg 1994;32:234–41.

88. Suominen S, Asko-Seljavaara S, Kinnunen J, et al. Abdominal wall competence after free trans-

verse rectus abdominus myocutaneous flap harvest: a prospective study. Ann Plast Surg 39:299–34.

89. Kind GM, Rademaker AW, Mustoe TA. Abdominal wall recovery following TRAM flap: a functional outcome study. Plast Reconstr Surg 1997;99:417–28.

90. Kroll SS, Schusterman MA, Reece GP, et al. Abdominal wall strength, bulging, and hernia after TRAM flap breast reconstruction. Plast Reconstr Surg 1995;96:616–9.

91. Fitoussi A, Le Taillandier M, Biffaud JC, et al. Functional evaluation of the abdominal wall after raising a rectus abdominus myocutaneous flap. Ann Chir Plast Esthet 1997;42:138–46.

92. Hartrampf CR Jr, Bried JT. General considerations in TRAM flap surgery. In: Hartrampf CR, editor. Breast reconstruction with living tissue. New York: Raven Press; 1991. p. 33–70.

93. Kroll SS, Marchi M. Comparison of strategies for preventing abdominal wall weakness after TRAM flap breast reconstruction. Plast Reconstr Surg 1992;89:1045–51.

94. Kroll SS, Gherardini G, Martin JE, et al. Fat necrosis in free and pedicled TRAM flaps. Plast Reconstr Surg 1998;102:1502–7.

95. Shestak KC. Bipedicle TRAM flap reconstruction. In: Spear S, editor. The breast: principles and art. Philadelphia: Lippincott-Raven; 1998. p. 535–46.

96. Petit JY, Rietjens M, Ferreira MA, et al. Abdominal sequellae after pedicled TRAM flap breast reconstruction. Plast Reconstr Surg 1997;99:723–9.

97. Jensen JA. Is double pedicle TRAM flap reconstruction of a single breast within the standard of care? Plast Reconstr Surg 1989;102:586–7.

98. Spear SL, Hartrampf CR Jr. The double pedicle TRAM flap and the standard of care. Plast Reconstr Surg 1998;100:1592–3.

99. Maxwell GP. Iginio Tansini and the origin of the latissimus dorsi musculocutaneous flap. Plast Reconstr Surg 1980;65:686–92.

100. Hammond DC, Fisher J. Latissimus dorsi musculo-cutaneous flap breast reconstruction. In: Spear S, editor. The breast: principles and art. Philadelphia: Lippincott-Raven; 1998. p. 477–90.

101. Taylor GI, Townsend P, Corlett R. Superiority of the deep circumflex iliac vessels as the supply for free groin flaps. Clinical work. Plast Reconstr Surg 1979;64:745–59.

102. Elliott LF, Hartrampf CR Jr. The Rubens flap. The deep circumflex iliac artery flap. Clin Plast Surg 1998;25:283–91.

103. Fugino T, Harashina T, Endomoto K. Primary breast reconstruction after a standard radical mastectomy by a free flap transfer. Plast Reconstr Surg 1976;58:372–4.

104. Shaw WW. Superior gluteal free flap breast reconstruction. Clin Plast Surg 1998;25:267–74.

105. Elliott LF, Beegle PH, Hartrampf CR Jr. The lateral transverse thigh free flap: an alternative for autogenous-tissue breast reconstruction. Plast Reconstr Surg 1990;85:169–78.

106. Slavin SA. Reconstruction of the breast conservation patient. In: Spear S, editor. The breast: principles and art. Philadelphia: Lippincott-Raven; 1998 p. 221–38.

107. Beadle F, Silver B, Botnick L, et al. Cosmetic results following primary radiation therapy for early breast cancer. Cancer 1984;54:2911–8.

108. Kroll SS, Singletary SE. Repair of partial mastectomy defects. Clin Plast Surg 1998;25:303–10.

109. Grisotti A. Immediate reconstruction after partial mastectomy. Oper Tech Plast Reconstr Surg 1994;1:1–12.

110. Petit JY, Rietjens M, Garusi C, et al. Integration of plastic surgery in the course of breast conserving surgery for cancer to improve cosmetic results and radicality of tumor excision. Recent Results Cancer Res 1998;152:202–11.

111. Little JW, Spear SL. The finishing touches in nipple–areola reconstruction. Perspect Plast Surg 1988;2:1–17.

112. Bostwick J III. Creating a nipple. In: Berger K, Bostwick J III, editors. A women's decision. St. Louis: Quality Medical Publishing; 1994.

12

Adjuvant Systemic Therapy of Early Breast Cancer

GERSHON Y. LOCKER, MD

The modern era of breast cancer treatment began over 100 years ago with the development of surgical techniques that emphasized the need for total resection of tumor. Nevertheless, despite gross total excision, many patients with seemingly localized disease suffered relapse or distant recurrence and died of their cancer. This was presumably due to the growth of microscopic tumor unappreciated at the time of initial therapy. The need for additional, adjuvant therapy after surgery led to numerous randomized controlled trials (RCTs) addressing the problem. The role of adjuvant systemic therapy in increasing survival and decreasing mortality has been established by these studies and confirmed by overview meta-analyses. The basis for this success is the recognition of and adherence to the principles of adjuvant therapy, which are that (1) local treatments do not cure all patients with seemingly localized cancer; (2) populations at high risk of relapse can be identified; (3) patterns of relapse and failure are understood; (4) palliative therapy against overt macroscopic tumor can potentially eradicate occult microscopic disease; (5) the value of adjuvant therapy has been validated in RCTs; (6) the choice of adjuvant therapy considers the biology of the tumor and of the patient and; (7) the benefits of treatment outweigh the toxicity and risks of therapy.

Halstead in the late 19th century appreciated that not all patients with early breast cancer were cured by surgery. Regrettably this fact remains so even today. It is only in the last 30 years, however, that the other principles of adjuvant therapy were applied to the treatment of early breast cancer leading to the improvement of outcome.

IDENTIFICATION OF POPULATIONS AT HIGH RISK OF RELAPSE

Although not every women with early stage, "localized" breast cancer is rendered cancer free by local treatment, many women are. It is critical, if additional treatments are to be used, that they be directed at women at highest risk of recurrence. Indiscriminate administration of adjunctive therapies runs the risk of unnecessarily exposing those already cured to toxicity, morbidity and, with some aggressive approaches, even mortality from treatment. Choice of patients to be treated is critical in the development of successful adjuvant therapy. For women with early stage, operable breast cancer, the single most important prognostic feature for recurrence and death is the presence or absence of tumor metastases in the axillary lymph nodes.[1,2] Patients with no axillary nodal metastases have a 70 to 75 percent chance of long-term disease-free survival (DFS) when treated with surgery alone. Patients with any number of nodal metastases have a 25 to 30 percent chance of long-term survival.[3] The risk of recurrence and death increases with the number of involved nodes. Women with more than 10 nodes involved have an extremely poor prognosis, less than a 20 percent cure rate as shown in most studies. From the beginning of the era of adjuvant therapy trials, patients with involved axillary nodes were identified as the highest-risk group and were the subjects of adjuvant approaches. As systemic adjuvant therapies for node-positive disease became accepted, attention turned to improving the prognosis of the 30 percent of node-negative cases destined to have recurrences and die. Multiple studies have shown that in these women, the size of the primary tumor is the most important predictor of surgical outcome.[3] Women with tumors smaller than 1 cm in diameter and no involved nodes have better than a 90 percent chance of long-term DFS. Adjuvant therapy is not a major priority in this group and is not routinely given. On the other hand, women with tumors > 5 cm, despite having no nodal metastases, have a prognosis comparable to patients with axillary nodal spread. Clearly, women with large tumors, whatever the axillary status, are candidates for additional therapy beyond surgery. Other than nodal status and tumor size, the use of prognostic features to determine who should or should not be considered for adjuvant therapy is very controversial. While tumor grade may be helpful,[1] the variability of grading between pathologists makes it problematic. Hormone receptor status, proliferation markers (%S phase, thymidine labeling, Ki67), oncogene expression/mutation (c-erbB-2, p53) may be more reproducible and have also been correlated with outcome of local therapy.[4] Nevertheless, to date, none has been universally accepted as an independent predictor for the need for adjuvant treatment. The American Society of Clinical Oncology (ASCO) Tumor Marker Expert Panel, using criteria of evidence-based medicine, could not endorse any of these tumor markers by themselves as adequate to determine the need for additional therapy beyond breast surgery.[4] Some of the markers, however, may be of value in determining the type of adjuvant therapy to be used (hormone receptors, (c-erbB-2). Studies in the past and current practice use nodal status and tumor size as primary determinants of need for treatment. The other prognostic factors are used (often together) only when the need for, or the potential benefits of, systemic therapy after local treatment is unclear.

UNDERSTANDING PATTERNS OF RELAPSE AND FAILURE

There are multiple effective treatments of breast cancer. Which one is most appropriate to increase survival and cure rate after primary therapy of early disease is dependent on the nature of the failure. Is it due to inadequate control of the primary tumor, regional spread, or distant metastases? The Halstedian view of breast cancer spread was that of a prolonged period of local/regional disease before systemic dissemination. By implication, failure to cure might be due to incomplete surgery. As discussed in Chapter 11, multiple studies have failed to confirm the survival benefit of more aggressive versus less aggressive surgery. A recent meta-analysis of 3,400 women in randomized trials of more versus less extensive surgery found no difference in 10-year survival between the two approaches.[5] This was true whether or not the patients had axillary nodal involvement. Radiation therapy is another approach to local and regional control. If the Halstedian paradigm were true, local regional irradiation by killing residual tumor should increase the overall cure rate and survival. Again, most studies have failed to confirm survival benefit with irradiation of the chest wall/draining nodes, despite significantly decreasing local recurrence[5] (see also Chapter 16). In studies of local modalities, the decrease in local recurrence did not improve survival benefit, in part because of the development of distant recurrences. This refutation of the Halstedian theory strongly argues that failure to cure localized breast cancer with local therapies is due to the presence of unappreciated distant micrometastases, that are destined to grow and kill the patient. To improve surgical results, additional therapy must be directed to the systemic nature of breast cancer in high-risk women.

PALLIATIVE THERAPY AGAINST OVERT MACROSCOPIC TUMOR AND POTENTIAL ERADICATION OF OCCULT MICROSCOPIC DISEASE

A basic assumption underlying adjuvant systemic therapy of early breast cancer is that those therapies that may be only palliative against bulky macroscopic metastases might be curative against microscopic disseminated tumor that is assumed to be present in high-risk patients. To develop effective adjuvant systemic therapy of early disease, one must first identify effective and safe therapies for advanced-stage breast cancer.

Systemic therapy for overt advanced breast cancer began 100 years ago when Beatson observed shrinkage of locally extensive breast cancers after oophorectomy in premenopausal women.[6] This phenomenon is based on the trophic effect of estrogen on approximately half of all breast cancers studied. Removal of the ovaries leading to a drop in endogenous estrogen levels in younger women can arrest cancer growth and result in regression. Another approach to depriving breast cancers of estrogen effects is to block estrogen binding to the protein, estrogen receptor (ER), in the breast cancer cell cytoplasm. The receptor-estrogen complex mediates much of the effect of the hormone on the cell, and blocking the interaction, such as by removing estrogen, leads to regression of the hormone-dependent cancer.[7] Tamoxifen (Nolvadex) is the prototype competitive inhibitor of estrogen binding at its receptor. The ability to measure estrogen and progesterone receptors and thus predict responsiveness to endocrine therapy made hormonal treatment of overt, metastatic breast cancer a standard approach.[8] Oophorectomy in premenopausal women and tamoxifen in women of all ages cause significant regressions of clinically advanced estrogen and or progesterone receptor–containing breast cancers with generally acceptable toxicity. They were obvious candidates to be tried in the adjuvant setting after local therapy of early disease to treat occult micrometastases.

Unfortunately, not all breast cancers are estrogen dependent and responsive to hormonal manipulation. After the introduction of chemotherapeutic drugs in the 1940s and 1950s, multiple agents were identified that were able to cause temporary shrinkage of tumor in women with disseminated breast cancer. Melphelan (PAM), thiotepa (T), cyclophosphamide (C), methotrexate (M), fluorouracil (F), or vinblastine (V) have a 20 to 30 percent chance of causing transient regression of metastatic breast cancer when used alone.[9] In the late 1960s Cooper combined five drugs and reported higher regression rates.[10] This regimen was the forerunner of the cyclophosphamide methotrexate fluorouracil (CMF) combination regimen, which was in the 1970s the standard chemotherapeutic treatment of advanced disease (Table 12–1).[11] In the late 1970s, doxorubicin (Adriamycin[A]) was introduced and found to be the most active single agent against advanced breast cancer. It was soon combined with other drugs[11] (ex-cyclophosphamide adriamycin fluorouracil [ex-CAF]) and, in the 1980s, became the new standard treatment of overt metastatic disease (see Table 12–1). Finally, another class of drugs, the taxanes (paclitaxel–Taxol and docetaxel–Taxotere) were introduced in the last decade with activity comparable with that of doxorubicin in the palliation of advanced mammary cancer. All these drugs can be given safely, though they have significant toxicity. All were candidates for use in the adjuvant setting.

A recent trend in the treatment of metastatic breast cancer is the use of high-dose chemotherapy, either with cytokine support of the bone marrow or with stem cell or bone marrow storage and reinfusion ("bone marrow transplantation"). These therapies are based on the assumption of a dose-response curve for drug-induced cancer cell death. While still controversial in advanced breast cancer (and very toxic), such approaches are also candidates for evaluation against the poorest-risk, early-stage disease.

ADJUVANT THERAPY VALIDATED IN RANDOMIZED CONTROLLED TRIALS

Effective therapies of advanced breast cancer were long known and anecdotally used after surgery for early breast cancer, but their value as adjuncts to primary therapy was difficult to assess. Unlike in advanced disease, where tumor shrinkage after systemic treatment can be determined directly by observation or radiographically, when used to increase survival after treatment of early stage disease, there are no direct determinants of effectiveness. Cure in an individual patient with early-stage disease may have been achieved as a result of the systemic therapy or might have occurred even if it had not been given as a result of the local treatment. Recurrence may be a sign of failure of adjunctive therapy but might have been delayed because of it. The only way to truly evaluate the usefulness of additional treatments after primary therapy of breast cancer is by large RCTs. Initially, those trials randomized women with high-risk, early-stage disease to surgery alone or to surgery plus an experimental adjuvant therapy. As adjuvant treatments were proved effective, the next generation of trials randomized women to primary therapy plus "standard" adjuvant systemic treatment versus primary therapy plus "experimental" adjuvant treatment. The end point of such trials were disease-free interval (DFI) and DFS (the time to recurrence and percentage of patients alive without recurrence of cancer at any time point) and overall survival (time to death and percentage of patients alive at any time point). In general, the benefits of adjuvant systemic chemotherapy or hormonal therapies are more pronounced on DFS than overall survival

because once a patient relapses, there are effective palliative treatments to prolong life in advanced disease. Perhaps the most convincing effect of adjuvant treatment, however, is on the percentage of patients alive long after treatment. Multiple randomized trials have shown that systemic treatment of early-stage breast cancer significantly and reproducibly decreases the risk of death years after local therapy. This benefit persists with time, suggesting the likelihood of cure.

CHEMOTHERAPY

Single Agents

As in the case of advanced disease, the earliest trials of adjuvant chemotherapy were of single agents. The National Surgical Adjuvant Breast and Bowel Project (NSABP) conducted randomized trials in the 1950s and 1960s looking at a short course of thiotepa or fluorouracil after surgery versus surgery alone. Overall, there was no survival benefit to the chemotherapy, but there was a suggestion that thiotepa might have some benefit in premenopausal women.[12] The rationale for these studies was a belief that manipulation of the tumor during surgery might promote detachment and spread of its cells and that chemotherapy might kill the scattered cells. It was only with the realization that failure may be due to distant metastases already present at the time of surgery that trials of protracted chemotherapy were undertaken. The risk of toxicity of these more prolonged approaches led to restriction of the trials to women with node-positive disease. The critical single-agent study was done by the NSABP in the early 1970s. It randomized 349 women with node-positive disease to surgery alone or surgery plus 2 years of intermittent oral melphalan.[13] At 10 years, there was significant improvement in DFS and a trend toward improved overall survival in the chemotherapy group. The benefits, however, were confined to women under 50 years. At about the same time, randomized studies were showing the superiority of combination

Table 12–1. ADJUVANT SYSTEMIC THERAPY REGIMENS USED IN THE TREATMENT OF EARLY BREAST CANCER

Regimen	Indication	Frequency	Drugs	Dose
CMF	Poor prognosis node – or 1 to 3 + nodes (erbB-2 –)	Every 28 days × 6 months	Cyclophosphamide Methotrexate Fluorouracil	100 mg/M^2 po qd × 14 d 40 mg/M^2 IV dl and d8 600 mg/M^2 IV dl and d8
AC	Poor prognosis node – or 1 to 3 + nodes (erbB-2 + or –)	Every 21 days × 4 treatments	Cyclophosphamide Doxorubicin	600 mg/M^2 IV dl 60 mg/M^2 IV dl
CAF	4 or more + nodes	Every 28 days × 6 months	Cyclophosphamide Doxorubicin Fluorouracil	100 mg/M^2 po qd × 14d 30 mg/M^2 IV dl and d8 600 mg/M^2 IV dl and d8
AC→ Paclitaxel	4 or more + nodes	Every 21 days × 4 treatments	AC given × 4 as above Followed by Paclitaxel	175 mg/M^2 3 h IV infusion
Tamoxifen	Receptor (ER or PR)-containing tumors • Postmenopausal node ± • Premenopausal node –	Daily for 5 years		20 mg po daily

chemotherapy over single-agent therapy in the treatment of metastatic breast cancer. Would the same be true for adjuvant therapy?

Combination Cyclophosphamide Methotrexate Fluorouracil Therapy and Meta-analyses

In the early 1970s Bonadonna at the National Cancer Institute in Milan evaluated CMF given 2 weeks on and 2 weeks off for 12 months ("classic CMF").[14] Three hundred and eighty-six women with node-positive disease were randomized to surgery ± CMF. As with the PAM trial, patients on CMF had a statistically significant improvement in DFS and a trend toward improved overall survival. Again the benefit was confined to premenopausal women with no significant benefit for postmenopausal patients.[14] Treatment with CMF (and its variants) became the standard adjuvant therapy for premenopausal women with node-positive disease (see Table 12–1). Although there are several ways of administering CMF (eg, classic monthly: po C × 14 days + IV MF day 1 and 8; all IV every 3 weeks), several studies support the classic 28-day program as being the most effective.[15,16] On the other hand, in a subsequent randomized study, Bonadonna found that 6 months of CMF to be as efficacious as 1 year of drugs.[17] Six months of

CMF remains a standard adjuvant systemic therapy for early-stage breast cancer today.

Almost immediately after the adoption of adjuvant chemotherapy for node-positive premenopausal women, several questions arose: was combination chemotherapy truly better than single-agent therapy? Is there really only a disease-free but not overall survival benefit to adjuvant chemotherapy? What is the optimal duration of therapy? Is it of any benefit in poor-risk, node-negative disease? Was it truly of no value in postmenopausal women? Each of these issues was evaluated in individual randomized trials. Nevertheless, it became increasingly difficult, even with relatively large studies, to definitively come up with answers, as results were often conflicting.

In 1985, 1990,[18] and 1995,[19] a consortium of breast cancer researchers, the Early Breast Cancer Trialists' Collaborative Group (EBCTCG) conducted meta-analyses, using primary data from multiple randomized trials of adjuvant chemotherapy to address these issues. The 1990 overview looked at 13 studies (enrolling ~3,400 women) comparing single-agent versus combination chemotherapy.[18] There was greater benefit with polychemotherapy, a relative 17 ± 5 percent decrease in yearly risk of death due to breast cancer compared with single-agent therapy, reinforcing the widely held clinical impression. The 1995 overview, consequently, looked only at combination chemotherapy regimens, It reviewed prolonged chemotherapy versus no chemotherapy in 47 trials encompassing 18,000 women; longer versus shorter chemotherapy in 6,100 patients in 11 trials; CMF versus anthracycline (doxorubicin or epirubicin)–based combinations in 6,000 women in 11 trials.[19] For all studies, there was a statistically significant benefit in polychemotherapy versus no chemotherapy in terms of recurrence (relative decrease of 24%, $p < .00001$) and also survival (relative decrease in mortality of 15%, $p < .00001$). Chemotherapy was not just delaying recurrence. Comparisons of standard durations of adjuvant CMF-like regimens (6 months) with more prolonged durations found no significant survival benefit to more prolonged therapy,[19] confirming Bonadonna's results.[17] The benefits of chemotherapy in the 1995 overview was seen in all nodal groups.[19] In trials of combination chemotherapy versus control, mortality was cut by the same relative amount in both node-positive and node-negative patients. Given the differences in the risk of death in the two groups, the absolute benefit, however, was different. In women under age 50 years, the absolute decrease in death at 10 years was 12.4 percent ($p < .00001$) in the node-positive group and 5.7 percent ($p < .02$) in the node-negative group. Finally, despite the many seemingly negative trials, polychemotherapy was found to be of value in postmenopausal women but only in the 50- to 69-year-old age group.[19] For node-positive women over 50 years, chemotherapy decreased the rate of death from any cause by an absolute 2.3 percent ($p = .002$), far less than in younger women. For node-negative older women, however, the absolute decrease in rate of death (6.4% $p < .005$) was comparable with that in younger women. The paradox of chemotherapy having a greater absolute benefit in postmenopausal node-negative women than in node-positive ones is unexplained. As a result of the multiple studies that comprised the EBCTCG overviews, by 1990, in premenopausal women, adjuvant chemotherapy, particularly CMF, became standard for both node-positive and high-risk, node-negative breast cancers. In postmenopausal women, chemotherapy was reserved for receptor-negative patients because of the perceived lesser benefit and increased toxicity. It was also being used for high-risk operable male breast cancer.[20]

Doxorubicin

The suggestion that doxorubicin-based chemotherapy was more effective than CMF in the palliation of advanced breast cancer[11] led to the use of combinations containing the drug as adjuvant therapy particularly in poor prognostic groups, such as those with multiple positive nodes. The 1995 overview analyzed 11 CMF versus anthracycline (doxorubicin or epirubicin) polychemotherapy trials.[19] At 5 years after surgery, anthracycline combinations decreased recurrence by an absolute 3.2 percent ($p = .006$) and mortality by an absolute 2.7 percent ($p = .02$). Individual trials themselves have been contradictory, but there are some general trends. The NSABP Protocol B15 showed that in node-positive women, a short four-treatment course of IV doxorubicin/cyclophosphamide (AC) (see Table 12–1) was equivalent to the effect of classic CMF for 6 months.[21] Furthermore, the AC regimen was effective and well tolerated in postmenopausal women. It is now widely used as an alternative to CMF for poor prognosis node-negative and 1- to 3-node–positive adjuvant therapy.[21] Its popularity is based on the briefer duration of treatment (3 versus 6 months), less overall toxicity and lower risk of permanent menopause in younger women. Studies comparing CMF with CAF (doxorubicin substituted for methotrexate) have been harder to interpret. They have suffered from using the inferior all-IV 3-weekly CMF in the control arm or using epirubicin as their anthracycline drug. The Southwest Oncology Group (SWOG), however, did conduct a study of standard CMF versus CAF (± tamoxifen) in node-negative women. Their preliminary report was of a small but statistically significant 2 percent improvement in survival ($p = .03$) for the CAF groups compared with the CMF groups,[22] similar to the 1995 meta-analysis results.[19] Whether such a small benefit in a relatively good prognosis group warrants the excess toxicity is questionable. The difference, however, would be clinically significant in the high-risk multinode-positive patient. If the final results of this study continue to show the difference, it would support CAF × 6 as an alternative for adjuvant chemotherapy for women with four or more positive lymph nodes.

Investigational Approaches

Unfortunately, even with aggressive doxorubicin-based chemotherapy, the prognosis remains poor for women with many axillary nodes involved.[19] Another approach to improving the results was the use of multiple non–cross-resistant agents as adjuvant therapy. Studies looking at CMF variants alternating with doxorubicin regimens have not consistently shown benefit.[21,23,24] The introduction of the taxanes, which are highly active and not cross-resistant with doxorubicin, offer greater hope of improving outcomes. Several studies are evaluating doxorubicin based regimens ± paclitaxel or docetaxel. The Cancer and Acute Leukemia Group (CALGB) reported the preliminary results of CALGB 9344, which found that the addition of four doses of paclitaxel after AC × 4 (see Table 12–1) in node-positive women decreased recurrence rate by 22 percent and death by 26 percent. The absolute decrease in mortality at 18 months was 2 percent ($p = .039$).[25] While it is too soon to state that AC × 4 → paclitaxel × 4 is the standard therapy for node-positive disease (or if it is better than CAF × 6), the data suggest a role for the taxanes. It is reasonable to consider AC→ paclitaxel as an alternative to CAF in high-risk situations where the toxicity of prolonged doxorubicin administration is a concern (Table 12–2).

The assumption that there is a dose-response relationship to tumor cell kill and the development of cytokine and stem cell bone marrow support has lead to a series of studies looking at higher-or more-intense-dose adjuvant chemotherapy regimens. These studies are of three types. Some escalate drugs two to four times the conventional dosage and use cytokine support (escalated conventional dose). Others escalate drug doses minimally but give drugs at briefer intervals (dose-dense therapy). There are few studies that address this concept. The third approach uses massive (5- to 10-fold) dose escalation and requires stem cell support ("bone marrow transplant"). Only for the escalated conventional dose approach are final results of randomized trials available. They are very disappointing. The NSABP trials B-22[26] and B-25[27] randomized node-positive patients to conventional AC × 4 or to regimens containing higher doses of cyclophosphamide (up to four-fold escalation with GCSF). There was no disease-free or overall survival benefit to the higher-dose schedules. The CALGB 9344 trial randomized conventional AC × 4 (± paclitaxel) versus AC × 4 (± paclitaxel) with the doxorubicin escalated by 25 or 50 percent. There was no benefit to the higher-dose doxorubicin regimens compared with those containing conventional AC.[25] To date, there is no convincing evidence to support escalated standard-dose adjuvant chemotherapy.

While high-dose chemotherapy with stem cell transplant is widely employed in some centers as adjuvant therapy for women with 10 or more involved nodes, data to support it are incomplete. Proponents of the approach cite vastly superior survival results in women undergoing the technique compared with historical controls receiving conventional chemotherapy. Critics believe the superiority compared with historical controls is due to patient selection and cite a small randomized study that found no benefit in the approach.[28] The Eastern Cooperative Oncology Group (ECOG) has completed a study in women with 10 or

Table 12–2. GUIDELINES FOR THE CHOICE OF ADJUVANT SYSTEMIC THERAPY

Node-Tumor-Receptor Status	Premenopausal	Postmenopausal	Over Age 70 Years
Axillary node negative: tumor < 1 cm	No Rx*‡	No Rx*‡	No Rx*‡
Axillary node negative: tumor > 1 cm or Poor prognosis receptor positive	Tamoxifen or CMF† or AC or tamoxifen + AC	Tamoxifen or tamoxifen + AC*	Tamoxifen
Axillary node negative: tumor > 1 cm or Poor prognosis receptor negative‡	CMF† or AC	AC or CMF†	Chemo Rx on individual basis*
Axillary node positive: 1 to 3 + nodes Receptor positive	CMF† or AC ± Tam	Tamoxifen ± AC* (or CMF†)	Tamoxifen
Axillary node positive: 1 to 3 + nodes Receptor negative‡	CMF† or AC	AC (or CMF†)	Chemo Rx on individual basis
Axillary node positive: ≥ 4 + nodes Receptor positive	CAF or AC→ paclitaxel ± tamoxifen	Tamoxifen + CAF or AC→ paclitaxel	Tamoxifen (± chemo Rx on individual basis)
Axillary node positive: ≥ 4 + nodes Receptor negative‡	CAF or AC→ paclitaxel	CAF or AC→ paclitaxel	Chemo Rx on individual basis

* If multiple prognostic markers adverse consider Rx
† If c-erbB-2 overexpressed doxorubicin based chemotherapy should be used
‡ Consider Tamoxifen as chemopreventive agent
Rx = therapy; CMF = cyclophosphamide, methotrexate, fluorouracil; AC = adriamycin, cyclophosphamide; CAF = cyclophosphamide, adriamycin, fluorouracil.

more positive nodes of CAF × 6 versus CAF × 6 followed by high-dose chemotherapy with stem cell reinfusion. The CALGB trial is also conducting a study in 10 or more node-positive patients. They are randomized to CAF followed by low-dose consolidation chemotherapy or by the same drugs given in high doses with stem cell support. For women with four to nine nodes involved, SWOG is conducting a study of sequential high conventional dose doxorubicin→ paclitaxel→ cyclophosphamide therapy versus AC × 4 followed by high-dose chemotherapy with stem cells. The latter trial, unfortunately, suffers from not having a truly standard control arm. Hopefully, when the longterm results of these large studies are reported, we will know what role (if any) high-dose chemotherapy with stem cell support has in the adjuvant treatment of early breast cancer.

HORMONAL THERAPY

Tamoxifen

Multiple events in the late 1970s led to the development of tamoxifen as the most widely prescribed drug for the adjuvant systemic therapy of early breast cancer. Tamoxifen was shown to be an effective and safe therapy of metastatic breast cancer in postmenopausal women.[29] Estrogen receptor could be used to predict response of metastatic disease.[8] Initial reports of randomized trials of adjuvant chemotherapy in early breast cancer found minimal benefit in postmenopausal women compared with younger women.[13,14] Trials in the United Kingdom and Scandinavia began looking at adjuvant tamoxifen after surgery in node-positive postmenopausal breast cancer patients. In 1983, Baum reported preliminary results of one of the studies. Tamoxifen given after surgery decreased recurrence and increased survival.[30] Since then over 50 randomized trials have been conducted looking at the role of adjuvant tamoxifen in 37,000 women. As with chemotherapy, the EBCTCG conducted meta-analysis overviews of the tamoxifen trials, most recently in 1995.[31] Tamoxifen was beneficial in node-positive and node-negative disease, in postmenopausal and premenopausal patients. Although any duration of therapy was beneficial, longer durations were more beneficial than briefer duration. Only for women with tumors not containing ER was there no benefit.[31] For all women given tamoxifen, there was a 26 percent relative decrease in recurrence, a 14 percent relative decrease in death, and, at 10 years after surgery, an absolute decrease of 3.7

percent in death from any cause, compared with women not getting the drug ($p < .00001$).[31] For women with tumors containing hormone receptor and receiving 5 years of tamoxifen, the absolute decrease in death at 10 years was 5.6 percent for node-negative tumors and 10.9 percent for node-positive tumors.[31] In the 1990s, tamoxifen became standard adjuvant therapy for all postmenopausal women with node-positive and poor-prognosis, node-negative breast cancers containing hormone receptor.

Several controversies persist in the use of adjuvant tamoxifen. One is the duration of therapy; the other is its role in premenopausal women. While the meta-analysis and individual randomized trials favor 5 years of therapy,[31] two studies of 5 years versus more than 5 years in predominantly node-negative women found no benefit to additional years of therapy.[32,33] The ECOG, however, found that more than 5 years of tamoxifen added to adjuvant chemotherapy in women with receptor containing tumors was more beneficial than only 5 years of the drug.[34] In general, the standard approach is to give node-negative women 5 years of tamoxifen; for node-positive women, 5 years is suggested, but individualizing duration of therapy on the basis of risk of recurrence and toxicity is widely done. The Oxford Group is conducting a trial (ATLAS), which is directly addressing the optimal duration of adjuvant tamoxifen therapy.

In the United States, chemotherapy is the predominant form of adjuvant systemic therapy used in premenopausal women. This is not surprising since many younger women have breast cancers that do not contain hormone receptor and are unlikely to benefit from adjuvant tamoxifen. Yet NSABP trial B-14 found tamoxifen to be an effective therapy in premenopausal axillary node-negative women.[35] The meta-analysis looking at 5 years of tamoxifen found no significant difference in the benefit of tamoxifen between younger and older patients.[31] This emphasizes that in hormone receptor-positive breast cancer (particularly node-negative disease), tamoxifen can be con-

sidered an alternative to chemotherapy in premenopausal women. Tamoxifen is also of value in receptor-positive male breast cancer.[36]

Oophorectomy and Gonadotropin Releasing Hormone Analogue

The sporadic use of adjuvant oophorectomy after breast cancer surgery in younger women was continued by surgeons for many years in the hope of preventing recurrence. Randomized trials looking at its value date back 50 years.[37] Unfortunately, these early trials suffer from the lack of hormone responsiveness of most breast cancers in premenopausal women and they predate our ability to predict responsiveness with hormone receptor measurements. The EBCTCG conducted overview meta-analyses of adjuvant oophorectomy in 1985, 1990, and 1995. The most recent overview encompassed 12 trials randomizing 2,100 women to surgical or radiation oophorectomy versus no castration.[38] In women under the age of 50 years, oophorectomy resulted in an 18 percent relative decrease in recurrence, an 18 percent relative decrease in death, and, at 15 years after surgery, an absolute decrease of 6.3 percent in death from any cause, compared with women not getting the procedure ($p < .001$).[38] The relative benefit was the same in node-negative and node-positive patients.[38] These results are very similar to the chemotherapy meta-analysis results. Furthermore, in a Scottish trial, adjuvant CMF was compared with oophorectomy in premenopausal women with node-positive disease.[39] There was no difference seen in the overall result. In women with receptor-positive tumors, the trend was the superiority of castration; in receptor-negative disease CMF appeared better.

In the United States, adjuvant surgical castration is rarely done these days, with tamoxifen the preferred adjuvant hormonal approach in younger women (if any hormonal approach is used). The introduction of gonadotropin-releasing hormone (GnRH) analog has the potential to change this practice. These drugs, when given by slow-release depot injection, continually stimulate the pituitary, eventually depleting it of FSH and LH. This results in the cessation of ovarian function, achieving a bio-chemical oophorectomy.[7] The GnRH analog, goserelin (Zoladex) and leuprolide (Lupron) have antitumor activity comparable with oophorectomy and with tamoxifen against overt hormone-responsive metastatic disease in premenopausal women.[40] Furthermore, their action on the ovary is reversible. Currently, the European "ZEBRA" study is comparing adjuvant goserelin with chemotherapy in premenopausal women. Despite its proven efficacy as adjuvant therapy in younger women, oophorectomy is unlikely to be widely accepted in the United States.

Other Hormonal Approaches

Several other hormonal therapies have activity against metastatic breast cancer and have been evaluated as adjuvant therapy in early disease. Toremifene (Fareston) is a derivative of tamoxifen with a similar mechanism of action and activity against disseminated disease.[7] It is being evaluated in randomized trials against tamoxifen as adjuvant therapy in older women. Progestins lower endogenous estrogen levels in postmenopausal women and cause tumor regression in many women with advanced disease.[7] Medroxyprogesterone has been studied as adjuvant therapy in randomized trials, with negative results.[41,42] Aromatase inhibitors (AI) inhibit the enzyme that catalyzes the conversion of androgen to estrogen. They, too, lower serum (and intracellular) estrogen levels in older women and are effective hormonal therapies of metastatic breast cancer.[7] Aminoglutethimide, one of the first-generation aromatase inhibitors, however, was no better than placebo in an adjuvant trial after surgery in postmenopausal women.[43] New classes of more potent and selective aromatase inhibitors have been recently introduced for the treatment of advanced disease and are being evaluated as

adjuvant therapy. The ATAC trial is a multinational randomized double-blinded study in postmenopausal women of adjuvant tamoxifen versus the new AI anastrozole (Arimidex) versus the combination for 5 years. Another trial looks at women that have received 5 years of tamoxifen and are then being randomized to no further therapy or treatment with the AI letrozole (Femara). The results of the toremifene, arimidex, and letrozole trials and a European trial of the AI formestane are not yet known. To date, other than tamoxifen and oophorectomy, there are no standard hormonal adjuvant therapies.

COMBINED CHEMOHORMONAL THERAPY

The 1995 EBCTCG overviews looked at the relative benefits of adjuvant combined chemohormonal therapy versus single-modality treatment.[19,31,38] There was a suggestion that in women aged 50 to 69 years, tamoxifen plus chemotherapy decreased the annual risk of death by 10 percent compared with tamoxifen alone.[31] The issue was prospectively studied in newer trials. The NSABP, SWOG, and the International Breast Cancer Study Group, each found benefit in their studies of combined therapy versus tamoxifen alone in postmenopausal women;[44–46] the National Cancer Institute (NCI) of Canada did not.[47] While it is premature to suggest that all postmenopausal women with receptor-positive cancer should receive chemotherapy and tamoxifen; certainly, it is appropriate in selected high-risk women under the age of 70 years. The best way to combine the two, simultaneously or sequentially, still remains unresolved.

For women under the age 50 years, the 1995 overview suggested that the addition of oophorectomy to adjuvant chemotherapy was of borderline benefit, with a nonstatistically significant decrease of 10 percent in the annual mortality.[38] Furthermore, the ECOG recently reported the preliminary results of a randomized study in premenopausal women with hormone-sensitive, node-positive breast cancer. Women were randomized to receive CAF × 6 or CAF × 6 + 2 years of goserelin or CAF × 6 + goserelin + tamoxifen. The results are preliminary. It seems unlikely that adding goserelin to adjuvant chemotherapy improves results in premenopausal women in whom the chemotherapy already achieved a chemical castration but may be of value in younger women who are still menstruating. Unfortunately, the meta-analyses did not address these issues.[31] The addition of tamoxifen in the ECOG trial seemed beneficial in older women in whom chemotherapy led to menopause. Although not conclusively proven effective, chemotherapy plus tamoxifen is often given to premenopausal women with receptor-positive early breast cancer, usually because the chemotherapy has rendered them menopausal or more recently for chemopreventive reasons (vide infra).

NEOADJUVANT THERAPY

Increasingly, lumpectomy plus radiation has become the desired standard of local therapy for early breast cancer. Unfortunately, tumor or breast size in many women make lumpectomy cosmetically or technically not feasible. The gratifying results with initial chemotherapy in the treatment of locally inoperable breast cancer (such as inflammatory carcinoma) led to trials of preoperative chemotherapy in the hope of shrinking operable but large tumors to the point that breast conservation could be accomplished. Bonadonna's group in Milan, in two trials using several preoperative chemotherapy regimens, was able to perform breast preservation surgery (quadrentectomy) in 66 percent of women with tumors > 5 cm.[48] No one preoperative chemotherapy regimen was clearly superior.[48] Building on these findings, the NSABP investigated whether preoperative chemotherapy, besides shrinking the primary tumor, might also be more effective as an adjuvant systemic therapy than postoperative chemother-

apy. The NSABP trial B-18 randomized women to receive four cycles of preoperative AC or four cycles of postoperative therapy.[49,50] In women with tumors > 5 cm in diameter, there was a near-doubling of the breast conservation rate with neoadjuvant chemotherapy.[50] Nevertheless, there was no difference in overall distant recurrence and survival.[49] A new NSABP trial (B-27) is asking the same questions but looking at AC ± docetaxel given in various neoadjuvant and/or adjuvant combinations. In patients with large hormone receptor-positive breast cancers, neoadjuvant tamoxifen has been shown to be as effective as chemotherapy in shrinking the tumor to facilitate breast conservation.[51] It should be considered in patients that are not candidates for chemotherapy because of age or infirmity. For now, neoadjuvant therapies remain an effective way to facilitate breast conservation but not to improve survival over that achieved with postoperative adjuvant treatment.

DUCTAL CARCINOMA IN SITU

Although the primary role of adjuvant systemic therapy is to treat occult distant disease, there may also be a local benefit, at least in ductal carcinoma in situ trial (DCIS). The NSABP trial B-24 randomized 1,804 women with DCIS treated with lumpectomy plus radiation to no further therapy or to 5 years of tamoxifen.[52] At 5 years, tamoxifen decreased the risk of the development of invasive breast cancer in the treated breast by 47 percent (2.1% versus 3.4% in control, $p = .04$) and of all breast cancer events (ipsilateral and contralateral) by 34 percent (8.8% versus 13% in control, $p = .007$).[52] These results apply only to women who had lumpectomy/radiation for DCIS. They are not relevant to women treated with mastectomy. While the absolute magnitude of the benefit was small, certainly tamoxifen should be considered in many women with DCIS treated with breast conservation, particularly those with high-risk pathology.

THE CHOICE OF ADJUVANT THERAPY AND THE BIOLOGY OF THE TUMOR AND OF THE PATIENT

Despite the successes of adjuvant chemotherapy and hormonal therapy, many patients that receive such treatments have recurrences and die. To optimize results, when choosing treatment, tumor and patient biology must be taken into account. This is most apparent in the use of hormonal therapy. Although there is a small but real response rate with tamoxifen in metastatic hormone receptor-negative breast cancer, the 1995 meta-analysis found no significant benefit to adjuvant tamoxifen in women with receptor-poor tumors.[31] It is, therefore, critical that hormone receptor be measured in any patient with newly diagnosed breast cancer.[4] Although there was some controversy in the past as to whether hormone receptor status is also of value in predicting response to chemotherapy, it is now known that no such relationship exists.[19] On the other hand, there is preliminary data that suggest the presence of an overexpressed c-erbB-2 oncogene in breast cancers may have predictive value in the choice of chemotherapy.[53,54] The NSABP trial found that melphalan with fluorouracil + doxorubicin was more effective adjuvant therapy than melphalan with fluorouracil alone. However, when the data were reanalyzed, the benefit was only seen in patients whose tumors overexpressed c-erbB-2.[53] The CALGB trial randomized women to three different dose-intense CAF regimens. The two higher-dose regimens (both within the range of standard dosage) were superior to the low-dose regimen; however, an analysis of the data by c-erbB-2 status found the difference to be present only in the subset of oncogene overexpressor.[54] These data suggest that if adjuvant chemotherapy is to be given in the presence of c-erbB-2 overexpression, it should contain doxorubicin at full dose. What is not clear is whether lack of c-erbB-2 overexpression predicts the effectiveness of nondoxorubucin-containing regimens. While there are suggestions that c-erbB-2 overexpression may predict unresponsiveness to adjuvant tamoxifen,[55,56] recent studies are not supportive.[57,58]

Though the biology of the tumor is important, so too is the biology of the patient in the choice of adjuvant systemic therapy. Age is the most important factor. There is little data on the efficacy of chemotherapy in patients over the age of 70 years; of the 19,000 reviewed in the EBCTCG chemotherapy overview, there were only 600 women over 70 years. They could draw no conclusion as to the value of chemotherapy in that age group.[19] Chemotherapy should be reserved for women over 70 years with poor prognostic tumors containing no hormone receptor, with a reasonable life expectancy, and that are physiologically in excellent health. It is important to emphasize, however, that being over 70 years should not a priori exclude a woman from consideration of chemotherapy. In the younger postmenopausal groups, chemotherapy is clearly beneficial alone or when added to tamoxifen. Nevertheless, it should not be universally given. The EBCTCG trial analyzed the same randomized trials where they found a survival benefit to chemotherapy plus tamoxifen in women 50 to 69 years but found no increase in "quality (of life)–adjusted survival" compared with tamoxifen alone.[59] The implication is not that chemotherapy should not be given to women age 50 to 69 years but rather that its use in addition to tamoxifen should be limited to high-risk, poor-prognosis patients, despite calls to the contrary. The administration of adjuvant systemic therapy cannot be considered a standardized process. It must always be individualized.

BENEFITS VERSUS TOXICITY AND RISKS OF THERAPY

The acute toxicities of adjuvant systemic therapy of early breast cancer are significant but generally well tolerated and are easily justified given the potential benefit. The toxicities of chemotherapy can be divided into those of the CMF-like regimens and those of the doxorubicin regimens. All chemotherapies used as adjuvant treatment cause significant myelosuppression, with leukopenia generally clinically more significant than anemia or thrombocytopenia. In the NSABP trials of classic CMF × 6, the incidence of neutropenia less than 2,000 was ~ 10 percent and severe infection about 1 percent.[21] With AC × 4, it is 4 percent severe neutropenia and 2 percent severe infection.[21] With 6 months of CAF, the risk of leukopenia and infection is higher. Thrombocytopenia is seen in less than 1 percent of patients in most regimens.[21] Doxorubicin-containing regimens are more emetogenic than CMF; however, the incidence of severe vomiting is rapidly dropping with the introduction of serotonin antagonists. Alopecia is nearly universal with doxorubicin and is seen in about 40 percent of CMF patients.[21] Diarrhea is rarely seen with either regimens; the use of serotonin antagonist antiemetics is associated with constipation (and mild headache). Cystitis is seen in about 1 percent of patients receiving cyclophosphamide-containing regimens and correlates with longer durations of therapy.[21] Other rare side effects of both regimens include mucositis, thromboembolic events, and, for doxorubicin, extravasation skin ulceration.

The most common chronic chemotherapy toxicity is the cessation of menses and induction of menopause in premenopausal women. This is more common with 6 months of CMF (and CAF) than with AC × 4. In one study, amenorrhea was seen in 68 percent of women on CMF and 34 percent of women on AC.[60] Symptomatic cardiomyopathy is a rare complication seen with doxorubicin-containing regimens. The risk is less than 1 percent with cumulative doxorubicin doses less than 350 mg/M^2.[61] The cumulative dose with AC × 4 is 240/m^2; with CAF, it is 360/m^2. The risk is increased with age, left chest wall irradiation, and prior heart disease. Chemotherapy agents are carinogenic in experimental systems. Nev-

ertheless, the incidence of second malignancies has been low. The ECOG estimated the risk of secondary leukemia or myelodysplasia after its CMF adjuvant regimens to be less than 0.2 percent similar to that of the general population.[62] Bonadonna could find no increased risk of malignancy in long-term follow-up of his adjuvant CMF patients.[63] The M.D. Anderson Hospital, in reviewing its adjuvant doxorubicin programs, found the risk of secondary leukemia or myelodysplasia to be 0.2 to 0.5 percent.[64] There is some suggestion that concomitant high-dose cyclophosphamide may increase the doxorubicin leukemia risk.[65] Other than menopause in younger women, long-term complications of adjuvant chemotherapy are infrequent.

Tamoxifen is a selective estrogen receptor modular (SERM) and so may be antiestrogenic or estrogenic, depending on its interaction with the individual tissue receptor. Its toxicity profile reflects this duality. The most common acute tamoxifen side effects are menopausal symptoms. In the NSABP trial B-14, hot flashes were seen in about two-thirds of patients, about a third had weight gain, fluid retention, and vaginal discharge, and a quarter experienced nausea, and weight loss.[35] Irregular menses were seen in a fourth of premenopausal women.[35] The only significant acute toxicities were rare thromboembolic events: deep vein thrombosis in 0.8 percent and pulmonary embolus in 0.4 percent. Mood swings and depression are unusual. Very-high-dose tamoxifen may cause retinal changes, but these are rarely seen with conventional doses. There are reports of cataracts in patients on the drug.[66] In a large review of ocular toxicity from the NSABP, there were no cases of vision-threatening eye toxicity with tamoxifen.[66]

There is an increased risk of developing uterine cancer in women receiving tamoxifen (2/1,000/y of therapy versus 1/1,000/y in control).[67] In the 1995 meta-analysis, 10 years after breast surgery, women on 5 years of the drug had a 1.1 percent risk of uterine malignancy compared with 0.3 percent for those who did not receive the drug.[31] Furthermore, most reported cases were early stage and highly curable,[68,69] although fatal cases of uterine cancer have been reported.[70] In contrast to the uterine cancer effects are thoses of tamoxifen on the development of contralateral breast cancer. Multiple studies have found that tamoxifen given to prevent recurrence of previous breast cancer significantly decreases the risk of developing new contralateral breast cancer.[68] The 1995 overview found a 47 percent decrease in the risk of contralateral malignancy in women receiving 5 years of the drug.[31] This effect of tamoxifen was confirmed by the Breast Cancer Prevention Trial (NSABP P-1), which found a virtually identical decrease in the development of new breast cancers in high risk women without a history of the disease.[71] This effect would suggest that even in women with a history of receptor-negative breast cancer, tamoxifen might be considered not to prevent recurrence but to decrease the risk of new malignancy.

Other beneficial effects of adjuvant tamoxifen include an estrogenic-like decrease in bone loss in postmenopausal women,[72–74] decrease in cholesterol,[75] and, in some studies, decreased cardiac mortality.[76–78] Overall, the risk/benefit ratio strongly favors tamoxifen's use as adjuvant therapy for hormone receptor-containing early-stage breast cancer.

SUMMARY

The addition of adjuvant chemotherapy or hormonal therapies to local treatment significantly decreases recurrence and mortality in women with axillary node-positive or high-risk, node-negative, operable breast cancer. The choice of therapy should be individualized on the basis of the perceived risk of recurrence, particularly as determined by nodal status and tumor size, patient age and general health, and the presence or absence of hormone (estrogen or progesterone) receptor in the tumor. Some general guidelines are reasonable (see Table 12–2). For all postmenopausal women with receptor-containing tumor warranting adjuvant therapy (node + or −), tamoxifen should be given for 5 years. If at particularly high risk, such as with multiple positive nodes or an extremely large tumor, the addition of chemotherapy (AC × 4) should be considered if the patient is in good health and has a reasonable life expectancy. For receptor-negative postmenopausal women with node-positive or high-risk, node-negative disease, chemotherapy (CMF or AC × 4 or for multiple nodes AC × 4→ paclitaxel × 4 or CAF) should be administered. The borderline efficacy of CMF in postmenopausal women make doxorubicin-containing regimens preferable if cardiac function permits. Chemotherapy should be used cautiously in women over 70 years. In the United States, for premenopausal women with positive nodes, adjuvant chemotherapy is standard. For patients with 1 to 3 positive nodes, AC or CMF is widely used. For women with four or more involved nodes, CAF × 6 is the standard. Recent data suggest that the addition of taxanes to doxorubicin regimens also has a role in this group (AC × 4→ paclitaxel × 4) and may supplant CAF.[25] If the patient's tumor is receptor positive, tamoxifen is frequently added to chemotherapy, but the data to support this are limited. Nevertheless, if the chemotherapy renders a woman menopausal or there is great concern about contralateral breast cancer, few would fault the addition of tamoxifen to chemotherapy for node-positive, premenopausal, receptor-positive, breast cancer adjuvant therapy. In Europe, such women might undergo oophorectomy as an alternative to chemotherapy ± tamoxifen.[39] For high-risk, node-negative premenopausal women, there are several alternatives. If the tumor is hormone receptor positive, tamoxifen, CMF, or AC (or chemotherapy + tamoxifen) are acceptable. If receptor negative, chemotherapy with CMF or AC is used. Although the SWOG trial suggested the superiority of CAF in this group of patients,[22] the added toxicity is likely to limit the use of this combination in node-negative women. The use of high-dose chemotherapy with stem cell support should be considered investigational, even for patients with 10 or more involved nodes. Neoadjuvant therapies are appropriate in an attempt to achieve breast conservation but have not been proved a more effective adjuvant systemic therapy than postoperative treatment.[49] Delay of local treatment (surgery and/or radiation) for the administration of neoadjuvant[49] or adjuvant therapy[79] does not negatively impact outcome. For women with high-risk DCIS treated with lumpectomy plus radiation, tamoxifen therapy should be considered on the basis of the preliminary results of NSABP trial B-24.[52] Whenever possible, women with early-stage breast cancer should be encouraged to enroll in RCTs of adjuvant therapies. Only with such studies will further progress be made in reducing mortality in women with breast cancer.

REFERENCES

1. Contesso H, Mouriesse H, Friedman S, et al. The importance of histologic grade in long-term prognosis of breast cancer: a study of 1,010 patients, uniformly treated at the Institut Gustave-Roussy. J Clin Oncol 1987;5;1378–6.
2. Fisher ER, Gregorio RM, Fisher B, et al. The pathology of invasive breast cancer. A syllabus derived from findings of the National Adjuvant Breast Project. Cancer 1975;36:1–85.
3. Donegan WL. Tumor-related prognostic factors for breast cancer. CA Cancer J Clin 1997;47:28–51.
4. Tumor Marker Guideline Panel, American Society Clinical Oncology. Clinical practice guidelines for the use of tumor markers in breast and colorectal cancer. J Clin Oncol 1996;14:2843–77.
5. Early Breast Cancer Trialists' Collaborative Group. Effects of radiotherapy and surgery in early breast cancer. An overview of the randomized trials. N Engl J Med 1995;333:1444–55.
6. Beatson GT. On the treatment of inoperable cases of carcinoma of the mamma: suggestion for a new method of treatment with illustrative cases. Lancet 1996;2:104–7.
7. Locker GY. Hormonal therapy of breast cancer. Cancer Treat Rev 1998;24:221–40.
8. Desombre ER, Carbone PP, Jensen EV, et al. Special Report. Steroid receptors in breast cancer. N Engl J Med 1979;301:1011–2.
9. Hoogstraten B, Fabian C. A reappraisal of single drugs for advanced breast cancer. Cancer Clin Trials 1979;2:101–98.
10. Cooper RG. Combination chemotherapy in hormone resistant breast cancer. Proc Am Assoc Cancer Res 1963;10:15.
11. Bull JM, Tormey DC, Li SH, et al. A randomized comparative trial of adriamycin versus methotrexate in combination drug therapy. Cancer 1978;41:1649–57.
12. Fisher B, Ravdin RG, Ausman RK, et al. Surgical adjuvant chemotherapy in cancer of the breast: results of a decade of cooperative investigations. Ann Surg 1968;168:337–56.
13. Fisher B, Carbone P, Economou SG, et al. L-Phenylalanine mustard (L-PAM) in the management of primary breast cancer. A report of early findings. N Engl J Med 1975;292:117–22.
14. Bonadonna G, Brusamolino E, Valagussa P, et al. Combination chemotherapy as an adjuvant treatment in operable breast cancer. N Engl J Med 1976;294:405–10.
15. Engelsman E, Rubens RD, Klign JGM. Comparison of the classical CMF with a three weekly intravenous CMF schedule in postmenopausal patients with advanced breast cancer: an EORTC study. Proceedings of the 4th EORTC Breast cancer Working Conference 1987;1:1.
16. Goldhirsch A, Colleoni M, Coates AS, et al. Adding adjuvant CMF chemotherapy to either radiotherapy or tamoxifen: are all CMF's alike? the International Breast Cancer Study Group (IBCSG). Ann Oncol 1998;9:489–93.
17. Tancini G, Bonadonna G, Valgussa P, et al. Adjuvant CMF in breast cancer: comparative 5 year results of 12 versus 6 cycles. J Clin Oncol 1983;1:2–10.
18. Early Breast Cancer Trialists' Collaborative Group. Systemic treatment of early breast cancer by hormonal, cytotoxic, or immune therapy: 133 randomized trials involving 31,000 recurrences and 24,000 deaths among 75,000 women. Lancet 1992;339:1–15, 71–85.
19. Early Breast Cancer Trialists' Collaborative Group. Polychemotherapy for early breast cancer: an overview of the randomized trials. Lancet 1998;352:930–42.
20. Bagley CS, Wesley MN, Young RC, Lipmann ME. Adjuvant chemotherapy in males with cancer of the breast. Am J Clin Oncol 1987;6:45–50.

21. Fisher B, Brown AM, Dimitrov NV, et al. Two months of doxorubicin-cyclophosphamide with and without interval reinduction therapy compared with 6 months of cyclophosphamide, methotrexate, and fluorouracil in positive-node breast cancer patients with tamoxifen-nonresponsive tumors: results from the NSABP B-15. J Clin Oncol 1990;8:1483–96.

22. Hutchins L, Green S, Ravdin P, et al. CMF versus CAF with and without tamoxifen in high risk node-negative breast cancer patients and a natural history follow-up study in low-risk node negative patients: first results of Intergroup Trial INT 102. Proc Am Soc Clin Oncol 1998;17:1a.

23. Moliterni A, Bonadonna G, Valagussa P, et al. Cyclophosphamide, methotrexate and fluorouracil with and without doxorubicin in the adjuvant treatment of resectable breast cancer with one to three positive axillary nodes. J Clin Oncol 1991;9:1124–30.

24. Tormey DC, Gray R, Abeloff MD, et al. Adjuvant therapy with a doxorubicin regimen and long term tamoxifen in premenopausal breast cancer patients: an ECOG trial. J Clin Oncol 1992 1992;10:1848–56.

25. Henderson IC, Berry D, Demetri G, et al. Improved disease-free and overall survival from the addition of sequential paclitaxel but not from the escalation of doxorubicin dose in the adjuvant chemotherapy of patients with node-positive primary breast cancer. Proc Am Soc Clin Oncol 1998;17:101a.

26. Fisher B, Anderson S, Wickerham DL, et al. Increased intensification and total dose of cyclophosphamide in a doxorubicin-cyclophosphamide regimen for the treatment of primary breast cancer: findings from National Surgical Adjuvant Breast and Bowel Project B-22. J Clin Oncol 1997;15:1858–69.

27. Wolmark N, Fisher B, Anderson S. The effect of increasing dose intensity and cumulative dose of adjuvant cyclophosphamide in node positive breast cancer: results of NSABP B-25. Breast Cancer Res Treat 1997;46:26.

28. Rodenhuis S, Richel DJ, van der Wall E, et al. A randomized trial of high-dose chemotherapy and haematopoetic progenitor-cell support in operable breast cancer with extensive axillary node involvement. Lancet 1998;352:515–21.

29. Mouridsen H, Palshof T. Tamoxifen in advanced breast cancer. Cancer Treat Rev 1978;5:131–41.

30. Baum M. Brinkley DM, Dosset JA, et al. Improved survival among patients treated with adjuvant tamoxifen after mastectomy for early breast cancer [letter]. Lancet 1983;2(8347):450.

31. Early Breast Cancer Trialists' Collaborative Group. Tamoxifen for early breast cancer: an overview of the randomized trials. Lancet 1998;351:1451–67.

32. Fisher B, Dignam J, Bryant J, et al. Five versus more than five years of tamoxifen therapy for breast cancer patients with negative lymph nodes and estrogen receptor-positive tumors. J Natl Cancer Inst 1996;88:1529–42.

33. Stewart HJ, Forrest AP, Everington D, et al. Randomized comparison of 5 years of adjuvant tamoxifen with continuous therapy for operable breast cancer. The Scottish Cancer Trials Breast Group. Br J Cancer 1996;74:297–9.

34. Tormey DC, Gray R, Falkson G. Postchemotherapy adjuvant tamoxifen therapy beyond five years in patients with lymph node-positive breast cancer. Eastern Cooperative Oncology Group. J Natl Cancer Inst 1996;88:1828–33.

35. Fisher B, Costantino J, Redmond C. A randomized clinical trial evaluating tamoxifen in the treatment of patients with node negative breast cancer who have estrogen receptor positive tumors. N Engl J Med 1989;320:479–84.

36. Ribeiro G, Swindell R. Adjuvant tamoxifen for male breast cancer. Br J Cancer 1992;65:252–4.

37. Cole MP. A clinical trial of an artificial menopause in carcinoma of the breast. INSERM 1975;55:143.

38. Early Breast Cancer Trialists' Collaborative Group. Ovarian ablation in early breast cancer: an overview of randomized trials. Lancet 1996;348:1189–96.

39. Scottish Cancer Trials Breast Group and ICRF Breast Unit. Adjuvant ovarian ablation versus CMF chemotherapy in premenopausal women with pathological stage II breast carcinoma: the Scottish trial. Lancet 1993;341:1293–8.

40. Davidson NE. Ovarian ablation as treatment for young women with breast cancer. J Natl Cancer Inst Monographs 1994;16:95–9.

41. Focan C, Beaudin M, Salamon E. Adjuvant high dose medroxyprogesterone for early breast cancer: 13 years update of a multicenter randomized trial. Eur J Oncol 1998;(Suppl 1):34.

42. Pannuti F, Martoni A, Cilenti G, et al. Adjuvant therapy for operable breast cancer with medroxyprogesterone acetate alone in post-menopausal patients or in combination with CMF in premenopausal patients. Eur J Cancer Clin Oncol 1988;24:423–9.

43. Jones AL, Powles TJ, Law M, et al. Adjuvant

aminoglutethimide for postmenopausal patients with primary breast cancer: analysis at 8 years. J Clin Oncol 1992;10:1547–52.

44. Fisher B, Dignam J, DeCillis A, et al. The worth of chemotherapy and tamoxifen (TAM) over TAM alone in node negative patients with estrogen-receptor positive invasive breast cancer: first results from NSABP B-20 [abstract]. Proc Ann Meet Am Soc Clin Oncol 1997;16:1a.

45. Albain K, Green S, Osborne CK, et al. Tamoxifen (T) versus cyclophosphamide, adriamycin and 5-FU plus either concurrent or sequential T in post-menopausal receptor (+), node (+) breast cancer: a Southwest Oncology Group phase III intergroup (SWOG-8814, INT-0100) [abstract]. Proc Ann Meet Am Soc Clin Oncol 1997;16:128a.

46. International Breast Cancer Study Group. Effectiveness of adjuvant chemotherapy in combination with tamoxifen for node-positive postmenopausal breast cancer patients. J Clin Oncol 1997;15:1385–94.

47. Pritchard KI, Paterson AH, Fine S, et al. Randomized trial of cyclophosphamide, methotrexate and fluorouracil chemotherapy added to tamoxifen as adjuvant therapy in postmenopausal women with node-positive estrogen and/or progesterone receptor-positive breast cancer: a report of the National Cancer Institute of Canada Clinical Trials Group. J Clin Oncol 1997;15:2302–11.

48. Bonadonna G, Valagussa P. Primary chemotherapy in operable breast cancer. Semin Oncol 1996;23:464–74.

49. Fisher B, Bryant J, Wolmark N, et al. Effect of preoperative chemotherapy on the outcome of women with operable breast cancer. J Clin Oncol 1998;16:2672–85.

50. Fisher B, Brown A, Mamounas E, et al. Effect of preoperative chemotherapy on local-regional disease in women with operable breast cancer: findings from NSABP B-18. J Clin Oncol 1997;15:2483–93.

51. Willsher PC, Robertson JFR, Chan SY, et al. Locally advanced breast cancer: early results of a randomized trial of multimodal therapy versus initial hormone therapy. Eur J Cancer 1997;33:45–9.

52. Wolmark N, Dignam J, Fisher B. The addition of tamoxifen to lumpectomy and radiotherapy in the treatment of ductal carcinoma in situ (DCIS): preliminary results of NSABP protocol B-24. Breast Cancer Res Treat 1998;50:227.

53. Paik S, Bryant J, Park C, et al. ErbB-2 and response to doxorubicin in patients with axil-

lary lymph node-positive, hormone receptor-negative breast cancer. J Natl Cancer Inst 1998;90:1361–70.

54. Thor AD, Berry DA, Budman DR, et al. ErbB-2, p53, and efficacy of adjuvant therapy in lymph node-positive breast cancer. J Natl Cancer Institute 1998;90:1346–60.

55. Borg A, Caldetorp B, Ferno M, et al. ErbB-2 amplification is associated with tamoxifen resistance in steroid-receptor positive breast cancer. Cancer Lett 1994;81:137–44.

56. Carlomagno C, Perrone F, Gallo C, et al. C-erbB-2 overexpression decreases the benefit of adjuvant tamoxifen in early-stage breast cancer without axillary node metastases. J Clin Oncol 1996;14:2702–8.

57. Soubeyran I, Quenel N, Coindre JM, et al. PS2 protein: a marker improving prediction of response to neoadjuvant tamoxifen in post-menopausal breast cancer. Br J Cancer 1996;74:1120–5.

58. Berns EM, Foekens JA, van Staveren IL, et al. Oncogene amplication and prognosis in breast cancer: relationship with systemic treatment. Gene 1995;159:11–8.

59. Gelber RD, Cole BF, Goldhirsch A, et al. Adjuvant chemotherapy plus tamoxifen compared with tamoxifen alone for postmenopausal breast cancer: meta-analysis of quality-adjusted survival. Lancet 1996;347:1066–71.

60. Bines J, Oleske DM, Cobleigh MA. Ovarian function in premenopausal women treated with adjuvant chemotherapy for breast cancer. J Clin Oncol 1996;14:1718–29.

61. Von Hoff D, Layard MW, Basa P, et al. Risk factors for doxorubicin-induced congestive heart failure. Ann Int Med 1979;91:710–7.

62. Tallman MS, Gray R, Bennett JM, et al. Leukemogenic potential of adjuvant chemotherapy for early-stage breast cancer: the ECOG experience. J Clin Oncol 1995;13:1557–63.

63. Valagussa P, Tancini G, Bonadonna G. Second malignancies after CMF for resectable breast cancer. J Clin Oncol 1987;5:1138–42.

64. Diamandidou E, Buzdar AU, Smith TL, et al. Treatment-related leukemia in breast cancer patients treated with fluorouracil-doxorubicin-cyclophosphamide combination adjuvant chemotherapy: the University of Texas M.D. Anderson Cancer Center experience. J Clin Oncol 1996;14:2722–30.

65. DeCillis A, Anderson A, Bryant J, et al. Acute myeloid leukemia and myelodysplastic syndrome on NSABP B-25: an update. Proc Am Soc Clin Oncol 1997;16:130a.

66. Gorin MB, Day R, Costantino JP, et al. Long-term tamoxifen citrate use and potential ocular toxicity. Am J Ophthalmol 1998;125:493–501.

67. Jordan VC, Assikis VJ. Endometrial carcinoma and tamoxifen: clearing up a controversy. Clin Cancer Res 1995;1:467–72.

68. Rutqvist LE, Johansson H, Signomklao T, et al. Adjuvant tamoxifen therapy for early stage breast cancer and second primary malignancies. J Natl Cancer Inst 1995;87:645–51.

69. Fisher B, Costantino JP, Redmond CK, et al. Endometrial cancer in tamoxifen-treated breast cancer patients: findings from the National Surgical Adjuvant Breast and Bowel Project (NSABP) B-14. J Natl Cancer Inst 1994;86:527–37.

70. Magriples U, Naftolin F, Schwartz PE, Carcangiu ML. High-grade endometrial carcinoma in tamoxifen-treated breast cancer patients. J Clin Oncol 1993;11:485–90.

71. Fisher B, Costantino JP, Wickerham DL, et al. Tamoxifen for the prevention of breast cancer: report of the NSABP P-1 study. J Natl Cancer Inst 1998;90:1371–88.

72. Love RR, Mazess RB, Barden HS, et al. Effects of tamoxifen on bone mineral density in postmenopausal women with breast cancer. N Engl J Med 1992;326:852–6.

73. Kristen B, Ejlertsen B, Dalgaard P, et al. Tamoxifen and bone metabolism in postmenopausal low-risk breast cancer patients: a randomized study. J Clin Oncol 1994;12:992–7.

74. Powles TJ, Hickish T, Kanis JA, et al. Effect of tamoxifen on bone mineral density measured by dual-energy x-ray absorptiometry in healthy premenopausal and postmenopausal women. J Clin Oncol 1996;14:78–84.

75. Love RR, Wiebe DA, Feyzi JM, et al. Effects of tamoxifen on cardiovascular risk factors in postmenopausal women after 5 years of treatment. J Natl Cancer Inst 1994;86:1534–9.

76. McDonald CC, Alexander FE, Whyte BW, et al. Cardiac and vascular morbidity in women receiving adjuvant tamoxifen for breast cancer in a randomized trial. The Scottish Cancer Trials Breast Group. Br Med J 1995;311:977–80.

77. Costantino JP, Kuller LH, Ives DG, et al. Coronary heart disease mortality and adjuvant tamoxifen therapy. J Natl Cancer Inst 1997;89:776–82.

78. Rutqvist LE, Mattsson A. Cardiac and thromboembolic morbidity among post menopausal women with early-stage breast cancer in a randomized trial of adjuvant tamoxifen. The Stockholm Breast Cancer Study Group. J Natl Cancer Inst 1993;85:1398–406

79. Recht A, Come SE, Henderson IC, et al. The sequencing of chemotherapy and radiation therapy after conservative surgery for early-stage breast cancer. N Engl J Med 1996;334:1356–61.

EARLY-STAGE BREAST CANCER

Mastectomy and Breast Conservation Therapy: Equivalent Survival

Several randomized clinical trials have confirmed equivalent survival data when lumpectomy and breast radiotherapy are compared to modified radical mastectomy for early-stage invasive breast cancer. Local recurrence rates after conservative surgery and radiotherapy range from 3 to 19 percent (Table 13–1).[14–20] It should be noted that the study from the NCI had the highest rate of local recurrence but did not require negative pathologic resection margins, the significance of which is discussed below. This same study was the only trial to show a significant advantage to mastectomy with respect to local recurrence. Despite a broad range of entry criteria (acceptable tumor size ranged from 2 to 5 cm), the data are remarkably consistent. The most important finding was the equivalent overall survival between treatment arms in all studies. Local recurrence in the mastectomy-treated patients ranged from 4 to 14 percent. Equivalent survival between extensive surgery and limited surgery plus radiotherapy was confirmed in a meta-analysis of randomized trials in breast cancer. Also, a threefold reduction in local recurrence was demonstrated with the addition of radiotherapy to local excision.[21]

There are large retrospective reviews correlating these results.[22] These studies have also been useful in identifying prognostic features from patients with breast cancer treated with conservative surgery and radiotherapy. It is very safe to conclude that the data supports the use of breast conservation therapy for the treatment of early-stage invasive breast cancer.

Risk Factors for Local Recurrence

Among patients treated with breast conservation therapy, several risk factors have been identified that predict for local recurrence. These have been classified as patient-related, tumor-related, and treatment-related factors. If a risk factor was associated with a prohibitively high recurrence rate, this would be a contraindication to BCT only if the same factor was not a risk factor for recurrence after mastectomy. For example, several series have shown age of diagnosis to be a predictive indicator for local recurrence after BCT, with younger patients being at higher risk.[23–26] However, one cannot conclude that young age is a contraindication for BCT, because other studies have shown the same population of young patients to be at higher risk for local recurrence after mastectomy.[27,28]

PATHOLOGIC VARIABLES

Table 13–2 lists several factors that are or at one time were thought to be factors predictive for local recurrence. Multicentricity in more than one quadrant of the breast is a contraindication to BCT. Several authors have concluded that the risk for local failure is significantly higher in

Table 13–1. BREAST CONSERVATION THERAPY COMPARED WITH MASTECTOMY: RANDOMIZED TRIALS

Trial	Follow-up (years)	Local Recurrence (%)			Survival (%)		
		Mastectomy	BCT	*p* Value	Mastectomy	BCT	*p* Value
NSABP B-06[14]	12	8	10	ns	59	63	ns
NCI[15,16]	10	6	19	.01	75	77	ns
Milan[17]	18	4	7	ns	65	65	ns
EORTC[18]	14	14	17	ns	61	54	ns
Danish[19]	—	4	3	ns	82	79	ns
IGR[20]	15	14	9	ns	65	73	ns

NS = not significant.

patients with documented disease in more than one quadrant of the breast.[29–31] This likely indicates the presence of residual tumor burden throughout the breast after local excision that cannot be controlled with radiotherapy doses of 45 to 50 Gy. Since mastectomy for multicentric disease is *not* associated with an increased risk of local recurrence,[32] it is the standard of care for patients with defined multicentricity.

Historically, it was thought that patients with an extensive intraductal component (EIC) associated with their invasive tumor were at significant risk for recurrence.[33,34] This condition has been defined as intraductal carcinoma occupying ≥ 25 percent of the area encompassed by invasive tumor as well as the surrounding stroma of the resected specimen. However, when this risk factor was re-evaluated in association with negative surgical resection margins, it was found that if negative margins for both invasive and noninvasive components could be obtained, no increase in local recurrence was observed.[35,36]

The presence of lobular carcinoma in situ (LCIS) within the tumor specimen likewise has no impact on the probability of local recurrence.[37] However, these patients may be at higher risk for development of a second subsequent cancer in the contralateral breast. Infiltrating lobular histology behaves differently than infiltrating ductal histology. Although the natural history of lobular carcinoma may differ

Table 13–2. RISK FACTORS FOR LOCAL RECURRENCE AFTER BREAST CONSERVATION THERAPY

Risk Factor	Current Literature Support
Young age at diagnosis[23–27]	Y
Multicentricity[29–32]	Y
Extensive intraductal component[35,36]	N
LCIS found in specimen[37]	N
Infiltrating lobular histology[38]	N
Subareolar location[39–41]	N
Paget's disease[42]	N
Pathologic grade[43]	N
Family history[44,45]	N
Positive surgical margins[47,51]	Y

LCIS = lobular carcinoma in situ.

(larger size at presentation, higher hormonal receptor positivity, decreased axillary involvement), there is no difference in local control in patients with infiltrating lobular histology treated with local excision and radiotherapy.[38]

Patients with centrally located tumors were initially thought to be unsuitable for BCT due to cosmetic concerns about tumors near the nipple-areolar complex.[30] There was also a concern that involvement of major breast ducts might be associated with more diffuse disease. However, recent analysis of tumors within 2 cm of the nipple-areolar complex show no increased risk of local failure when treated with breast conservation therapy, provided negative resection margins are achieved.[39] Good to excellent cosmesis can be achieved in this scenerio.[40,41]

Patients with Paget's disease of the nipple were previously considered poor candidates for BCT because of its significant association with separate palpable infiltrating malignancies. For patients with Paget's disease and no palpable malignancy, the concern was the possibility of microscopic invasive disease. This concern is probably less valid today with newer mammographic technologies. Moreover, it has been shown that if patients presenting with Paget's disease of the breast without an associated palpable mass are treated with local excision and radiotherapy, there is no increased risk of recurrence.[42]

Tumor size and histologic grade have prognostic significance for survival, risk of axillary involvement, and the development of distant metastatic disease. However, local control may not be impacted by either the size or histologic grade of the primary lesion. Most retrospective studies find no significant difference in local control for T1 or T2 tumors. Recent studies fail to correlate higher grade tumors with increased local recurrence.[43]

PATIENT VARIABLES

Significant family history of breast cancer is not a contraindication for BCT. There is no higher risk of local failure in patients with a history of breast cancer in a first-degree relative. In fact, several studies have shown that patients with breast cancer who have a first-degree relative with the disease may have an increased overall survival.[44,45] This observation may correlate with evolving data showing a good prognosis with BRCA1 genetic overexpression.[46]

Young age at diagnosis is associated with an increased local recurrence rate. The studies differ in the age at which risk of recurrence is significantly higher, but all conclude young age to be a risk factor. Because these same patients are at higher risk for local failure after mastectomy, young age is not a contraindication to BCT.[24–27] In addition, there is no impact on overall survival for younger patients treated with breast preservation therapy.

THERAPEUTIC VARIABLES

Surgical Factors

The principal surgical factor correlated with increased local–regional recurrence after BCT is an inability to resect the lesion with clear pathologic margins. Definition of a "clear margin" varies. While the absence of tumor at the inked margin of the resected specimen is defined by some authors as a negative margin, others have differentiated between negative and close margins by using 1 to 3 mm to define a negative margin. These distinctions notwithstanding, there appears to be a consistently significant increase in local recurrence with diffusely positive margins compared to "negative" margins. The recurrence rate for diffusely positive margins approaches 30 percent, compared to 2 to 10 percent for negative margins. Thus, the presence of diffusely positive pathologic lumpectomy margins is an indication for re-excision. If re-excision is not possible, mastectomy should be performed. Surgical margins classified as negative, close, focally positive, or more than focally positive correlate with a 2, 3, 9, and 28 percent risk of local recurrence, respectively (Table 13–3).[47–49]

Focally positive and close margins appear to be associated with a risk of local recurrence that is intermediate between diffusely positive and negative margins. In some studies, this intermediate risk of recurrence is statistically significant, implying re-excision should be performed.[50] However, other studies do not show significance related to close or focally positive margins.[51] The presence of two or more positive margins has been shown to be predictive of higher local failure compared to one.[52] Of particular note, proper evaluation of resection margins is essential, as one-third of patients with focally positive shaved margins are negative when inked margins are properly evaluated.

The amount of tumor at the margin of a surgical specimen correlates with the risk of diffuse involvement in the breast.[53] There is a strong correlation between the extent of involvement of surgical margins and residual tumor burden in the subsequently re-excised specimen. The risk of residual disease is a continuum based upon distance from the tumor, with margin distance determined within the context of cosmetic outcome.[54] Standard doses of radiotherapy are less likely to control a breast with a significant microscopic tumor burden. Although boost doses of radiotherapy to the surgical bed are believed to increase local control, definitive evidence is meager. One study looked at the effect on local control with both re-excision and boost doses of radiotherapy.[55] There was a statistically significant increase in local control with re-excision for close, indeterminate, or positive margins compared to no re-excision. There was no difference in local control for these same patients when evaluated by total dose delivered to the tumor site, indicating that re-excision for questionable margin status was more important than boost irradiation. This supports the notion that the best radiation in the world cannot compensate for inadequate surgery. The presence of a focally positive margin appears to be significant and should also be re-excised. Although the significance of close resection margin probably depends more on the underlying definitions, re-excision does not appear necessary. Ideally, negative margins should be obtained to optimize local control.

The anticipated cosmetic outcome after lumpectomy is critical to the surgical selection of patients for BCT. The pressure of a large tumor-to-breast ratio is likely to lead to a less satisfactory cosmetic outcome from the point of view of both patient and physician. Excision of a major proportion of breast tissue to obtain negative margins (usually greater than a quadrant) is a relative contraindication to BCT. Cosmetic evaluation of the breast is very subjective, with many layers of complexity in terms of self-esteem and sensuality. While studies comparing lumpectomy to quadrantectomy have shown better local control with quadrantectomy followed by radiotherapy, in general lumpectomy plus radiotherapy provides equivalent local control, with better cosmesis from the point of view of both patient and physician.[56,57]

Radiation Therapy Factors

Certain collagen vascular diseases, such as scleroderma and systemic lupus erythematosus, have been associated with an increase in acute skin and subcutaneous toxicity to standard doses of radiotherapy and may be related to inadequate repair of sublethal radiation injury. However, a retrospective review of patients with collagen vascular disease showed that only patients with scleroderma exhibited prohibitive toxicity. Patients with other collagen vascular diseases did not experience prohibitive toxicity and could be considered candidates for BCT.[58]

The potentially deleterious effects of radiotherapy on the developing fetus prohibit patients in the first two trimesters of pregnancy from being candidates for BCT. Estimated cumulative fetal doses of 3 to 4 Gy are delivered with tangential radiotherapy.[59] Because there is no known threshold dose for mutagenesis, radiotherapy is an absolute contraindication during the first two trimesters. Long-term effects of radiation during the third trimester are unclear.

Boost to Lumpectomy Site

Two questions exist regarding the use of irradiation to the lumpectomy site in conjunction with whole breast irradiation. First, is a boost necessary? Most centers treat the whole breast with fraction sizes of 180 cGy to a total dose of 45 to 50 Gy followed by a boost to the tumor site of an additional 10 to 15 Gy. Protocols established by the National Surgical Adjuvant Breast Project (NSABP) routinely treat at 200 cGy per day to a total dose of 50 Gy with no boost to the tumor site. The principal rationale for boost irradiation is that it can be delivered safely without major cosmetic detriment. In a large retrospective study, 17 percent of patients who did not receive a boost showed local failure, compared to 11 percent for those

Table 13–3. MARGINS OF EXCISION CORRELATED TO RATE OF LOCAL RECURRENCE

Study	Margin Status (%)					
	Negative	Positive	Close	Indeterminate	Focally involved	More than Focally involved
Anscher et al[47]	10	2		10		
Gage et al[51]	2	16	3		9	28
Heimann et al[49]	2	11				
Ryoo* et al[48]	6	13	8			
Smitt et al[63]	2	18†				
Solin* et al[62]	10	8	14	13		
Spivack et al[50]	3.7	18				

*Boost radiation delivered based on margin status.
†Combined data on close or positive margins.

who did.[60] On the other hand, another study randomizing patients to a boost after whole breast radiation versus no boost found increased local control in boosted patients.[61] However, patients treated with a boost had a worse cosmetic outcome, with a statistically significant increase in telangiectasia formation. Unfortunately, the dose per fraction in the study was 250 cGy for both the whole breast and boost portions of treatment—this represents a higher fractional dose than is routinely used in the United States.

The second question is whether an increased radiation boost can compensate for close or positive resection margins. The data on this show mixed results. Retrospective data are often confounded by the routine use of an increased boost dose to patients with close margins. On the one hand, there are studies showing that the increasing dose used to boost close margins increased local control.[62] On the other hand, studies demonstrate that patients with positive margins have higher local recurrence rates with or without a boost.[63] The issue may be resolved by a current EORTC study randomizing patients with inadequate surgical margins to boost doses of 10 and 25 Gy.

Systemic Therapy Factors

Two conclusions can be gleaned from data on the addition of chemotherapy to BCT. Chemotherapy added to lumpectomy and radiotherapy in patients at high risk for development of metastatic disease reduces the risk of ipsilateral breast recurrence to as low as 2.6 percent.[64] On the other hand, chemotherapy cannot substitute for radiotherapy in BCT. Local recurrence in patients treated with local excision and chemotherapy has been shown to be significantly higher than that for standard lumpectomy and radiotherapy.[65]

Tamoxifen and Local Control

Tamoxifen benefits estrogen-receptor positive patients both in terms of overall survival and local control. Three randomized trials evaluating the addition of tamoxifen to BCT have shown local control and event-free survival to be significantly improved in tamoxifen-treated patients. Tamoxifen reduces ipsilateral and contralateral recurrences.[66–69] There is currently a randomized trial is underway to evaluate the omission of breast radiation in elderly women with estrogen-receptor positive tumors treated with excision and tamoxifen.

Cytologic Factors and Local Recurrence

New cytologic and genetic factors are being identified and associated with breast cancer prognosis. The majority of these studies to date are small retrospective series and have not influenced the choice of therapy. Case control studies looking at the overexpression of insulin-like growth factor-I receptor (IGF-IR) and *HER-2/neu* indicate that overexpression may predict for an increased risk of local recurrence.[70,71] In these studies, the tumor tissue of all patients who had experienced local recurrence at a single institution were evaluated for overexpression of these newly described markers. Case controls were drawn from those patients treated who did not experience local recurrence. Overexpression of IGF-IR and *HER-2/neu* was found significantly more frequently in patients who experienced recurrence. Although *HER-2/neu* overexpression negatively impacted disease-free survival in patients treated with tamoxifen and radiotherapy,[72] this effect was not seen in patients treated with chemotherapy.

The impact on local control, however, is unclear. Several studies show that patients with the germ-line mutations *BRCA1* or *BRCA2* may experience statistically significant improvement in survival.[73] Overexpression of *p53* has been associated with poor response to tamoxifen, but no data exist on its role with radiotherapy or local control.[74] The "tumor suppressor" gene *p53* is thought to confer radioresistance by a loss of apoptosis in response to radiation. The possibility of radioresistance has been raised in a preliminary study of patients treated with BCT or mastectomy and postoperative radiotherapy.[75] Finally, the presence of angiogenesis as measured by microvessel count has been shown to be prognostically significant for survival. Those patients with node-negative cancers and a low mean vessel count (MVC) had excellent overall survival, but the impact on local recurrence was not indicated.[76] However, laboratory studies have shown a synergistic effect between angiogenesis inhibitors and radiotherapy.[77]

Lumpectomy Alone

The NSABP B-06 trial determined that the risk of local recurrence after local excision alone was as high as 35 percent, compared to 10 percent when combined with radiotherapy. An alternative view of this data is that 65 percent of patients will not experience local recurrence after lumpectomy alone. Therefore, the majority of patients treated with radiotherapy would not have local recurrence in the absence of radiation. Attempts have been made to identify subsets of patients with early stage breast cancer who do not require radiotherapy. Six studies listed in Table 13–4 prospectively randomized patients to excision versus excision plus radiotherapy.[78–81] Although all studies have shown a significant increase in local recurrence in the patients who did not receive radiation, none showed a statistically significant survival advantage with radiotherapy.

The stress of tumor recurrence on the patient as well as the low morbidity of tangential breast radiation must be considered when evaluating these results. Although no survival advantage was documented, local recurrence may be predictive of subsequent increased mortality. Also, a significant number of patients who experience recurrence after local excision alone choose mastectomy at the time of recurrence, regardless of survival data.

Within these studies, subset analyses were performed to identify patients with favorable prognostic features, since these patients may benefit least from the addition of radiotherapy.[82,83] The two favorable prognostic factors identified were advancing age of the patient and small tumor size. In patients with T1 tumors and advancing ages, the local recurrence risk ranged from 4 to 16 percent. Of note, the Uppsala study compared patients > 50 years old with T1 tumors to all others and found a recurrence rate of "only" 15.9 percent.[84] However, such a local recurrence is probably unacceptable since the addition of radiation likely reduces the risk of recurrence to < 5 percent. Of note, some studies were unable to identify subsets of patients who did not benefit from radiotherapy.[85] As indicated above, there is currently a prospective trial for patients > 70 years old with T1 tumors evaluating the omission of radiation in patients receiving tamoxifen, based on the subset analysis of the prior studies and knowledge of the impact of tamoxifen on local control. Outside of a trial setting, the omission of radiation therapy from breast conserving therapy is not presently indicated. Interestingly, practice patterns in the treatment of patients > 65 years old have been shown to differ from younger patients, with this population more likely to be treated with local excision and no radiotherapy.[86,87] The ongoing study may justify these practice patterns.

DUCTAL CARCINOMA IN SITU

The increasing acceptance of screening mammography has led to a dramatic increase in the incidence of ductal carcinoma in situ (DCIS), or intraductal carcinoma. Historically, pathologic evaluation of intraductal carcinoma showed focality in the majority of cases. However, Holland showed intraductal foci of intraductal disease remote from the primary site in 40 percent of patients.[88] Thus, the rationale for radiotherapy to the remaining breast following local excision appears appropriate for the majority of patients with intraductal cancer. There was a subset of patients on NSABP B-06

Table 13–4. COMPARISON OF LUMPECTOMY VERSUS LUMPECTOMY PLUS RADIOTHERAPY: RANDOMIZED TRIALS

Trial	Follow-up (years)	Local Recurrence (%)			Survival (%)		
		No XRT	XRT	*p* Value	No XRT	XRT	*p* Value
NSABP B-06[14]	12	35	10	+	58	62	ns
Scottish trial[69]	5	28	6	+	85	88	ns
Ontario[78]	8	35	11	+	90	91	ns
Milan[79,80]	5	18	2	+	92	92	ns
Uppsala[81]	5	18	2	+	90	91	ns

XRT = external beam radiation therapy.

identified as having in situ histology. The local recurrence rate in patients undergoing excision without radiotherapy was 43 percent, versus 7 percent in patients receiving radiation.[89,90]

The largest prospective study of DCIS is the NSABP randomized study B-17 comparing local excision alone with local excision plus radiotherapy.[91,92] There was a significant decrease in local recurrence in the radiation arm but no difference in overall survival. The addition of radiation reduced the noninvasive cancer recurrence from 10.4 to 7.5 percent. Invasive cancer recurrences were reduced from 10.5 to 2.9 percent. Importantly, of those with recurrence in the local excision-only arm, half the recurrences were invasive. Other retrospective series confirm these findings.[93–95] Thus, the standard of care for patients with DCIS who are eligible for breast sparing treatment is local excision followed by radiotherapy.

Several centers have attempted to identify subgroups of patients with an extremely low risk for recurrence after local excision. Tumor grade, particularly the presence of comedocarcinoma, is a significant predictor of local recurrence. The Van Nuys Prognostic Index (VNPI) has been proposed, using 155 patients treated with local excision alone.[96,97] There is a score given to each of three factors: tumor grade, size of disease, and extent of negative surgical margins. The result of a low VNPI appears to be predictive for decreased local recurrence.[98] There is presently a single-arm nonrandomized study underway evaluating low-risk patients for local recurrence after local excision alone. As

an entry criteria, a minimum of 3 mm negative surgical margins are required.

The impact of local recurrence for DCIS does not appear to have an impact on survival.[99,100] However, the potentially devastating emotional trauma the patient experiences with recurrence should be balanced against the very low risk of radiation complications. Decreased mortality from breast cancer is likely the result of earlier detection of earlier-stage disease, particularly DCIS. The reported 75 percent reduction in subsequent development of invasive breast cancer for patients with DCIS treated with postexcisional radiotherapy supports this conclusion.

RADIOTHERAPY FOR LOCALLY ADVANCED BREAST CANCER

Early studies of local-regional radiotherapy following mastectomy for locally advanced disease showed reduced recurrences in the axilla, supraclavicular fossa, and chest wall. However, these patients experienced an increase in nonbreast cancer-related mortality that negated the survival advantage.[101,3]

Cardiac toxicity due to chest wall radiotherapy is purported to be the causative factor in the increase in nonbreast cancer-related mortality. Concerns about cardiac morbidity from radiotherapy in the face of potentially cardiotoxic adriamycin-based chemotherapy led to decreased use of postmastectomy radiotherapy. Technical factors in historically quoted studies may explain the high incidence of radiation cardiac toxicity. The principle factor is the use of an en face internal mammary and supraclavicular portal, often referred to as a "hockey stick" port. Other considerations are related to dosimetry, such as the use of orthovoltage energy radiotherapy. The energy delivered with orthovoltage radiation is lower in energy, less penetrating, therefore leading to greater inhomogeneity of dose. Comparative dosimetric analysis has shown the dose to the heart to be significantly higher with orthovoltage than with modern megavoltage radiotherapy.[102,103]

When patients treated with orthovoltage radiotherapy were excluded from analysis, a survival benefit of approximately 10 percent was seen in the patients receiving chest wall radiotherapy.[104] Recently, two prospective randomized studies reported results showing survival advantage from the addition of local–regional radiotherapy after mastectomy and chemotherapy for node-positive premenopausal breast cancer patients. Both studies show an improvement in survival of 8 to 10 percent.[105,106] Both studies have shown a benefit to radiating all patients, regardless of the number of lymph nodes involved. Although patients with one to three nodes positive and four or more nodes positive both showed benefit from radiation in subgroup analysis, routine regional lymph node radiotherapy in all patients with positive nodes is not generally accepted practice (Table 13–5).

There has been criticism of the studies for inadequate evaluation of the axilla. Many patients had small numbers of axillary lymph nodes excised. The patient with only one positive node excised may have had other involved nodes in the undissected axilla. Thus, a proportion of the patients thought to have one to three nodes positive may have actually had four or more involved nodes. Prior studies have shown this population of patients to be at lower risk for local–regional recurrence. There was also criticism that the local recurrence rates in these studies were inordinately high compared to prior studies.[107]

Prior retrospective studies have evaluated the role of radiotherapy following mastectomy for locally advanced breast cancer. Studies have looked at recurrence patterns in patients treated with mastectomy alone.[108] Results have shown that patients with four or more nodes positive, large primary tumors > 5 cm, pectoral fascia, or skin involvement are at greatest risk of local recurrence after mastectomy, as high as 25 to 30 percent. Chest wall radiotherapy in these patients reduces local recurrence to < 10 percent. Recurrence patterns show the chest wall and supraclavicular fossa to be the most common sites of recurrence, with axillary recurrence seen less frequently. Patients with tumors < 2 cm and negative axillary lymph nodes have local recurrence risk of < 10 percent and would not appear to benefit from radiotherapy.[109] Patients with tumors between two and five centimeters or one to three involved axillary lymph nodes are at intermediate risk, the role of radiotherapy is controversial in these patients because of modest potential benefit.[110]

Extracapsular extension (ECE) of tumor in axillary lymph nodes is a potential risk factor for regional recurrence. It is likely to be associated with other poor prognostic indicators, such as multiple positive axillary nodes. While shown to be significant on univariate analysis,

Table 13–5. POSTOPERATIVE CHEST WALL RADIOTHERAPY FOLLOWING MASTECTOMY

Treatment indicated[108–110]
    Tumor greater than 5 cm or
    Positive surgical margins or
    Four or more positive axillary lymph nodes

Treatment to be considered[112]
    Premenopausal patients with one to three positive nodes
        Inclusion of internal mammary nodes controversial

Treatment not indicated
    All patients with
        Tumor less than five centimeters and
        Negative margins and
        No positive lymph nodes
    Postmenopausal patients with
        One to three positive lymph nodes

Treatment not indicated based on recent literature[113]
    Patients with extracapsular extension of lymph node involvement

Treatment guidelines differ
    Male patients with breast cancer

ECE was not found to predict for regional failure on multivariate analysis.[111,112]

The recently published trials showing a survival benefit to radiotherapy after mastectomy included the internal mammary nodes. The argument for treatment is that persistent microscopic involvement after chemotherapy is still potentially curable with regional radiotherapy. Theoretically, untreated microscopically involved nodes may lead to development of distant disease. Currently, there is an EORTC study underway evaluating the efficacy of treating internal mammary nodes; efficacy and toxicity data, however, will not be available for 15 or more years.

Detecting involved internal mammary nodes is difficult. The region is not clinically evaluable as are the axilla or supraclavicular fossa. Computed tomography scanning can detect grossly enlarged nodes but not microscopic disease in normal-sized nodes. Sentinel lymph node mapping, on the other hand, may resolve this issue.[113]

MULTIMODALITY THERAPY FOR LOCALLY ADVANCED BREAST CANCER

Neoadjuvant chemotherapy is the subject of intense clinical investigation for tumor downstaging before surgery. Patients who otherwise would not be candidates for breast conservation therapy may experience a significant reduction in tumor burden after neoadjuvant therapy allowing for local excision with negative margins. Response rates are reported to be approximately 65 to 75 percent.[114–116] Studies have shown no detriment to overall survival when compared to standard postoperative treatment. Complete clinical response may define a more favorable subgroup than a partial response although this has not been universally noted.[117]

What is the optimal therapy for women experiencing a complete response? In one study, those patients who had a complete clinical response to chemotherapy who then received radiotherapy to the breast without

surgery had a higher local recurrence rate than those with partial response, local excision, and subsequent radiotherapy.[118] Residual disease, although not clinically detectable, may still be extensive in these patients. In a prospective evaluation of mastectomy specimens in patients who had a complete clinical response to neoadjuvant chemotherapy and radiation therapy, residual disease ranging from 0.6 to 6.5 cm was confirmed in all specimens.[119]

What is the role of postmastectomy radiotherapy in patients who can not undergo BCT after chemotherapy? Clinical staging often underestimates the extent of disease when compared to pathologic staging. Neoadjuvant therapy only confounds the issue. Should regional lymphatic irradiation be used in all patients with locally advanced disease? There is currently an intergroup trial evaluating neoadjuvant therapy that prohibits chest wall radiotherapy after mastectomy, regardless of pathologic findings. In light of the recent data showing a survival advantage in selected patients treated with postmastectomy radiotherapy, this approach is difficult to justify.

The sequencing of chemotherapy and radiotherapy in all stages has been studied in detail. Current practice focuses on systemic therapy as the top therapeutic priority since it has the greatest impact on survival. Concurrent chemotherapy and radiotherapy are prohibitively toxic. Although there are data showing a detrimental impact on local control from delaying radiotherapy more than 6 months after surgery,[120] a randomized trial comparing upfront chemotherapy followed by radiation versus upfront radiotherapy followed by chemotherapy concluded that delaying chemotherapy increased distant metastases and adversely affected survival. Although delayed radiotherapy increases local failure, a significant percentage of patients experiencing local recurrence can be salvaged.[121]

TECHNIQUES OF RADIOTHERAPY

Breast irradiation after local excision is generally administered with megavoltage photon energies of 4 to 10 MV to deliver 45 to 50.4 Gy to the whole breast at 180 cGy per fraction. Tangential portals are established from midline to midaxilla using wedge filters and a half beam block or independent jaws to minimize pulmonary radiation. Many centers deliver a boost to the tumor bed using electron beam radiation for an additional 900 to 1500 cGy. Alternatively, NSABP protocols prescribe 5000 cGy at 200 cGy per fraction, with an optional boost. Superiorly, the tail of the breast is encompassed while excluding the humoral head. Inferiorly, a reasonable margin of 1.5 to 2.0 cm below the inframammary fold is standard. The chest wall curvature necessitates treatment of a small volume of lung tissue. If the maximum width of lung tissue treated is < 2 cm, the risk of pulmonary injury is exceptionally low (Figure 13–1).[122]

The boost treatment volume generally encompasses the surgical bed with margins. Some centers advocate the use of clips at the time of surgery to outline the surgical bed for boost treatment.[123] Electron energies of 6 to 15 MeV are used, depending on the depth needed to encompass the tumor bed. The use of interstitial implants for the boost treatment has been supplanted in recent years.

Three-dimensional treatment planning is a major development in the delivery of radiotherapy. As the contour of the breast is irregular, there is potential for significant inhomogeneity of dose. Using CT scanning of the treatment volumes, technology exists to determine dose delivery in three dimensions with modifications to maximize homogeneity of dose throughout the breast tissue.

RADIOTHERAPY COMPLICATIONS

Dosimetric analyses of historic treatment techniques show an average of 25 percent of the cardiac volume received at least 50 percent of the prescribed dose. With modern treatment energies, 5.7 percent of the cardiac volume receives this same dose.[124] Serum troponin measurements during radiotherapy, a measure of cardiac injury, revealed no significant elevation in one study.[125] Patients treated for left-sided tumors who also had internal mammary nodes treated with modern techniques were evaluated after ten years for possible late effects to the heart. Thallium stress tests revealed no statistical evidence of increased abnormality when compared to the general population.[126] No increased rate of myocardial infarction or cardiac-related deaths was seen in retrospective reviews of patients treated with tangential radiation.[127,128]

Other reported complications from breast radiation include lymphedema, rib fracture, brachial plexopathy, pulmonary fibrosis, carcinogenesis, and contralateral breast cancer. Standard surgical therapy for invasive breast cancer includes level I and II axillary dissection, which has a finite risk of arm edema of 10 to 15 percent.[129,130] The addition of radiotherapy may increase the risk to as high as 20 percent. The measured incidence of arm edema likely differs from the incidence of clinically significant arm edema. One study showed a direct relationship between the incidence of arm edema and the number of lymph nodes dissected.[131] There is less risk of lymphedema in a level I and level II selective dissection than in a full axillary dissection. It is hoped that sentinel node biopsy will eliminate this complication for patients with histologically negative nodes. Any risk of lymphedema after sentinel node biopsy has yet to be determined. Brachial plexopathy is a complication in patients receiving supraclavicular radiation. The delivered dose is the significant

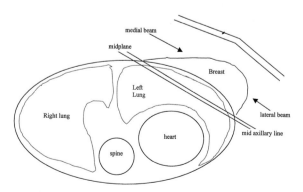

Figure 13–1. Cross-sectional representation of tangential radiation portals for breast conservation therapy.

risk factor as the incidence is reported to be < 2 percent if 50 Gy is delivered, versus 5 percent if > 50 Gy is given.[122] Rib fracture possibly related to beam energy has been reported after breast and chest wall radiotherapy. The incidence is very low (< 0.5 percent), but 4 MV photons may be associated with a higher incidence (2.2 percent) than are higher energy beams.[122]

The chief rationale for the use of BCT over mastectomy is cosmesis. Poor cosmesis should be considered a complication of treatment. In general, 75 to 85 percent of patients and treating physicians report good to excellent cosmesis after lumpectomy and radiotherapy. Factors that may affect cosmesis include delivery of concurrent chemotherapy, type and extent of surgery, and the dose of radiotherapy delivered.[132,133]

Two series have shown that radiotherapy delivered after breast augmentation can lead to capsular contracture in 30 percent of patients. Although radiation following breast reconstruction is very well tolerated,[134,135] the reported contracture rate for the general population is 5 to 10 percent. Subcutaneous implantation is associated with a higher risk of contracture than are subpectoral implants. Postmastectomy radiotherapy after transverse rectus abdominus myocutaneous (TRAM) flap breast reconstruction can be delivered effectively without cosmetic compromise.[136]

The carcinogenic potential of ionizing radiotherapy is rare and the latent period long. Follow-up intervals > 20 years are usually necessary to see carcinogenic effects. Most large retrospective series report scattered cases of sarcoma developing in the treated field years after treatment. Lymphangiosarcoma has been reported in patients who experience significant lymphedema in the treated breast or ipsilateral arm. Osteosarcomas are found to be most common within the treated field, with an overall incidence of sarcoma development of 0.2 percent and a median latency of 11 years.[137,138]

Patients with breast cancer are at higher risk for developing a contralateral breast cancer than is the general population. Whether radiotherapy further increases that risk is the subject of debate. Current technology virtually eliminates dose to the contralateral breast with tangential radiotherapy. However, the half-beam block technique described earlier allowed for up to 400 to 500 cGy to be delivered to the contralateral breast. Hazard analysis of historical series revealed a small increased risk in irradiated patients compared to patients treated with surgery alone.[139]

LOCAL RECURRENCE

Local recurrence has been shown to predict for subsequent distant metastases, having an impact on survival.[140] These data must be considered in "very low risk" patients evaluated for omission of radiotherapy. Salvage treatment with mastectomy after ipsilateral breast recurrence in patients treated with BCT offers subsequent disease-free survival in 40 to 70 percent of affected patients. Axillary recurrences are rare but subsequent survival is lower (25 to 30 percent).[141] Failure in the supraclavicular fossa has a dismal prognosis.[142] Short interval to recurrence is likely to be predictive of subsequent distant disease.[143]

There is a question whether development of cancer in a treated breast many years after BCT represents relapse or a new primary cancer. It has been postulated that the location of the recurrence in relation to the primary, the time interval between incidents, and the presence or absence of diffuse disease in the surrounding stroma may distinguish between recurrence and a new primary. The presence of a lesion near the original tumor site with disease in the surrounding stroma presenting relatively shortly after initial diagnosis more likely represents recurrent disease than does a remote lesion presenting in normal surrounding tissue after a long interval.[144] Differences in DNA content detectable by flow cytometry are more likely in a second primary malignancy than in a recurrent tumor. The subsequent treatment of the disease may differ, particularly in patients exposed to systemic treatment.

Standard therapy for patients experiencing recurrence in an irradiated breast is mastectomy. However, there are limited data on the retreatment of patients with further excision and reirradiation; 62 percent of patients were salvaged and treatment was well tolerated, as 15 out of 16 patients received 5000 cGy with no reported deleterious effect.[145]

The majority of patients who experience recurrence after local excision and no radiotherapy are treated with and often choose mastectomy over re-excision and radiotherapy as salvage treatment. If the overall goal of breast conserving treatment is breast retention, therapy should optimize the patient's wish, even at the expense of potential over-treatment.

CONCLUSION

Breast conservation therapy consisting of local excision and breast radiotherapy should be the treatment of choice for the majority of patients with early invasive and in situ carcinoma. Radiotherapy to the breast has been shown to be effective in improving local and regional control, with minimal complications. The incidence of intraductal and early stage breast cancer may continue to increase as mammographically detected lesions become more predominant. Radiotherapy delivery may become more selective as methods are improved to identify patients at high and low risk for local recurrence. However, with the very small risk of complication from treatment, the number of patients not receiving radiotherapy should remain very small. Recent data regarding postmastectomy radiotherapy indicate that subgroups of patients with locally advanced disease achieve a survival benefit from the addition of postmastectomy radiation. Modern radiotherapy techniques minimize cardiac injury. Identifying patients with significant risk for local failure, optimizing local treatment in these patients, and evaluating the impact on overall cure are areas for current and future investigation.

REFERENCES

1. Fletcher GH. Local results of irradiation in the primary management of localized breast cancer. Cancer 1972;29:545–51.
2. National Institutes of Health Consensus Development Panel. Consensus statement: treatment of early-stage breast cancer. J Natl Cancer Inst Monogr 1992;11:15.
3. Cuzick J, Stewart H, Peto R, et al. Overview of randomized trials of adjuvant radiotherapy in breast cancer. Recent Results Cancer Res 1988;111:109–29.
4. Cuzick J, Stewart H, Rutqvist L, et al. Cause-specific mortality in long-term survivors of breast cancer who participated in trials of radiotherapy. J Clin Oncol 1994;12:447–53.
5. Recht A, Bartelink H, Fourquet A, et al. Postmastectomy radiotherapy: questions for the twenty-first century. J Clin Oncol 1998;16:2886–9.
6. Lipsztein R, Dalton JF, Bloomer WD. Sequelae of breast irradiation. JAMA 1985;253:3582–4.
7. Garfinkel L, Boring C, Heath C Jr. Changing trends: an overview of breast cancer incidence and mortality. Cancer 1994;74 Suppl:222–7.
8. Bland KI, Menck HR, Scott-Connor CE, et al. The National Cancer Data Base 10-year survey of breast cancer treatment at hospitals in the United States. Cancer 1998;83:1263–73.
9. Bjurstrum N, Bjorneld L, Duffy SW, et al. The Gothenberg Breast Screening Trial. First results on mortality, incidence, and mode of detection for women 39–49. Cancer 1997;80:2091–9.
10. Garne J, Aspegren K, Balldin G, Ranstam J. Increasing incidence of and declining mortality from breast cancer. Cancer 1997;79:69–74.
11. Nattinger AB, Gottlieb MS, Hoffman RG, et al. Minimal increase in the use of breast-conserving surgery from 1986 to 1990. Med Care, 1996;34:479–89.
12. Kotwall CA, Covington DL, Rutledge R, et al. Patient, hospital, and surgeon factors associated with breast conserving surgery. A statewide analysis in North Carolina. Ann Surg 1996;224:419–26.
13. Morrow M, Bucci C, Rademaker A. Medical contraindications are not a major factor in the under utilization of breast conserving therapy. J Am Coll Surg 1998;186:269–74.
14. Fisher B, Anderson S, Redmond CK. Reanalysis and results after 12 years of follow-up in a randomized clinical trial comparing total mastectomy with lumpectomy with or without irradiation in the treatment of breast cancer. N Engl J Med 1995;333:1456–61.

15. Lichter AS, Lippmann ME, Danforth DN Jr, et al. Mastectomy versus breast conserving therapy in the treatment of stage I and II carcinoma of the breast: a randomized trial at the National Cancer Institute. J Clin Oncol 1992;10:976–83.

16. Jacobson JA, Danforth DN, Cowan KH, et al. Ten-year results of a comparison of conservation with mastectomy in the treatment of stage I and II breast cancer. N Engl J Med 1995;332:901–11.

17. Veronesi U Luini A, Galimberti V, Zurrida S. Conservation approaches for the management of stage I/II carcinoma of the breast: Milan Cancer Institute Trials. World J Surg 1994;18:70–5.

18. Van Dongen JA, Bartelink H, Fentiman IS, et al. Randomized clinical trial to assess the value of breast-conserving therapy in stage I and II breast cancer: EORTC 10801 trial. J Natl Cancer Inst 1992;11:15–8.

19. Blichert-Toft M, Rose C, Anderson JA, et al. Danish randomized trial comparing breast conservation therapy with mastectomy: six years of life table analysis. J Natl Cancer Inst Monogr 1992;11:19–25.

20. Arriagada R, Le MG, Rochard F, Contesso G. Conservative treatment versus mastectomy in early breast cancer: Patterns of failure with 15 years of follow-up data. Institut Gustave-Roussy Breast Cancer Group. J Clin Oncol 1996;14:1558–64.

21. Early breast cancer trialists' Collaborative Group. Effects of radiotherapy and surgery in early breast cancer. N Engl J Med 1995;333:1444–55.

22. Winchester DJ, Menck HR, Winchester DP. The National Cancer Data Base report on the results of a large non-randomized comparison of breast preservation and modified radical mastectomy. Cancer 1997;80:162–7.

23. Cowen D, Jacquemier J, Houvenaeghel G, et al. Local and distant recurrence after conservative management of "very low risk" breast cancer are dependant events: a 10-year follow-up. Int J Radiat Oncol Biol Phys 1998;41: 801–7.

24. Elkhuizen PH, Van de Vijver MJ, Hermans J, et al. Local recurrence after breast conserving therapy for invasive cancer; high incidence in young patients and association with poor survival. Int J Radiat Oncol Biol Phys 1998;40: 859–67.

25. Fowble BL, Schultz DJ, Overmoyer B, et al. The influence of young age on outcome in early stage breast cancer. Int J Radiat Oncol Biol Phys 1994;30:23–33.

26. Kim SH, Simkovich-Heerdt A, Tran KN, et al. Women 35 years of age have higher locoregional relapse rates after undergoing breast conservation therapy. J Am Coll Surg 1998;187:1–8.

27. Matthews RH, McNeese MD, Montague ED, Oswald MJ. Prognostic implications of age in breast cancer patients treated with tumorectomy and irradiation or with mastectomy. Int J Radiat Oncol Biol Phys 14:659–63.

28. Donegan WL, Perez-Mesa CM, Watson FR. A biostatistical study of locally recurrent breast carcinoma. Surg Gyn Obstet 1966;122:329.

29. Fowble B. Radiotherapeutic considerations in the treatment of primary breast cancer. J Natl Cancer Inst Monogr 1992;11:49–58.

30. Recht A, Harris JR. Selection of patients with early stage breast cancer for conservative surgery and radiation. Oncology 1990;4:23–30.

31. Leopold K, Recht A, Schnitt SJ, et al. Results of conservative surgery and radiation therapy for multiple synchronous cancers of one breast. Int J Radiat Oncol Biol Phys 1989;16:11–16.

32. Fowble B, Yeh I, Schultz DJ, et al. The role of mastectomy in patients with stage I–II breast cancer presenting with gross multifocal or multicentric disease or diffuse calcifications. Int J Radiat Oncol Biol Phys 1993;27:567–73.

33. Kurtz J. Factors influencing the risk of local recurrence in the breast. Eur J Cancer 1992;28:660–6.

34. Schnitt SJ, Connolly J, Khettry V, et al. Pathologic findings on reexcision of the primary site in breast cancer patients considered for treatment by primary radiation therapy. Cancer 1997;59: 675–81.

35. Hurd TC, Sneige N, Allen PK, et al. Impact of extensive intraductal component on recurrence in patients with stage I or II breast cancer treated with breast conservation therapy. Ann Surg Oncol 1997;4:119–24.

36. Schnitt SJ, Abner A, Gelman R, et al. The relationship between microscopic margins of resection and the risk of local recurrence in patients with breast cancer treated with breast-conserving surgery and radiation therapy. Cancer 1994;74:1746–51.

37. Moran M, Haffty BG. Lobular carcinoma in situ as a component of breast cancer: the long-term outcome in patients treated with breast-conserving therapy. Int J Radiat Oncol Biol Phys 1998;40:353–8.

38. Schnitt SJ, Connolly JL, Recht A, et al. Influence of infiltrating lobular histology on local tumor control in breast cancer patients treated with conservative surgery and radiotherapy. Cancer 1989;64:448–54.

39. Haffty BG, Wilson LD, Smith R, et al. Subareolar breast cancer: long-term results with conservative surgery and radiation therapy. Int J Radiat Oncol Biol Phys 1995;33:53–7.

40. Bussieres E, Guyon F, Thomas L, et al. Conservation treatment in subareolar breast cancers. Eur J Surg Oncol 1996;22:267–70.

41. Dale PS, Giulliano AE. Nipple-areolar preservation during breast-conserving therapy for subareolar breast carcinomas. Arch Surg 1996;131:430–3.

42. Pierce LJ, Haffty BG, Solin LJ, et al. The conservative management of Paget's disease of the breast with radiotherapy. Cancer 1997;80:1065–72.

43. Nixon AJ, Schnitt SJ, Gelman R, et al. Relationship of tumor grade to other pathologic features and to treatmetn outcome of patients with early stage breast cancer. Cancer 1996;78:1426–31

44. Chabner E, Nixon A, Gelman R, et al. Family history and treatment outcome in young women after breast-conserving surgery and radiation therapy for early-stage breast cancer. J Clin Oncol 1998;16:2045–51.

45. Malone KE, Daling JR, Weiss NS, et al. Family history and survival of young women with invasive breast carcinoma. Cancer 1996;78:1417–25.

46. Porter D, Cohen B, Wallace M, et al. Breast cancer incidence, penetrance and survival in probable carriers of BRCA1 gene mutation in families linked to BRCA1 on chromosome 17q12-21. Br J Surg 1994;81:1512–15.

47. Anscher MS, Jones P, Prosnitz LR, et al. Local failure and margin status in early stage breast carcinoma treated with conservative surgery and radiation therapy. Ann Surg 1993;218:22–8.

48. Ryoo MC, Kagan AR, Wollin M, et al. Prognostic factors for recurrence and cosmesis in 393 patients after radiotherapy. Radiology 1989;172:555–9.

49. Heimann R, Powers C, Halpern HJ, et al. Breast preservation in stage I and II carcinoma of the breast. The University of Chicago experience. Cancer 1996;78:1722–30.

50. Spivack B, Khanna MM, Tafra L, et al. Margin status and local recurrence after breast-conserving surgery. Arch Surg 1994;129: 952–6.

51. Gage I, Schnitt SJ, Nixon AJ, et al. Pathologic margin involvement and the risk of recurrence in patients treated with breast-conserving surgery. Cancer 1996;78:1921–8.

52. DiBiase SJ, Komarnicky LT, Schwartz GF, et al. The number of positive margins influences the outcome of women treated with breast preservation of early stage breast carcinoma. Cancer 1998;82:2212–20.

53. Guidi AJ, Connolly JL, Harris JR, Schnitt SJ. The relationship between shaved margin and inked margin status in breast excision specimens. Cancer 1997;9:1568–73.

54. Holland R, Veling SH, Mravunac M, Hendriks JH. Histologic multifocality of Tis, T1-2 breast carcinomas. Implications for clinical trials of breast conserving surgery. Cancer 1985:56: 979–90.

55. Wazer DE, Schmidt-Ullrich RK, Ruthazer R, et al. Factors determining outcome for breast-conserving irradiation with margin-directed dose escalation to the tumor bed. Int J Radiat Oncol Biol Phys 1998;40:851–8.

56. Fagundes MA, Fagundes HM, Brito CS, et al. Breast-conserving surgery and definitive radiation: a comparison between quadrantectomy and local excision with special focus on locoregional control and cosmesis. Int J Radiat Oncol Biol Phys 1993;27:553–60.

57. Veronesi U, Volterrani F, Luini A, et al. Quadrantectomy versus lumpectomy for small breast cancer. Eur J Cancer 1990;26:671–3.

58. Ross J, Hussey D, Mayr N, Davis CS. Acute and late reactions to radiation therapy in patients with collagen vascular diseases. Cancer 1993; 71:3744–52.

59. Antypas C, Sandilos P, Kouvaris J, et al. Fetal dose during breast cancer radiotherapy. Int J Radiat Oncol Biol Phys 1998;40:995–9.

60. Clark RM, Wilkinson RH, Miceli PN, MacDonald WD. Breast cancer: experiences with conservation therapy. Am J Clin Oncol 1987;10:461–8.

61. Romestaing P, Lehingue Y, Carrie C, et al. Role of 10-Gy boost in the conservative treatment of early breast cancer: results of a randomized clinical trial in Lyon, France. J Clin Oncol 1997;15:963–8.

62. Solin LJ, Fowble BL, Schultz DJ, Goodman RL. The significance of pathology margins of tumor excision on the outcome of patients treated with definitive irradiation for early stage breast cancer. Int J Radiat Oncol Biol Phys 1991;21:279–87.

63. Smitt MC, Nowels KW, Zdeblick MJ, et al. The importance of the lumpectomy surgical margin status in long-term results of breast conservation. Cancer 1995;76:259–67.

64. Fisher B, Digham J, Mamounas E, et al. Sequential methotrexate and fluorouracil for the treatment of node-negative breast cancer patients with estrogen receptor-negative tumors: eight-year results from the National Surgical Adjuvant Breast and Bowel Project (NSABP) B-13 and

first report of findings from NSABP B-19 comparing methotrexate and fluorouracil with conventional cyclophosphamide, methotrexate, and fluorouracil. J Clin Oncol 1996;14:1982–92.

65. Fisher BJ, Parera FE, Cooke AL, et al. Long-term follow-up of axillary node positive breast cancer patients receiving adjuvant systemic therapy alone: patterns of recurrence. Int J Radiat Oncol Biol Phys 1997;38:541–50.

66. Fisher BJ, Perera FE, Cooke AL, et al. Long-term follow-up of axillary node positive breast cancer patients receiving adjuvant tamoxifen alone: patterns of recurrence. Int J Radiat Oncol Biol Phys 1998;42:117–23.

67. Cooke AL, Parera F, Fisher B, et al. Tamoxifen with and without radiation after partial mastectomy in patients with involved nodes. Int J Radiat Oncol Biol Phys 1995;31:777–81.

68. Dalberg K, Johansson H, Johansson U, Rutqvist LE. A randomzed trial of long term adjuvant tamoxifen plus postoperative radiation therapy versus radiation therapy alone for patients with early stage breast cancer treated with breast conserving surgery, Stockholm Breast Cancer Study Group. Cancer 1998;82:2204–11.

69. Forrest P, Stewart H, Everington D, et al. Randomized controlled trial of conservation therapy for breast cancer: 6-year analysis of the Scottish trial. Scottish Cancer Trials Breast Group. Lancet 1996;348:708–13.

70. Turner BC, Haffty BG, Narayanam L, et al. Insulin-like growth factor-I receptor overexpression mediates cellular radioresistance and local breast cancer recurrence after lumpectomy and radiation. Cancer Res 1997;57:3079–83

71. Haffty BG, Brown F, Carter D, Flynn S. Evaluation of HER-2 neu oncoprotein expression as a prognostic indicator of local recurrence in conservatively treated breast cancer: a case-control study. Int J Radiat Oncol Biol Phys 1996;35: 751–7.

72. Sjogren S, Inganas M, Lindgren A, et al. Prognostic and predictive value of c-erbB-2 overexpression in primary breast cancer, alone and in combination with other prognostic markers. J Clin Oncol 1998;16:462–9.

73. Gaffney DK, Brohet KM, Lewis CM, et al. Response to radiation therapy and prognosis in breast cancer patients with BRCA1 and BRCA2 mutations. Radiother Oncol 1998;47:129–36.

74. Formenti SC, Dunnington G, Uzieli B, et al. Original p53 status predicts for pathological response in locally advanced breast cancer treated preoperatively with continuous infusion 5-fluorouracil and radiation therapy. Int J Radiat Oncol Biol Phys 1997;39:1059–68.

75. Berns M, Klijn J, van Putten WL, et al. P53 protein accumulation predicts poor response to tamoxifen therapy of patients with recurrent breast cancer. J Clin Oncol 1998;16:121–7.

76. Gorski DH, Mauceri HJ, Salloum RM, et al. Potentiation of the antitumor effect of ionizing radiation by brief concomitant exposures to angiostatin. Cancer Res 1998;58:5686–9.

77. Heimann R, Ferguson D, Powers C, et al. Angiogenesis as a predictor of long-term survival for patients with node negative breast cancer. J Natl Cancer Inst 1998;88:1764.

78. Clark RM, Whelan T, Levine M, et al. Randomized clinical trial of breast irradiation following lumpectomy and axillary dissection for node-negative breast cancer. An update. J Natl Cancer Inst 1996;88:1659–64.

79. Veronesi U. Breast cancer trials on conservative surgery. Eur J Surg Oncol 1995;21:231–3.

80. Veronesi U, Luini A, Del Vecchio M, et al. Radiotherapy after breast preserving surgery in women with localized cancer of the breast. N Engl J Med 1993;328:1587–91.

81. Liljegren G, Holmberg L, Adami HO, et al. Sector resection with or without postoperative radiotherapy for stage I breast cancer. Five year results of a clinical trial. J Natl Cancer Inst 1994;86:717–22.

82. Nemoto T, Patel JK, Rosner D, et al. Factors affecting recurrence in lumpectomy without irradiation for breast cancer. Cancer 1991;67: 2079–82.

83. Morrow M, Harris JR, Schnitt SJ. Local control following breast-conserving surgery for invasive breast cancer: results of clinical trials. J Natl Cancer Inst 1995;87:1669–73.

84. Liljegren G, Lindgren A, Bergh J, et al. Risk factors for local recurrence after conservative treatment in stage I breast cancer. Definition of a subgroup not requiring radiotherapy. Ann Oncol 1997;8:235–41.

85. Schnitt SJ, Hayman J, Gelman R, et al. A prospective study of conservative surgery alone in the treatment of selected patients with stage I breast cancer. Cancer 1996;77:1094–1100.

86. Solin LJ, Schultz DJ, Fowble BL. Ten year results of the treatment of early-stage breast carcinoma in elderly women using breast-conserving surgery and definitive breast irradiation. Int J Radiat Oncol Biol Phys 1995;33:45–51

87. Merchant TE, McCormick B, Yahalom J, Borgen P. The influence of older age on breast cancer

treatment decisions and outcome. Int J Radiat Oncol Biol Phys 1996;34:565–70.

88. Holland R, Hendricks JH, Vebeek AL, et al. Extent, distribution and mammographic histological correlations of breast ductal carcinoma in situ. Lancet 1990;335:519–22.

89. Fisher B, Anderson S. Conservative surgery for the management of invasive and non-invasive carcinoma of the breast: NSABP trials. National Surgical Adjuvant Breast and Bowel Project. World J Surg 1994;18:63–9.

90. Fisher B, Constantino J, Redmond C, et al. Lumpectomy compared with lumpectomy and radiation therapy for the treatment of intraductal breast cancer. N Engl J Med 1993;328:1581–6.

91. Fisher B, Dignam J, Wolmark N, et al. Lumpectomy and radiation therapy for the treatment of intraductal breast cancer: findings from the National Surgical Adjuvant Breast and Bowel Project B-17. J Clin Oncol 1998;16:441–52.

92. Fisher E, Constantino J, Fisher B. Pathologic findings from the National Surgical Adjuvant Breast Project (NSABP) protocol B-17. Intraductal carcinoma (ductal carcinoma in situ). Cancer 1995;75:1310–9.

93. Fowble B, Hanlon AL, Fein DA, et al. Results of conservative surgery and radiation for mammographically detected ductal carcinoma in situ (DCIS). Int J Radiat Oncol Biol Phys 1997;38:949–57.

94. Solin LJ, Kurtz J, Fourquet A, et al. Fifteen-year results of breast conserving surgery and definitive breast irradiation for the treatment of ductal carcinoma in situ of the breast. J Clin Oncol 1996;14:754–63.

95. Vicina FA, Lacerna MD, Goldstein NS, et al. Ductal carcinoma in situ detected in the mammographic era: an analysis of clinical, pathologic, and treatment related factors affecting outcome with breast-conserving therapy. Int J Radiat Oncol Biol Phys 1997;39:627–35.

96. Silverstein MJ, Lagios MD, Craig PH, et al. A prognostic index for ductal carcinoma in situ of the breast. Cancer 1996;77:2267–74.

97. Silverstein MJ, Lagios MD. Use of predictors to plan therapy for DCIS of the breast. Oncology 1997;11:393–406.

98. Lagios MD, Silverstein MJ. Ductal carcinoma in situ. The success of breast conservation therapy: a shared experience of two single institutional non-randomized prospective studies. Surg Oncol Clin North Am 1997;6:385–92.

99. Winchester DP, Strom EH. Standards for diagnosis and management of ductal carcinoma in situ of the breast. CA-A 1998;48:108–28.

100. Silverstein MJ, Lagios MD, Martino S, et al. Outcome after invasive local recurrence in patients with ductal carcinoma in situ of the breast. J Clin Oncol 1998;16:1367–73.

101. Auquier A, Rutqvist LE, Host H, et al. Post-mastectomy megavoltage radiotherapy: the Oslo and Stockholm trials. Eur J Cancer 1992;28:433–7.

102. Gagliardi G, Lax I, Soderstrom S, et al. Prediction of excess risk of long-term cardiac mortality after radiotherapy of stage I breast cancer. Radiother Oncol 1998;46:63–71.

103. Kuske R. Adjuvant chest wall and nodal irradiation: maximize cure, minimize late toxicity [editorial]. J Clin Oncol 1998;16:2579–82.

104. Arriagada R, Rutqvist LE, Mattson A, et al. Adequate locoregional treatment for early breast cancer may prevent secondary dissemination. J Clin Oncol 1995;13:2869–78.

105. Overgaard M, Hansen PS, Overgaard J, et al. Postoperative radiotherapy in high-risk premenopausal women with breast cancer who receive adjuvant chemotherapy. N Engl J Med 1997;337:949–55.

106. Ragaz J, Jackson SM, Le N, et al. Adjuvant radiotherapy and chemotherapy in node-positive premenopausal women with breast cancer. N Engl J Med 1997;337:956–62.

107. Recht A, Bartelink H, Fourquet A, et al. Postmastectomy radiotherapy: questions for the twenty-first century. J Clin Oncol 1998;16:2886–9.

108. Fowble B, Gray R, Gilchrist K, et al. Identification of a subgroup of patients with breast cancer and histologically positive axillary lymph nodes receiving adjuvant chemotherapy who may benefit from postoperative radiotherapy. J Clin Oncol 1988;6:1107–17.

109. Fowble B. Post-mastectomy radiotherapy: then and now. Oncology 1997;11:213–31.

110. Kozeniowski S. "One to three" or "four or more"? Selecting patients for post-mastectomy radiation therapy. Cancer 1997;80:1357–8.

111. Fisher BF, Perera F, Cooke A, et al. Extracapsular axillary node extension in patients receiving adjuvant systemic therapy: an indication for radiotherapy? Int J Radiat Oncol Biol Phys 1997;38:551–9.

112. Donegan WL, Stine SB, Samter TG. Implications of extracapsular nodal metastases for treatment and prognosis of breast cancer. Cancer 1993;72:778–82.

113. Krag D, Weaver D, Ashikaga T, et al. The sentinel node in breast cancer. N Engl J Med 1998;339:941–6.

114. Fisher B, Bryant J, Wolmark N, et al. Effect of preoperative chemotherapy on the outcome of women with operable breast cancer. J Clin Oncol 1998;16:2672–85.

115. Fisher B, Brown A, Mamounas E, et al. Effect of preoperative chemotherapy on local-regional disease in women with operable breast cancer: findings from National Surgical Adjuvant Breast and Bowel Project B-18. J Clin Oncol 1997;15:2483–93.

116. Jacquillat C, Weil M, Baillet F, et al. Results of neoadjuvant chemotherapy and radiation therapy in the breast conserving treatment of 250 patients with all stages of infiltrative breast cancer. Cancer 1990;66:119–29.

117. Brenin DR, Morrow M. Breast conservation surgery in the neo-adjuvant setting. Semin Oncol 1998;25:13–18.

118. Ellis P, Smith I, Ashley S, et al. Clinical, prognostic and predictive factors for primary chemotherapy in operable breast cancer. J Clin Oncol 1998;16:107–14.

119. Mumtaz H, Davidson T, Spittle M, et al. Breast surgery after neoadjuvant treatment. Is it necessary? Eur J Surg Oncol 1996;22:335–41.

120. Bucholz TA, Austin-Seymour MM, Moe RE, et al. Effect of delay in radiation in the combined modality treatment of breast cancer. Int J Radiat Oncol Biol Phys 1993;26:23–5.

121. Recht A, Come SE, Henderson IC, et al. The sequencing of chemotherapy and radiation therapy after conservative surgery for early-stage breast cancer. N Engl J Med 1996;334:1356–61.

122. Pierce S, Recht A, Lingos T, et al. Long-term radiation complications following conservative surgery (CS) and radiation therapy (RT) in patients with early stage breast cancer. Int J Radiat Oncol Biol Phys 1992;23:915–23.

123. Fein DA, Fowble BL, Hanlon AL, et al. Does the placement of surgical clips within the excision cavity influence local control for patients treated with breast-conserving surgery and irradiation. Int J Radiat Oncol Biol Phys 1996;34:1009–17.

124. Geynes G, Gagliardi G, Lax I, et al. Evaluation of irradiated heart volumes in stage I breast cancer patients treated with postoperative adjuvant radiotherapy. J Clin Oncol 1997;15:1348–53.

125. Hughes-Davies L, Sacks D, Rescigno J, et al. Serum cardiac troponin T levels during treatment of early-stage breast cancer. J Clin Oncol 1995;13:2582–4.

126. Cowen D, Gonzague-Casabianca L, Brenot-Rossi I, et al. Thallium-201 perfusion scintigraphy in the evaluation of late myocardial damage in left-side breast cancer treated with adjuvant radiotherapy. Int J Radiat Oncol Biol Phys 1998;41:809–15.

127. Rutqvist LE, Liedberg A, Hammar N, Dalberg K. Myocardial infarction among women with early-stage breast cancer treated with conservative surgery and breast irradiation. Int J Radiat Oncol Biol Phys 1998;40:359–63.

128. Nixon AJ, Manola J, Gelman R, et al. No long-term increase in cardiac related mortality after breast-conserving surgery and radiation therapy using modern techniques. J Clin Oncol 1998;16:1374–9.

129. Hoe AL, Iven D, Royle GT, Taylor I. Incidence of arm swelling following axillary clearance for breast cancer. Br J Surg 1992;79:261–2.

130. Siegel BM, Mayzel KA, Love SM. Level I and II axillary dissection in the treatment of early-stage breast cancer. An analysis of 259 consecutive patients. Arch Surg 1990;125:1144–7.

131. Kiel KD, Rademaker AW. Early-stage breast cancer: arm edema after wide excision and breast irradiation. Radiology 1996;198:279–83.

132. Taylor ME, Perez CA, Halverson KJ, et al. Factors influencing cosmetic results after conservation therapy for breast cancer. Int J Radiat Oncol Biol Phys 1995;31:756–64.

133. Olivotto IA, Weir LM, Kim-Sing C, et al. Late cosmetic results of short fractionation for breast conservation. Radiother Oncol 1996;41:7–13.

134. Victor SJ, Brown DM, Horwitz EM, et al. Treatment outcome with radiation therapy after breast augmentation or reconstruction in patients with primary breast carcinoma. Cancer 1998;82:1303–9.

135. Ryu J, Yahalom J, Shank B, et al. Radiation therapy after breast augmentation or reconstruction in early or recurrent breast cancer. Cancer 1990;66:844–7.

136. Hunt KK, Baldwin BJ, Strom EA, et al. Feasibility of postmastectomy radiotherapy after TRAM flap breast reconstruction. Ann Surg Oncol 1997;4:377–84.

137. Karlsson P, Holmberg E, Johansson KA, et al. Soft tissue sarcoma after treatment for breast cancer. Radiother Oncol 1996;38:25–31.

138. Pendlebury SC, Bilous M, Langlands AO. Sarcomas following radiation therapy for breast cancer: a report of three cases and a review of the literature. Int J Radiat Oncol Biol Phys 1995; 31:405–16.

139. Boice JD, Harvey EB, Blettner M, et al. Cancer in the contralateral breast after radiotherapy for breast cancer. N Engl J Med 1992;326:781–5.

140. Touboul E, Buffat L, Belkacemi Y, et al. Local

recurrences and distant metastases after breast-conserving surgery and radiation therapy for early breast cancer. Int J Radiat Oncol Biol Phys 1999;43:25–38.

141. Leborgne F, Leborgne JH, Ortega B, et al. Breast conservation treatment of early stage breast cancer: patterns of failure. Int J Radiat Oncol Biol Phys 1995;31:765–75.

142. Willner J. The role of radiation therapy in the multidisciplinary management of recurrent and metastatic breast cancer [correspondence]. Cancer 1995;75:902–3.

143. Haffty BG, Reiss M, Beinfield M, et al. Ipsilat- eral breast tumor recurrence as a predictor of distant disease: implications for systemic therapy at the time of local relapse. J Clin Oncol 1996;14:52–7.

144. Haffty BG, Carter D, Flynn SD, et al. Local recurrence versus new primary: clinical analysis of 82 breast relapses and potential applications for genetic fingerprinting. Int J Radiat Oncol Biol Phys 1993;27:575–83.

145. Mullen E, Deutsch M, Bloomer WD. Salvage radiotherapy for local failures of lumpectomy and breast irradiation. Radiother Oncol 1997; 42:25–9.

14

Carcinoma of the Breast in Men

PHILIP N. REDLICH, MD, PhD
WILLIAM L. DONEGAN, MD

Breast cancer is not entirely a disease of women. 0.7 percent of all cases of breast cancer in the United States occur in males. Men account for 0.9 percent of deaths from breast cancer. About 0.2 percent of cancers in males arise in the breast. An estimated 1,300 new cases of breast cancer in men are expected in the United States, in 1999, and 400 men will die of the disease. Breast cancer causes 0.14 percent of deaths from cancer in men.[1]

The earliest record of cancer of the breast, which dates from the Edwin Smith surgical papyrus, describes the disease in a man. This Egyptian antiquity, written circa 3000 to 2500 BC, indicates that no known treatment was successful for bulging tumors of the breast.[2] Holleb attributes the first documented case of male breast cancer to John of Arderne in England in the fourteenth century;[3] Meyskens attributes it to William Fabry of Germany in the sixteenth century.[4] Clinical descriptions of male breast cancer began to appear in medical journals in France and England in the early nineteenth century. Considered a curiosity, male breast cancer received little attention until later that century when collections of cases began to appear in the literature.[5] In 1883, Porier published a detailed description of the clinical evolution of breast cancer in males that leaves little room for improvement. In 1927, Wainwright in Pennsylvania was able to report on 418 collected cases.[5]

He described the poor prognosis associated with high histologic grade, cutaneous ulceration, and axillary node involvement. Postoperative mortality was 6.1 percent; only nineteen percent of 111 cases with complete follow-up survived 5 years. Wainwright concluded that the prognosis was not as good in men as in women.

Reports from numerous countries document the pervasiveness of male breast cancer. Because of the low incidence of breast cancer in men, information on the subject is based largely on case reports and retrospective analyses of data collected in medical centers and tumor registries over many years. Few individual physicians have personal experience with more than a small number of cases. Clinical trials of treatment are nonexistent for males, and in most respects, advances in treatment are translations from lessons learned about the disease in women, the prevalence of which has enabled controlled studies. As a consequence, guidelines for treatment of women are being used for males, and men are now receiving less radical operations and more effective systemic adjuvant therapy. Similarly, the role of hereditary factors and gene mutations are being explored in males.

It has recently come to be appreciated that breast cancer is similar in both sexes. Early reports emphasized differences, but accumulating information makes it clear there are more similarities than differences; this change is important not only for discovering causation but for application of treatment. While the etiology of breast cancer in both sexes is unknown, there is little reason to believe that it is different. Men and women are subject to similar environmental exposures. The pathology and clinical courses are parallel, and in similar circumstances, men and women prove equally curable. The older age of men at diagnosis, subareolar origin of the tumor, and presentation in more advanced stages with poorer overall prognosis can be attributed to the small size of the male breast and the scant notice it receives. Screening for early detection does not exist for men, but public and professional awareness of breast cancer in men, and appropriate application to men of the intensive research of the disease in women, should result in progress.

EPIDEMIOLOGY

The age-specific incidence and mortality of breast cancer rise steadily in males beginning in the third decade.[6] The disease has been diagnosed in teenagers, but cases usually begin to appear in the fourth decade of life, with the average age at diagnosis in large series clustering around 65 years, 5 to 8 years older than the average age of women at diagnosis.[7,8] Wide age ranges are reported, from 23 to 97 years.[9] In reports from various countries, the incidence in men parallels that of women.[10,11] High rates are reported in England and Wales and low rates in Japan and Finland. Black races in subSaharan Africa have a high frequency of affected males, often attributed to a high prevalence of liver disease which leads to alterations in estrogen metabolism. Males account for 7 percent of cases of breast cancer in Tanzania[12] and 9 percent of cases in Nigeria.[13] The lower average age at diagnosis in African countries also suggests an earlier onset.

Factors identified with high risk for men are fragmentary and sometimes controversial but suggest genetic, hormonal, and environmental influences. In many respects, they reflect the risk

patterns known for women (Table 14–1). Case control studies associate high risk variously with high socioeconomic status, higher levels of education, Ashkenazi Jewish descent, childlessness, obesity, limited exercise, tallness, and consumption of red meat.[14,15] Linkage between male breast cancer and exposure to low frequency magnetic fields has not been confirmed.[16]

From 11 to 27 percent of affected males report a family history of breast cancer.[17,18–20] Families with high rates of breast cancer sometimes include affected males; multiple males may be affected and males in more than one generation of such families have developed breast cancer.[21] Female descendents of males with breast cancer are at increased risk, indicating transmission through the male line. In males, inheritance of breast cancer risk has been linked to germline mutations in the BRCA2 gene on chromosome 13q12-13. Between 35 and 45 percent of familial breast cancer can be accounted for by BRCA2 mutations, often including families in which both males and females are affected. For females who are members of high-risk families, mutations in BRCA1 or BRCA2 carry an estimated 56 to 85 percent lifetime risk of breast cancer. Limited figures indicate that from 4 to 43 percent of males with breast cancer carry various mutations on chromosome 13q. Family history of breast cancer is usually present in reported series of male breast cancer patients with BRCA2 mutations but the frequency of a positive family history ranges up to 85 percent.[18,22,23] Mutations in the androgen-receptor (AR) gene associated with androgen insensitivity syndrome are also linked to male breast cancer.[24,25]

Men with Klinefelter's syndrome (obesity, hypogonadism, aspermatogenesis, increased urinary gonadotropins, and gynecomastia), identified by an XXY karyotype are estimated to have a 20- to 50-fold increase in risk for breast cancer and a 3 percent lifetime risk.[26–29] Nevertheless, cases of Klinefelter's syndrome are not regularly found in reported series of males with breast cancer; the frequency varies widely, from 0 to 7.5 percent.

Endocrine abnormalities are not often found in males with breast cancer, but available information suggests some role for excess estrogen or a deficiency of androgen. High levels of endogenous estrogens may result from obesity and liver cirrhosis, which are often associated with male breast cancer in Denmark and in African countries.[30,31] Testicular function declines with aging as the incidence of breast cancer rises. Breast cancer has been reported in three orchiectomized male transsexuals treated with estrogen to enhance breast development.[32,33] Crichlow cites four cases of breast cancer in men treated with estrogens for prostate cancer; more frequent than primary breast carcinoma, however, among men with prostatic carcinoma is metastatic involvement of the breast.[34] In one series, no breast cancers were seen in over 4,000 males treated with estrogens for prostate cancer, but durations of exposure may have been relatively short. Androgen deficiency is suggested by the frequent histories of orchitis, inguinal herniorrhaphy, mumps infections in adulthood, orchiectomy, and testicular injury among men with breast cancer.[35] Impaired testicular function may result from occupational exposure to high environmental temperatures and chemicals, which is reported by many affected men.

There have been a number of reports associating male breast cancer with chronic hyperprolactinemia. Such cases have included bilateral breast involvement[36a] and a history of prolactinoma and head injury.[36b] The precise role of prolactin and any associated endocrine disturbances is undetermined.

Case reports document primary breast cancer in men after exposure of the breast to ionizing radiation, in one case to treat pubertal gynecomastia.[37,38] Radiation is known to be carcinogenic for the breasts of women, particularly with exposure early in life. Women exposed to atomic radiation or to multiple fluoroscopies in the course of treatment for tuberculosis, or who have been irradiated for mastitis or treated with radiation for Hodgkin's disease, are known to be at increased risk. Reid and colleagues found a

Table 14–1. ASSOCIATIONS WITH INCREASED RISK FOR BREAST CANCER IN MEN

Genetic
    First-degree relatives with breast cancer
    Ashkenazi Jewish descent
    BRCA2 gene mutations
    Klinefelter's syndrome
    Androgen insensitivity
Environmental exposures
    Ionizing radiation
    Estrogens
Occupational exposures
    Soap and perfume workers
    Blast furnace workers and steelworkers
Reduced testicular function
    Mumps orchitis
    Inguinal herniorrhaphy
    Undescended testes
    Gynecomastia
Hyperprolactinemia
    Head trauma
    Hyperprolactinemia
Other
    High body weight early in life
    High socioeconomic status
    Higher education
    Childlessness

prior history of breast irradiation in 3.1 percent of 229 men with breast cancer.[9]

Ductal and lobular development of the male breast from genetic, environmental, or endogenous causes may place it at increased risk for carcinogenesis. Up to 40 percent of breast cancers in males are associated with gynecomastia. This relationship is inconclusive in view of the high frequency of gynecomastia in adult males. Noteworthy, however, is the parallel increase of breast cancer and gynecomastia in men with aging and the derivation of cancers from ductal and lobular elements when present. Ductal hyperplasia is often seen in association with ductal carcinoma in males, and in situ and invasive lobular carcinoma has been seen with Klinefelter's syndrome[39] and after chronic cimetidine stimulation of the male breast.[40] The presence of gynecomastia and the influences that produce it are often indistinguishable.

Of importance in the epidemiology of breast cancer in men is freedom of men from the unique reproductive functions of women that are so prominent in risk for breast cancer. The absence of these promoters is potentially useful in providing a less cluttered view of the disease. The fact remains that in the majority of men or women, no special risk feature is evident other than age. Avoiding potential mammary carcinogens and aspiring to a low-risk profile are some lessons in prevention derived from studies of breast cancer in males. Fortunately, ionizing radiation is no longer used to treat pubertal gynecomastia, acne, and other benign conditions of youth. Hormonal stimulation of the male breast and obesity are avoidable. Identification of individuals with an inherited high risk for breast cancer through genetic testing can permit more informed decisions about prophylactic mastectomy for men.[41]

PATHOLOGY

The same histologic types of breast cancer occur in men and women but the frequencies of these types vary (Table 14–2). Noninvasive ductal carcinoma has been described either in a

Table 14–2. HISTOLOGIC TYPES OF BREAST CANCER IN MEN

Noninvasive Carcinoma
    Ductal carcinoma in situ
    Lobular carcinoma in situ
    Paget's disease
    Papillary carcinoma in situ
Invasive Carcinoma
    Argyrophilic neuroendocrine carcinoma
    Colloid carcinoma
    Inflammatory carcinoma
    Intracystic papillary carcinoma
    Invasive ductal carcinoma
    Invasive lobular carcinoma
    Invasive papillary carcinoma
    Medullary carcinoma
    Mucinous carcinoma
    Oncocytic carcinoma
    Secretory carcinoma
Sarcoma
    Phyllodes tumor
    Fibrosarcoma
    Leiomyosarcoma
    Lymphosarcoma
    Myxoliposarcoma
    Osteosarcoma
    Spindle cell sarcoma

Adapted from Donegan WL, Redlich PN. Breast cancer in men. Surg Clin North Am 1996;76:343–63.

pure form or mixed with an invasive component.[42,43] Ductal carcinoma in situ (DCIS) comprises approximately 5 percent of all cases of male breast carcinoma but ranges as high as 17 percent in reported series.[43] The median age of occurrence of DCIS is usually the late 50s to mid-60s but has been reported in men under the age of 40 years. The most frequent histologic pattern is the papillary subtype, with the majority of cases being of low or intermediate grade. In a recent review of Paget's disease, this histologic type is characterized as presenting in the fifth to sixth decade of life and being associated with a palpable mass in 50 percent of cases.[44]

Virtually all known histologic types of invasive breast cancer have been identified in men. Invasive ductal carcinomas predominate, accounting for up to approximately 90 percent of cases. Also, special histologic types have been noted. Both invasive lobular carcinoma and lobular carcinoma in situ (LCIS) have been reported in men but are much less common than in women. Sarcomas comprise a minority of reported invasive breast cancers; there have been a variety of types noted (see Table 14–2). Metastatic cancer to the breast must be included in the differential diagnosis of breast masses. Lung carcinoma has been reported to metastasize to the male breast.[45]

CLINICAL PRESENTATION AND EVALUATION

The clinical features of male breast cancer have been well described in the literature[9,20,46–54] and recently summarized.[55] Signs and symptoms of male breast cancer are shown in Table 14–3. The mean age of patients presenting with this disease as noted above, is usually in the late 50s to mid-60s, with a range from the mid-20s to the early 90s. The most common presenting complaints are related to a breast mass, usually occurring in > 70 percent of cases, and axillary adenopathy, occurring in 30 to 50 percent of cases. For pure DCIS, a subareolar mass and nipple discharge were the two most common

Table 14–3. SIGNS AND SYMPTOMS OF MALE BREAST CANCER

Frequent
- Breast mass
- Axillary adenopathy
- Nipple retraction
- Nipple discharge
- Retraction of skin
- Ulceration of nipple or skin

Less Frequent
- Fixation to muscle
- Breast pain
- Inflammatory skin changes
- Skin discoloration

Table 14–4. STAGE OF DISEASE AT PRESENTATION

Stage	Frequency (%)
0	0–17
I	10–40
II	20–40
III	15–40
IV	10–15

symptoms in a recent series, occurring in 58 and 35 percent of patients, respectively.[43] In virtually all series, there is a report of significant delay in diagnosis of breast cancer in men. In early series, the mean duration of symptoms was > 14 months. In recent series, the mean duration is declining to a range of 3 to 6 months.[48,50,52,54] There is a history of trauma in many series, ranging from 5 to 10 percent of cases. Many series report the presence of gynecomastia associated with this disease in 7 to 23 percent of cases.[9,20,50] The mass is centrally located in the majority of cases and has an average diameter of 2.5 to 3.0 cm, with a range of 0.5 to 12 cm. Bilaterality of the disease is present in usually < 1 percent of cases, although in one series,[50] 7 percent of patients were found to have bilateral disease. Clinically suspicious axillary adenopathy is often found in these patients, ranging as high as 55 percent. The accuracy of the clinical exam is questionable, however, and pathologically proven metastases are usually more frequent. In some series, histologically proven axillary metastases occur as often as 70 percent of the time but more frequently are in the 40 to 60 percent range. The stage of disease at presentation is somewhat variable between reported series and may not be entirely comparable from series to series due to the large time spans involved and modification of staging systems over time. Stratification of patients by TNM stage at the time of presentation is presented in Table 14–4.

Evaluation of breast lesions includes the use of mammography, ultrasonography, fine needle aspiration cytology (FNAC), needle core biopsy, and open biopsy. Characteristics of male breast cancer on mammography include a mass eccentric to the nipple, spiculated margins, and microcalcifications (Figure 14–1).[56–58] Malignancy must be differentiated from gynecomastia, which often presents as an area of increased density positioned symmetrically in the retroareola region, but may obscure tumors.[56] Secondary radiologic signs of malignancy include architectural distortion, nipple and skin changes, and enlarged axillary nodes.[56] The ultrasound fea-

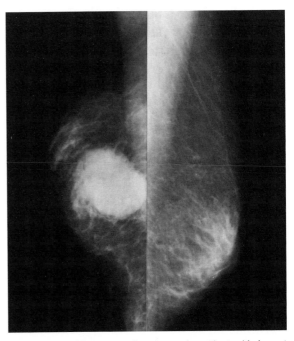

Figure 14–1. Mammography of a male patient with breast cancer. This 83 year-old man presented with a 4-month history of a right-breast mass. He had a 4.5 cm tumor, T2N1M0 (stage IIB), treated by modified radical mastectomy and adjuvant tamoxifen. He is free of disease 3 years later. Shown are the medial-lateral-oblique views of both breasts, the tumor being in the right breast on the left side of the figure.

tures of male breast cancer compared to other benign entities, including gynecomastia, lipoma, and fat necrosis have been reported.[58] Male breast cancer appears as a hypoechoic lesion with irregular margins with architectural distortion of surrounding normal breast tissue and subcutaneous fat. Ultrasound should be regarded as complimentary to mammography in the evaluation of the male breast.

The first diagnostic step in the evaluation of a male breast mass is often FNAC. Cytologic features of male breast cancer are similar to those seen in the female and allow this modality to be a reliable means of assessment.[59] Difficulties encountered using FNAC include epithelial hyperplasia associated with gynecomastia and the differentiation between primary and metastatic lesions of the breast.[59] Combined physical examination and FNAC for the evaluation of palpable breast masses in males has been studied.[60] This combination was found to be diagnostically accurate and resulted in a reduction of patient charges compared to routine open biopsy. In another series reviewing the diagnostic evaluation of over 700 male patients, the role of palpation, mammography, cytology, and ultrasound was evaluated. The combined palpation and mammography demonstrated a very high sensitivity for an accurate diagnosis.[61] Accurate diagnosis by cytology requires an experienced cytologist, the absence of which mandates either needle core biopsy or ultimately open biopsy of lesions. Open biopsy should be performed in all lesions where uncertainty exists regarding the diagnosis, both to confirm the diagnosis and obtain tissue for estrogen and progesterone receptor measurements. Receptor status is important as a prognostic indicator for survival and as an indicator for response to hormonal manipulation.[54,62]

PROGNOSTIC FACTORS

Overall survival for men with breast cancer in large series ranges from 53 to 70 percent at 5 years and 38 to 53 percent at 10 years.[52,63,64]

Observed survival of men is regularly inferior to that of women. The Winchesters and colleagues reported on 4,755 cases of male breast cancer obtained through the National Cancer Data Base and compared them with 624,174 cases of breast cancer in women.[7] The mean age of men, 64.7 years, was older than that of women, which was 60.9 years. Similar distributions of tumor grades were found. Men presented in more advanced stages than women, and 5-year survival was significantly lower. However, when adjusted for age and comorbidity, survival was equivalent.

The survival of men with breast cancer compared to women with breast cancer has been addressed in many series. An overall worse prognosis for men has been identified by a number of authors.[51,54,65] Other authors suggest that the prognosis in male breast cancer is no worse than that for women with comparable disease.[7,47,50,66] Guinee and colleagues suggested that the prognosis is the same for male and female patients when stratified on the basis of histologically positive nodes.[49] There has been a similar prognosis for male and female patients when analyzed by disease-specific survival, tumor size, and axillary node involvement reported by other authors as well.[50,52,66]

There are a number of influences unrelated to breast cancer itself that contribute to the unfavorable comparison of men and women. Among them are the older age at diagnosis and their shorter life expectancy after 65 years of age due to comorbid disease; men have higher rates of death from heart disease, second cancers, and stroke.[55] These confounding variables bias comparisons of observed survival and disease-free survival in favor of women.[7] More valid comparisons require the use of survival adjusted for natural mortality (adjusted survival) or of disease-specific survival (DSS).[7] Adjusted five-and ten-year survivals reported by Joshi and colleagues[67] were 76 and 42 percent, respectively and DSS of 74 percent at 5 years and 51 percent at 10 years were reported by Cutuli and colleagues.[52] Further detrimental to the survival of men is the high frequency of locally and regionally advanced disease and of disseminated disease, features in keeping with delay in diagnosis and not necessarily with inherently aggressive cancers.[7,67] Skin involvement is often present and involved axillary nodes are found in 45 to 65 percent of men with axillary dissections. When factors of stage and comorbidity are taken into account, however, investigators find little or no difference between the prognosis of males and females with breast cancer.[44,50,52,66,67]

The patient's TNM stage at diagnosis is important prognostically for men, and outcome by stage is largely not influenced by variations in local treatment (Figure 14–2). The current TNM staging system, derived from studying breast cancer in women, may not be entirely appropriate for men. Male cancers average 2.0 to 2.9 cm in diameter, but the diminutive breasts of men allow even small tumors to readily reach underlying muscle and overlying skin or nipple.[8,67] Pivot and colleagues found skin or muscle involvement in 45 percent of 85 cases; skin involvement was directly correlated with tumor size.[68] Forty-five percent of tumors < 2 cm in diameter had produced nodal metastases, and all tumors > 5 cm in diameter had produced nodal metastases. There was a similar prognosis for T3 and T4 tumors. These authors proposed a reduced T1, T2, and T4 classification for men.

Among traditional prognosticators, the presence of axillary metastases and primary tumor size are the most important features in undisseminated cases.[51,69,70,71] There is a direct correlation between the size of the primary tumor and the involvement of axillary lymph nodes that links these two clinical features.[68,71] Guinee and associates found a progressive drop in 5-year survival from 94 percent for cases with tumors 0 to 10 mm in diameter to 39 percent in cases with tumors > 51 mm in diameter.[49] Tumor size is important prognostically, independent of axillary node status. In node-negative cases, the relative risks of death associated with T0-T1, T2, and T3-T4 cases were 1.0, 2.0, and 3.2, respectively.[52]

The presence of axillary metastases is the single-most important prognostic indicator of survival for male breast cancer. Crichlow reported 5-year survivals of 79 and 28 percent for 143 patients without and with pathologic axillary metastases, respectively.[29] In a review of 397 nondisseminated cases, the 5-year DSS of 77 and 51 percent for cases with histologically uninvolved and involved nodes, respectively, were reported.[52] As in women, the absolute number of involved nodes is inversely related to survival. In 335 collected cases, Guinee and colleagues demonstrated that the 5-year survival for those with negative nodes was 90 percent, for one to three positive nodes was 73 percent, and for four or more positive nodes 55 percent.[49] Others have found the same relationship[53,54] (Figure 14–3). Unequal numbers of involved nodes contribute to varied prognoses reported for node-positive cases (see Figure 14–3). Skin and nipple involvement are identified with adverse survival (Figure 14–4).[67] Skin ulceration becomes insignificant, however, when tumor size is taken into consideration, and fixation to skin and chest wall are not important prognosticially when size and nodal status are taken into account.[49] There has been a statistically significant difference in survival based on histologic grade reported in one series, a worse survival associated with grade III versus grade II disease.[53]

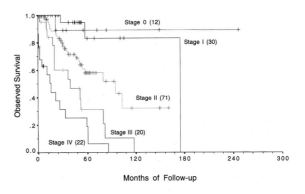

Figure 14–2. Survival of men with breast cancer stratified by TNM stage. Differences between the following stages reached statistical significance: 0 vs III, 0 vs IV, I vs II, I vs III, I vs IV, II vs III, II vs IV, and III vs IV. The number of cases is shown in parentheses. Reprinted with permission from Donegan WL, Redlich PN, Lang PJ, Gall MT. Carcinoma of the breast in males: a multi-institutional survey. Cancer 1998;83:498–509.

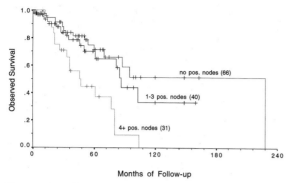

Figure 14–3. Survival by men with breast cancer stratified by number of axillary nodes with metastases. Differences between 0 vs 4+ positive nodes and 1–3 vs 4+ positive nodes reached statistical significance. The number of cases is shown in parentheses. Reprinted with permission from Donegan WL, Redlich PN, Lang PJ, Gall MT. Carcinoma of the breast in males: a multi-institutional survey. Cancer 1998;83:498–509.

The influence of steroid receptors on the prognosis of men is controversial. Estrogen receptor (ER) positivity, which is regularly more frequent in men than in women, is a weak but favorable prognostic sign for women. In men, ER positivity has been associated with both increased and decreased survival.[54,63,72] High tumor grade and aneuploidy are both associated with shortened survival.[63,73] Pich and colleagues found median survival significantly less for grade III than for grade II tumors.[74] Visfelt and Scheike graded 150 male breast carcinomas according to the degree of tubule formation, mitoses, and atypia and

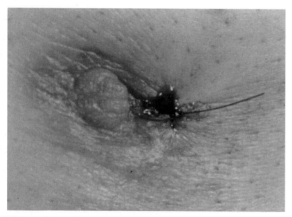

Figure 14–4. Direct involvement of the nipple in a man with breast carcinoma. The nipple is fixed to the underlying tumor, endurated, and retracted. The site of skin biopsy is marked by a stitch.

found 5-year survivals of 60, 40, and 5 percent in men with tumor grades of I, II, and III, respectively.[75] For diploid tumors, Pich and colleagues found a median survival of 77 months and only 38 months for aneuploid tumors[73] Mutation of *p53* cellular protein shortens median survival and disease-free survival.[73,76] The mean S-phase fraction of male breast cancers (7.2%) approximates that of females.[77] Winchester and colleagues found high S-phase fraction (SPF) to be a significant indicator of poor disease-free survival.[70] In a study of 27 male breast cancers, Pich and associates found that strong staining for argyrophilic nuclear organizer regions and for proliferating cell nuclear antigen were correlated with inferior survival.[74] The frequency of tumor markers with and without established prognostic significance are shown in Table 14–5.

TREATMENT OF LOCALIZED DISEASE

The treatment of male breast cancer localized to the breast and axillary nodes is mastectomy with axillary lymph node dissection.[55] In several recent series, modified radical mastectomy was the most common procedure performed, with from 34 to 76 percent of patients treated in this fashion.[8,20,50–52,54,65] In one multi-institutional survey, 82 percent of patients diagnosed since 1986 were treated by modified radical mastectomy.[54] Of 242 patients treated in the Department of Veterans' Affairs, 51 percent underwent modified radical mastectomy.[8] Other surgical procedures reported in these patients include radical mastectomy, simple mastectomy, and lumpectomies.

The use of radical mastectomy has decreased markedly in recent decades. No significant difference in outcome for patients who underwent radical mastectomy compared to modified radical mastectomy was found in a number of series.[20,78] The effect of the extent of mastectomy on the local regional recurrence rate is unclear, but a trend toward a lower local recurrence rate was identified for patients undergoing mastectomy versus lumpectomy.[52] Axillary dissection is considered part of the local–regional treatment of breast cancer. Cutuli and colleagues reported a statistically significant difference in the regional nodal recurrence rate of patients undergoing axillary dissection compared to those without dissection—1.2 percent of 320 patients with axillary dissection had a regional recurrence, compared to 13 percent of 77 patients without axillary dissection.[52]

Postoperative radiation therapy is frequently used as adjuvant therapy for male breast cancer. Its use, however, varies widely.[55] Some series suggest a decrease in the local–regional recurrence rate with the use of postoperative radiation therapy,[52,69] whereas no efficacy was noted in other series.[20,78] Chest wall radiation offers no survival benefit.[20,55,69] Overall, postoperative radiotherapy may reduce the local recurrence rate and should be considered as part of the overall treatment plan for cases at high risk for local or regional recurrence.[52,79]

Systemic adjuvant therapy, either chemotherapy, hormonal therapy, or both, is used for male patients based on the experience in female patients. The modality most often used for postoperative adjuvant hormonal therapy is tamoxifen.[46,50,80,81] Orchiectomy has been reported in a few series but is usually limited to only 3 percent of cases.[9,20,50] Tamoxifen is generally well tolerated by men, but side effects have been reported that, on occasion, may lead to termination of treatment.[80,81] Combination chemotherapy administered in an adjuvant setting has been used and reported by a number of authors.[9,52,54,55] Treatment with cyclophosphamide, methotrexate, and 5-fluorouracil (CMF) has been reported from the National Cancer Institute in a series of 24 patients with stage II disease. The projected 5-year survival rate was > 80 percent, representing an improvement over survival rates reported in other series.[82] In another report, 5-fluorouracil, doxorubicin, and cyclophosphamide (FAC) or CMF was administered in the adjuvant setting, with the projected 5-year survival > 85 percent.[83] Adverse effects of these chemotherapy regimens have been reported, limiting the ability of patients to tolerate all the planned treatments. In a recent series, Donegan and colleagues evaluated the effect of systemic adjuvant therapy, either chemotherapy, hormonal therapy, or combinations of both, on survival.[54] No improvement in overall survival was demonstrated; however, further analysis revealed

Table 14–5. TUMOR MARKERS IN MALE BREAST CANCERS

Marker	Frequency (%)	Prognosis	Reference
ER+	64–93	Controversial	Rayson,[94b] Willsher,[95] Joshi,[67] Bruce,[63] Cutuli[52]
PR+	73–96		Rayson,[94b] Willsher,[95] Joshi,[67] Cutuli[52]
pS2	50		Bruce[63]
Cathepsin D	46		Bruce[63]
AR+	95		Bruce[63]
HER2/neu+	21–45	Unfavorable	Rayson,[94b] Bines,[96] Willsher,[95] Joshi,[67] Bruce[63]
p53+	21–58	Unfavorable	Rayson,[94b] Bines,[96] Willsher,[95] Dawson,[97] Joshi[67] Bruce,[63] Anelli,[76] Pich[73]
MIB-1+	38–40	Unfavorable	Rayson,[94b] Willsher[95]
bcl-2+	93		Rayson[94b]
EGFR+	20		Willsher[95]
Mean SPF	7.2 (mean)	Highly unfavorable	Jonasson,[77] Winchester[70]
Grade III	33–73	Unfavorable	Willsher,[95] Jonasson,[77] Bruce,[63] McLachlan[53]
Aneuploidy	57	Unfavorable	Jonasson,[77] Pich[73]
Ki-ras	12		Dawson[97]
AgNOR+		Highly unfavorable	Pich[74]
pcna		Highly unfavorable	Pich[74]

ER = estrogen receptor protein; PR = progesterone receptor protein; AR = androgen receptor; EGFR = epidermal growth factor receptor; pS2 = estrogen-dependent protein; HER2/neu = transmembrane oncoprotein; Grade III = histologic grade; AgNOR = argyrophilic nucleolar organizer regions; pcna = proliferating cell nuclear antigen.

improved DSS in a subset of patients. Disease specific survival was improved in patients who were axillary lymph node positive with estrogen receptor positive tumors, although the number of patients with information regarding such systemic therapy was small.[54]

TREATMENT OF METASTATIC DISEASE

Many men with breast cancer present with metastatic disease, ranging from 11 to 16 percent in several recent series.[20,46,47,50,54] The pattern of spread in male patients is similar to that seen in female patients including local regional recurrences and metastases to bone, lung, liver, skin, and other areas.[9,20,50,51,53] The first-line palliative therapy used by most authors is hormonal therapy, most often with tamoxifen.[9,50,84,85] Reid and colleagues reported the use of hormonal therapy in 73 percent of patients treated for metastatic disease.[9] There has been a response rate of 25 to 58 percent to tamoxifen therapy reported in various series, the mean duration of response being 9 to 12 months, with few reported side effects. The response to tamoxifen seems to correlate with estrogen receptor status in that patients with receptor negative tumors show no response.[85,86] Historically, other hormonal treatments have been employed, including orchiectomy, adrenalectomy, and hypophysectomy. Response rates for orchiectomy are in the 30 to 60 percent range.[47,87–89] Response to secondary endocrine procedures have been reported in > 50 percent of cases.[87] Other hormonal manipulations, including androgen therapy and gonadotropin-releasing hormone agonist analogue therapy have been reported.[55] Systemic chemotherapy may be considered as a second-line palliative treatment, with an overall response rate of 30 to 40 percent.[28,62,87,90–92] Combination chemotherapy, such as CMF or doxorubicin-containing regimens, have been reported in various series and may be useful in patients who have failed prior therapies.[62,87,91,93]

CHANGES OVER TIME

During the last century, clinical acumen, classification systems, techniques of pathologic examination and methods for reporting the results of treating breast cancer have undergone extensive changes. True comparability of reporting between periods is unlikely, particularly when data are few and incomplete, as is the case for male breast cancer. Wainwright's review of collected cases diagnosed before 1927 provides one baseline against which to evaluate progress. By modern standards, it provides clear signs of delayed diagnosis and advanced disease.[5] The average symptomatic interval prior to diagnosis was 2.4 years. The modal age of cases was 60 to 64 years, with a mean of 52.6 years. Skin ulceration was observed in 38 percent of cases, and 68.9 percent of patients had involved axillary lymph nodes. Overall 5-year survival was only 19 percent.[20] While the age of men at the time of presentation has not declined convincingly, recent reports document shorter median symptomatic intervals of 3 to 8 months, suggesting an earlier diagnosis.[17,94a] Average tumor sizes stubbornly remain at 2.0 to 2.5 cm, but skin ulceration is now reported in only 12 to 13 percent of cases.[34,49] The rate of dissemination at diagnosis does not exceed that for females (in most reports 7 to 14 percent) and 2.9 to 5.6 percent of cases are now being diagnosed in situ—both favorable signs even in the absence of a concerted public screening effort.[49,55] The frequency of metastasis to axillary nodes generally remains high (45 to 51 percent), but in some reports the rate is as low as 33 percent.[34,52,55]

Favorable changes in managment of men have been less radical surgery and more frequent use of systemic adjuvant chemohormonal therapy. Men are now treated with modified radical mastectomy more often than with radical mastectomy, with no apparent detrimental effect and with improved cosmetic outcome. Chemotherapy, tamoxifen, or both, targeted at micrometastases, are an increasingly frequent component of primary treatment, with expectations that the benefits will parallel those for women. The indications are that these changes are improving the outlook for cure or extended survival of men. Current 5-year survivals of 47 to 51 percent overall, and as high as 76 percent in undisseminated cases, compare favorably with results reported early in the century. Some investigators have suggested that changes in therapy have resulted in little improvement in symptomatic interval, stage at diagnosis, or survival for men with breast cancer. In a report from the Mayo Clinic comparing the results from the period 1933 to 1958 with the period 1959 to 1983, fewer radical operations and a higher frequency of adjuvant systemic therapy were found in the more recent period, but not an improvement in median survival (5.5 years vs 6.3 years, respectively) or in 5-year disease-free survival of males with breast cancer (52 vs 47 percent).[20] In a more recent 10-year span from 1986 to 1995 compared with the period 1953 to 1985, investigators at the Medical College of Wisconsin noted a change of surgical treatment to modified radical mastectomy and increased use of systemic therapy and found improvement in 5-year observed survival of males treated in Wisconsin hospitals, from 42 to 59 percent ($p = .055$).[54] Stage for stage, the prognosis for men is comparable to, or somewhat inferior to, that for women. Truly accurate comparisons, however, are challenged by the need to control for multiple tumor-related and nontumor-related influences on outcome.

SUMMARY

Breast cancer in men is infrequent and occurs in an older population than does the disease in women. The disease in men is remarkably similar to the disease in women. Men present with advanced stages of disease more often than women, but a trend toward earlier diagnosis is evident. There is an increased awareness of the importance of family history and an association with *BRCA2* mutations. Analysis of treatment trends demonstrates the use of less radical surgery and increased use of systemic adjuvant therapy, especially in view of the high incidence of estrogen-receptor positivity of breast cancer in men compared to women. Important prognostic variables include stage, tumor size, and axillary node involvement. Also, survival decreases with increasing number of axillary nodes containing metastatic disease. Survival trends suggest improvement in the last one to two decades, although the length of this improvement is limited by the older male population with this disease. Though the survival of men is reported to be similar to women compared stage for stage, comorbidities in men, such as heart disease, strokes, and second malignancies, contribute to an overall survival that may be inferior to that found in women.

REFERENCES

1. Landis SH, Murray T, Bolden S, Wingo PA. Cancer Statistics, 1999. CA Cancer J Clin 1999; 49:8–31.
2. Breasted JH. The Edwin Smith surgical papyrus. Vol. I. Chicago: University of Chicago Press; 1930. p. 403–6.
3. Holleb AI, Freeman HP, Farrow JH. Cancer of the male breast. I and II. N Y State J Med 1968;68: 544,656.
4. Meyskens FL Jr, Tormey DC, Neifeld JP. Male breast cancer: a review. Cancer Treat Rev 1976;3:83–93.
5. Wainwright JM. Carcinoma of the male breast. Arch Surg 1927;14:836–59.
6. Cutler SJ, Young JL Jr (eds). Third National Cancer Survey: Incidence Data. National Cancer Institute Monograph 41. March 1975. DHEW Publication No (NIH) 75–787. US Department of Health, Education, and Welfare. Public Health Service. National Institutes of Health. National Cancer Institute, Bethesda, Maryland 20014. US Government Printing Office. Washington C.C. 20402. p. 106–107.
7. Winchester DJ, Bilimoria MM, Scott-Conarr CEH, Menck HR, Winchester DP. Male breast cancer: presentation, treatment, and survival (In press).
8. Schultz MZ, Coplin M, Radford D, Virgo KS, Johnson FE. Outcome of male breast cancer (MBC) in the Department of Veterans Affairs (DVA). Proc Annu Meet Am Soc Clin Oncol 1996;15:A257.

9. Reid C, Pintilie M, Goncalves S, et al. A review of 229 male breast cancer patients presenting to the Princess Margaret Comprehensive Cancer Centre. Proc Annu Meet Am Soc Clin Oncol 1997;16:A476.

10. Ewertz M, Homnberg L, Kajjalaninen S, et al. Incidence of male breast cancer in Scandinavia 1943–1982. Int J Cancer 1989;43:27–31.

11. Schottenfeld D, Lilienfeld AM, Diamond H. Some obervations on the epidemiology of breast cancer among males. Am J Pub Health 1963;52:890–7.

12. Amir H, Makwaya CK, Moshiro C, Kwesigabo G. Carcinoma of the male breast: a sexually transmitted disease? East Afr Med J 1996;73:187–90.

13. Hassan I, Mabogunje O. Cancer of the male breast in Zaria, Nigeria. East Afr Med J 1995;72:457–8.

14. Hsing AW, McLaughlin JK, Cocco P, et al. Risk factors for male breast cancer (United States). Cancer Causes Control 1998;9:269–75.

15. D'Avanzo B, LaVecchia C. Risk factors for male breast cancer. Br J Cancer 1995;71:1359–62.

16. Stenlund C, Floderus B. Occupational exposure to magnetic fields in relation to male breast cancer and testicular cancer: a Swedish case-control study. Cancer Causes Control 1997;8:184–91.

17. Donegan WL, Perez-Mesa CM. Carcinoma of the male breast. Arch Surg 1973;106;273–9.

18. Olsson H, Andersson H, Johansson O, et al. Population-based cohort investigations of the risk for malignant tumors in first-degree relatives and wives of men with breast cancer. Cancer 1993;71:1273–8.

19. Friedman LS, Gayther SA, Kurosaki T, et al. Mutation analysis of BRCA1 and BRCA2 in a male breast cancer population. Am J Hum Genet 1997;60:313–9.

20. Gough DB, Donohue JH, Evans MM, et al. A 50-year experience of male breast cancer: is outcome changing? Surg Oncol 1993:2:325–33.

21. Everson RB, Fraumeni JF Jr, Wilson RE. Familial male breast cancer. Lancet 1976 Jan 3; 9–14.

22. Couch FJ, Farid LM, DeShano ML, et al. BRCA2 germline mutations in male breast cancer cases and breast cancer families. Nat Genet 1996;13:123–5.

23. Haraldsson K, Loman N, Zhang QX, et al. BRCA2 germ-line mutations are frequent in male breast cancer patients without a family history of the disease. Cancer Res 1998;58:1367–71.

24. Hiort O, Naber SP, Lehners A, et al. The role of androgen receptor gene mutations in male breast carcinoma. J Clin Endocrinol Metab 1996;81:3404–7.

25. Poujol N, Lobaccaro JM, Chiche L, et al. Functional and structural analysis of R607Q and R608K androgen receptor substitutions associated with male breast cancer. Mol Cell Endocrinol 1997;130:43–51.

26. Klinefelter HF Jr, Reifenstein EC Jr, Albright F. Syndrome characterized by gynecomastia, aspermatogenesis without A-leydigism and increased excretion of follicle-stimulating hormone. J Clin Endocrinol 1942;2(11):615–27.

27. Hultborn R, Hanson C, Kopf I, et al. Prevalence of Klinefelter's syndrome in male breast cancer patients. Anticancer Res 1997;17(6D):4293–7.

28. Volm MD, Gradishar WJ. How to diagnose and manage male breast cancer. Contemp Oncol 1994;4:17–28.

29. Crichlow RW. Breast cancer in males. Breast, Diseases of the Breast 1976;Oct/Dec:2(4):12–16.

30. Casagrande JT, Hanisch R, Pike MC, et al. A case-control study of male breast cancer. Cancer Res 1988;48:1326–30.

31. Srensen HT, Friis S, Olsen JH, et al. Risk of breast cancer in men with liver cirrhosis. Am J Gastroenterol 1998;93:231–3.

32. Symmers WC. Carcinoma of the breast in transsexual individuals after surgical and hormonal interference with the primary and secondary sex characteristics. Br Med J 1968;2:83–5.

33. Pritchard TJ, Pankowsky DA, Crowe JP, et al. Breast cancer in a male-to-female transsexual. JAMA 1988;259:2278–80.

34. Crichlow RW, Kaplan EL, Keamey WH. Male mammary cancer: an analysis of 32 cases. Ann Surg 1972:175;489–94.

35. Mabuchi K, Bross DS, Kessler II. Risk factors for male breast cancer. J Natl Cancer Inst 1985;74:371–5.

36a. Karamanakos P, Apostolopoulos V, Fafouliotis S, et al. Synchronous bilateral primary male breast carcinoma with hyperprolactinemia. Acta Oncol 1996:35:757–9.

36b. Volm MD, Talamonti MS, Thangavelu M, Gradishar WK. Pituitary adenoma and bilateral male breast cancer: an unusual association. J Surg Oncol 1997:64:74–8.

37. Thompson DK, Li FP, Cassady Jr. Breast cancer in a man 30 years after radiation for metastatic osteogenic sarcoma. Cancer 1979;44:2362–5.

38. Lowell DM, Marineau RG, Luria SB. Carcinoma of the male breast following radiation. Cancer 1968;22:581–6.

39. Sanchez AG, Villanueva AG, Redondo C. Lobular carcinoma of the breast in a patient with Klinefelter's syndrome. Cancer 1986;57:1181–3.

40. San Miguel P, Sancho M, Enriquez JL, et al. Lobular carcinoma of the male breast associated with the use of cimetidine. Virchows Arch 1997;430:261–3.

44. Daltry IR, Eeles RA, Kissin MW. Bilateral prophylactic mastectomy: not just a woman's problem! Breast 1998;7:236–7.

42. Cutuli B, Dilhuydy JM, DeLafontan B, et al. Ductal carcinoma of the male breast: analysis of 31 cases. Eur J Cancer 1997;33:35–8.

43. Hittmair AP, Lininger RA, Tavassoli FA. Ductal carcinoma in situ (DCIS) in the male breast. Cancer 1998;83:2139–49.

44. Desai DC, Brennan EJ Jr, Carp NZ. Paget's disease of the male breast. Am Surg 1996;62:1068–72.

45. Muttarak M, Nimmonrat A, Chaiwun B. Metastatic carcinoma of the male and female breast. Australas Radiol 1998;42:16–9.

46. Ribeiro, G. Male breast carcinoma—A review of 301 cases from the Christies Hospital & Holt Radium Institute, Manchester. Br J Cancer 1985;51:115–9.

47. van Geel AN, van Slooten EA, Mavrunac M, Hart AAM. A retrospective study of male breast cancer in Holland. Br J Surg 1985;72:724–7.

48. Hultborn R, Friberg S, Hultborn KA. Male breast carcinoma. I. A study of the total material reported to the Swedish Cancer Registry 1958–1967 with respect to clinical and histopathologic parameters. Acta Oncol 1987;26:241–56.

49. Guinee VF, Olsson H, Moller T, et al. The prognosis of breast cancer in males. Cancer 1993;71:154–61.

50. Borgen PI, Wong GY, Vlamis V, et al. Current management of male breast cancer: a review of 104 cases. Ann Surg 1992;215:451–9.

51. Salvadori B, Saccozzi R, Manzari A, et al. Prognosis of breast cancer in males: an analysis of 170 cases. Eur J Cancer 1994;30A:930–5.

52. Cutuli B, Lacroze M, Dilhuydy JM, et al. Male breast cancer: results of the treatments and prognostic factors in 397 cases. Eur J Cancer 1995;31A:1960–4.

53. McLachlan SA, Erlichman C, Liu FF, et al. Male breast cancer: an 11 year review of 66 patients. Breast Cancer Res Treat 1996;40:225–30.

54. Donegan WL, Redlich PN, Lang PJ, Gall MT. Carcinoma of the breast in males: a multi-institutional survey. Cancer 1998;83:498–509.

55. Donegan WL, Redlich PN. Breast cancer in men. Surg Clin North Am 1996;76:343–63.

56. Dershaw DD, Borgen PI, Deutch BM, Liberman L. Mammogrphic findings in men with breast cancer. AJR 1993;160:267–70.

57. Cooper RA, Gunter BA, Ramanurthy L. Mammography in men. Radiology 1994;191:651–6.

58. Stewart RAL, Howlett DC, Hern FJ. Pictorial review: the imaging reatures of male breast disease. Clin Radiol 1997;52:739–44.

59. Sneige N, Holder PD, Katz RL, et al. Fine-needle aspiration cytology of the male breast in a cancer center. Diagn Cytopathol 1993;9:691–7.

60. Vetto J, Schimdt W, Pommier R, et al. Accurate and cost effective evaluation of breast masses in males. Am J Surg 1998;175:383–7.

61. Ambrogetti D, Ciatto S, Catarzi S, Muraca MG. The combined diagnosis of male breast lesions: a review of a series of 748 consecutive cases. Radiol Med 1996;91:356–9.

62. Bezwoda WR, Hesdorffer C, Dansey R, et al. Breast cancer in men: clinical features, hormone receptor status and response to therapy. Cancer 1987;60:1337–40.

63. Bruce DM, Heys SD, Payne S, et al. Male breast cancer: clinico-pathological features, immunocytochemical characteristics and prognosis. Eur J Surg Oncol 1996;22:42–6.

64. Caton J, Rearden T, Ellis R. Male breast cancer: the Department of Defense (DOD) experience. Proc Annu Meet Am Soc Clin Oncol 1995;14:A140.

65. Ciatto S, Iossa A, Bonardi R, Pacini P. Male breast carcinoma: review of multicenter series of 150 cases. Tumori 1990;76:555–8.

66. Borgen PI, Senie RT, McKinnon WM, Rosen, PP. Carcinoma of the male breast: analysis of prognosis compared with matched female patients. Ann Surg Oncol 1997;4:385–8.

67. Joshi MG, Lee AK, Loda M, et al. Male breast carcinoma: an evaluation of prognostic factors contributing to a poorer outcome. Cancer 1996;77:490–8.

68. Pivot X, Llombart-Cussac A, Rhor-Albarddo A, et al. Clinical staging for male breast cancer: an adaptation of the international classification (TNM). Proc Annu Meet Am Soc Clin Oncol 1997;16:A655.

69. Lartigau E, El-Jabbour JN, Dubray B, Dische S. Male breast carcinoma: a single centre report of clinical parameters. Clin Oncol 1994;6:162–6.

70. Winchester DJ, Goldschmidt RA, Khan SJ, et al. Flow cytometric and molecular prognostic markers in male breast carcinoma patients [abstract]. Presented at the 46th Annual Cancer

Symposium of the Society of Surgical Oncology; Los Angeles; 1993; March 18–21.

71. Yap HY, Tashima CK, Blumenschein GR, Eckles NE. Male breast cancer: a natural history study. Cancer 1979;44:748–54.

72. Winchester DJ. Male breast cancer. Semin Surg Oncol 1996;12:364–9.

73. Pich A, Margaria E, Chiusa L, et al. DNA ploidy and p53 expression correlate with survival and cell proliferative activity in male breast carcinoma. Hum Pathol 1996;27:676–82.

74. Pich A, Margaria E, Chiusa L. Proliferative activity is a significant prognostic factor in male breast carcinoma. Am J Pathol 1994;145:481–9.

75. Visfelt J, Scheike O. Male breast cancer. I. Histologic typing and grading of 187 Danish cases. Cancer 1973;32:985–90.

76. Anelli A, Anelli TF, Youngson B, et al. Mutations of the p53 gene in male breast cancer. Cancer 1995;75:2233–8.

77. Jonasson JG, Agnarsson BA, Thorlacius S, et al. Male breast cancer in Iceland. Int J Cancer 1996;65:446–9.

78. Hultborn R, Friberg S, Hultborn DA, et al. Male breast carcinoma. II. A study of the total material reported to the Swedish Cancer Registry 1958–1967 with respect to treatment, prognostic factors and survival. Acta Oncol 1987;26:327–41.

79. Schuchardt U, Seegenschmiedt MH, Kirschner MJ, et al. Adjuvant radiotherapy for breast carcinoma in men: a 20-year clinical experience. Am J Clin Oncol 1996;19:330–6.

80. Anelli TFM, Anelli A, Tran KN et al. Tamoxifen administration is associated with a high rate of treatment-limiting symptoms in male breast cancer patients. Cancer 1994;74:74–7.

81. Ribeiro G, Swindell R. Adjuvant tamoxifen for male breast cancer. Br J Cancer 1992;65:252–4.

82. Bagley CS, Wesley MN, Young RC, Lippman ME. Adjuvant chemotherapy in males with cancer of the breast. Am J Clin Oncol 1987;10:55–60.

83. Patel, HZ, Buzdar AU, Hortobagyi GN. Role of adjuvant chemotherapy in male breast cancer. Cancer 1989;64:1583–5.

84. Becher R, Höffken K, Pape H, Schmidt CG. Tamoxifen treatment before orchiectomy in advanced breast cancer in men. N Engl J Med 1981;305:169–70.

85. Ribeiro GG. Tamoxifen in the treatment of male breast carcinoma. Clin Radiol 1983;34:625–8.

86. Patterson JS, Batersby LA, Back BK. Use of tamoxifen in advanced male breast cancer. Cancer Treat Rep 1980;64:801–4.

87. Jaiyesimi IA, Buzdar AU, Sahin AA, et al. Carcinoma of the male breast. Ann Intern Med 1992;117;771–7.

88. Kantarjian H, Yap H-Y, Hortobagyi G, et al. Hormonal therapy for metastatic male breast cancer. Arch Intern Med 1983;143:237–40.

89. Patel JK, Nemoto T, Dao TL. Metastatic breast cancer in males: assessment of endocrine therapy. Cancer 1984;53:1583–5.

90. Kraybill WG, Kaufman R, Kinne D. Treatment of advanced male breast cancer. Cancer 1981;47:2185–9.

91. Sandler B, Carman C, Perry RR. Cancer of the male breast. Am Surg 1994;60:816–20.

92. Yap HY, Tashima CK, Blumenschein GR, et al. Chemotherapy for advanced male breast cancer. JAMA 1980;243:1739–41.

93. Lopez M, DiLauro L, Papaido P, et al. Chemotherapy in metastatic male breast cancer. Oncology 1985;452:205–9.

94a. Stierer M, Rosen H, Weitensfelder W, et al. Male breast cancer: Austrian experience. World J Surg 1995;19:687–92.

94b. Rayson D, Erlichman C, Wold LE, et al. Molecular markers in male breast cancer. Proc Annu Meet Am Soc Clin Oncol 1997;16:A477.

95. Willsher PC, Leach IH, Ellis IO, et al. Male breast cancer: pathological and immunohistochemical features. Anticancer Res 1997;17:2335–8.

96. Bines J, Goss B, Hussong J, et al. c-erbB2 and p53 overexpression as predictors of survival in patients with male breast cancer. Proc Annu Meet Am Soc Clin Oncol 1997;16:A558.

97. Dawson PJ, Schroer KR, Wolman SR. Ras and p53 genes in male breast cancer. Mod Pathol 1996;9:367–70.

15

Estrogen Replacement Therapy for Breast Cancer Survivors

WENDY R. BREWSTER, MD

PHILIP J. DiSAIA, MD

Ninety percent of women will live to the climacteric age, compared to only 30 percent 200 years ago. Attrition and aging of ovarian follicles results in termination of the maturation of granulosa cells, which are responsible for estrogen production. Sources of estrogen in the premenopausal woman are several fold, including direct production of estradiol by the ovaries as well as the extraglandular aromatization in adipose cells of androstenedione created in the adrenal glands and ovary. The hallmark of menopause is a drop in ovarian production of estriol and testosterone. Peripheral aromatization of other steroids not produced by the ovaries is an additional source of estrogen in all women. However, this source is not sufficient in most women to prevent the symptoms characteristic of estrogen deprivation.

Given the current population, 30 million women in the United States will spend approximately 40 percent of their lifetime in the postmenopausal period. These women have a lifetime risk of one in eight of developing breast cancer. Thus, a considerable number of American women are likely to have a history of breast cancer treatment and at the same time be potential candidates for hormone-replacement therapy. In the last decade, indications for chemotherapy as adjuvant treatment to surgery have widened and now encompass many more premenopausal women.[1] Adjuvant therapy for breast cancer includes the use of alkylating agents and other drugs that cause amenorrhea in 84 percent of women aged 35 to 44 years. Other studies indicate that this treatment causes permanent ovarian failure in 86 percent of women > 40 years of age.[2] As a result, a larger number of women will potentially be rendered menopausal in the fourth, and fifth decades of their lives, which has serious consequences in terms of the risk of cardiovascular disease and osteoporosis.

The major concern of many physicians in prescribing estrogen-replacement therapy (ERT) for breast cancer survivors is the theory that metastatic quiescent tumor foci might be activated and the "fire" of breast cancer ignited by the "fuel" estrogen. Other fears are that estrogen might cause a second primary in the already environmentally/genetically primed contralateral breast or might change breast density and mask new mammographic findings. These concerns are in part based upon epidemiologic studies demonstrating a relationship between duration of postmenopausal estrogen replacement and breast cancer.[3,4] Also, surgical oophorectomy is beneficial in a subset of premenopausal breast cancer patients, and estrogen withdrawal has also been observed to promote regression of metastatic breast cancer lesions.[5] Despite very limited clinical data to support these concerns, it remains standard practice to prohibit breast cancer survivors from receiving ERT.

The well-substantiated benefits of estrogen replacement therapy must be balanced against theoretical concerns. Arguments in support of the safety of ERT are based on several natural experiments and observations, discussed in detail below.

BENEFITS OF ESTROGEN REPLACEMENT THERAPY

Over the last two decades, overwhelming evidence has been accrued demonstrating that postmenopausal estrogen replacement protects against ischemic heart disease, osteoporosis, deterioration in cognitive function, colorectal cancer, and provides relief from vasomotor symptoms and urogenital atrophy. Multimodality screening has resulted in an increase in the incidence of breast cancer diagnoses; this increase, however, reflects more frequent detection of early-stage breast cancer. Because breast cancer survival is inextricably linked to early diagnosis, there are now more breast cancer survivors than ever. Morbidity and mortality associated with estrogen deprivation present serious health concerns. The risk/benefit ratio of estrogen replacement therapy (ERT) is an appropriate consideration for all patients.

Coronary Artery Disease

Cardiovascular disease is the leading cause of mortality among women in the United States. The number of deaths from diseases of the circulatory system in women in the United States is greater than the number who die from cancers of the breast, reproductive tract, and maternal morbidity combined. It is only during the reproductive years that more women die from malignancy than from cardiovascular disease. This is reversed past 60 years of age.

The endocrine influences of factors thought to be contributors to the risk of cardiovascular disease have been studied extensively. The literature is vast and has been well summarized in several recent reviews. Unopposed estrogen raises the serum level of high-density lipoprotein cholesterol, especially the HDL2 subfraction, and lowers the serum level of low-density lipoprotein cholesterol.[6] Other less well-studied factors that may influence cardiovascular health during treatment with estrogen, with or without progestin, include beneficial effects on the circulation, blood pressure, coagulation, and fibrinolysis.[7,8] Estrogen also has vasodilating properties mediated by the generation of prostacyclin in the cell membrane.

Many epidemiological studies have found that postmenopausal women who use estrogen are at a much lower risk for coronary disease than are nonusers. Observational studies suggest a 50 percent reduction in the risk of coronary heart disease among healthy postmenopausal women taking oral estrogen.[9]

In 1981, Henderson and colleagues recruited over 8,000 women from a retirement community in Laguna Hills, California called Leisure World. This is a stable community and very few individuals were lost to follow-up. Of this cohort, 57 percent reported estrogen use, 14 percent were current users at the time of the questionnaire, and 43 percent reported previous use. The incidence of mortality from acute myocardial infarction was statistically lower among current users and those who had used estrogen in the past compared to nonusers. The relative risk was 0.59, with the 95 percent confidence interval (CI) of 0.42 to 0.82.

Hunt[10] reported on a cohort of 4,544 women who had taken hormone replacement therapy continuously for at least 1 year at the time of recruitment. When compared with the general female population, mortality rates for ischemic heart disease among the cohort were significantly lower, with a relative risk of 0.41 and a 95 percent CI of 0.2 to 0.61. Bush[11] evaluated a cohort of 2,270 women, 593 of whom were estrogen users. The age-adjusted relative risk of death from cardiovascular disease was 0.34, with the 95 percent CI of 0.12-0.81.

Stampfer[12] evaluated postmenopausal estrogen therapy and cardiovascular disease in the Nurses' Health Study, with a 10-year follow-up. Women currently using postmenopausal hormone therapy accounted for 21.8 percent of the total follow-up time of 337,854 person-years. There was a reduction in the age-adjusted relative risk of fatal cardiovascular disease among current hormone users. In the same study, the age-adjusted risk of major coronary artery disease among current estrogen users was about half that of women who had never used estrogen, with a relative risk of 0.51 $p < .0001$. For former users, the age-adjusted relative risk (RR) was 0.91. When this was adjusted for other risk factors, the relative risk was 0.83. The relative risk of fatal cardiovascular disease was decreased in both current and former users.

The above studies were all based on postmenopausal estrogen use only. Given the fact that current medical recommendations call for the addition of a progestin to estrogen therapy in nonhysterectomized women, there is the valid concern that progestin therapy may negate the benefits gained by estrogen (Table 15–1).

The investigators in the Postmenopausal Estrogen/Progestin Interventions (PEPI) trial examined this issue.[13] They found, as had been confirmed in numerous previous studies, that unopposed estrogen decreased the risk factors for cardiovascular disease. However, estrogen given with medroxyprogesterone acetate or micronized progesterone hormone-replacement therapy (HRT) was associated with lower fibrinogen levels and improved lipoprotein profiles. No adverse effects on the rate of cardiovascular incidents were observed for HRT over ERT.

Grodstein[14] evaluated the effect of combined estrogen and progestin use and the risk of cardiovascular disease in the Nurses' Health Study. Among the 59,337 women enrolled, there were 770 casualties of myocardial infarction or deaths from coronary artery disease. There was a marked decrease in the risk of major coronary artery disease among women who took estrogen with progestin compared to that for women who did not use hormones. The multivariate-adjusted relative risk was 0.39, with the 95 percent CI of 0.19 to 0.78.

Osteoporosis

Postmenopausal women are at risk for loss of cancellous bone in the vertebrae and other long bones, which places them at increased risk for fracture. Bone mineral density decreases rapidly within 5 years of menopause due to estrogen deficiency. This ultimately results in microarchitectural deterioration and a progressive increased fracture risk. Postmenopausal untreated women may lose 35 percent of their cortical bone and up to 50 percent of their trabecular bone. It is estimated that 1.2 million major fractures per year in the United States in women are related to osteoporosis. Fifteen percent of postmenopausal women will suffer wrist fractures, and an even larger number will incur spinal compression fractures. Compression fractures of the vertebral bones may result in loss of stature, pulmonary restriction, and

Table 15–1. EPIDEMIOLOGIC STUDIES OF THE CARDIOVASCULAR BENEFITS OF POSTMENOPAUSAL ESTROGEN AND PROGESTERONE USE

Study	Design	Number	Results
Falkeborn et al.[41]	Prospective	227 MI cases 23,174 women	RR = 0.74 ever estrogen only RR = 0.50 ever combined therapy
Psaty et al[42]	Case-control	502 MI cases 1,193 controls	RR = 0.69 estrogen alone RR = 0.68 current combined therapy
Grodstein et al[14]	Prospective	770 MI cases 59,337 women	RR = 0.60 current estrogen alone RR = 0.39 current combined therapy

MI= myocardial infarction; RR = relative risk.

decreased ambulation. An estimated 40 percent of the women who will live to the age of 80 years will develop spinal fractures and 33 percent will experience a hip fracture.

Of concern is the morbidity and mortality associated with hip fractures in older women. Within this group, 12 to 20 percent will die within 6 months of the fracture, and half of the survivors require long-term nursing care. Osteoporotic fractures in the United States resulted in health care costs of $7 billion in 1986. This is estimated to increase to as much as $62 billion by the year 2020.

Alzheimer's Disease

As the population ages, Alzheimer's disease has emerged as a major health problem. After the age of 65 years, the prevalence of dementia and Alzheimer's disease doubles every 5 years; 30 to 50 percent of women older than 83 years may suffer from dementia of some sort.

Laboratory studies suggest that estrogen may affect Alzheimer's disease through several mechanisms. Estrogen has been shown to improve regional cerebral blood flow and to increase glucose utilization. It can also stimulate neurite growth and synapse formation in vitro. Under some circumstances, estrogen may modify neural sensitivity to neurotrophin and play a role in the reparative neuronal response to injury. One key histologic feature of Alzheimer's disease is the deposition of beta-amyloid protein in cores of neuritic plaques. Estrogen may promote the breakdown of the amyloid precursor protein to fragments less likely to accumulate as beta amyloid. Acetylcholine is a key neurotransmitter in learning and memory. Estrogen affects several neurotransmitter systems, including the cholinergic system. Finally, estrogen may modify inflammatory responses postulated to participate in neuritic plaque formation.[15]

Tang and colleagues examined the effect of a history of estrogen use on the development of Alzheimer's disease in 1,200 women.[16] These subjects were initially free of Alzheimer's disease, Parkinson's disease, and stroke and were part of a longitudinal study of aging and health in a New York community. Overall, 158 (12.5 percent) reported taking estrogen after the onset of menopause. The age of onset of Alzheimer's disease was significantly later in women who had taken estrogen than in those who did not, 78 years versus 73 years. Even after adjustment for differences in education and ethnic origin, the relative risk of Alzheimer's disease was significantly reduced in estrogen users over nonusers: 0.4, with a 95 percent CI of 0.22 to 0.85.

Even among postmenopausal women who are not demented, ERT may help maintain cognitive function.[17] Estrogen appears to have a specific effect on verbal memory skills in healthy postmenopausal women.[18,19]

The emotional, physical, social, and financial costs of Alzeimer's disease to patients, families, caregivers, and society are tremendous. The estimated total cost of the disease in 1991 was estimated to be $173,932 per case. The estimated prevalence cost for both men and women for that year was $67.3 billion.[20] The economic cost of care alone is greater than the cost of care for heart disease and cancer combined. If the use of estrogen could delay the onset of Alzheimer's disease by several years, there would be a substantial saving in both emotional and financial costs.

Colorectal Cancer

There have been > 20 retrospective studies of the risk of colon cancer and ERT, with more than 70 percent of these reports illustrating a statistically significant reduction in incidence with users versus nonusers. One proposed mechanism affecting this protection is that estrogen reduces the concentration of bile acids, and may limit carcinogenic action to the colon mucosa. It has been demonstrated that bile acid concentrations are higher in colon cancer cases than in control subjects, and it is known that estrogen decreases bile acid synthesis and secretion.[21] Estrogen receptors are present in both normal and cancerous colon mucosal cells, and there is laboratory evidence to suggest that estrogen may inhibit the growth of colon cancer cells.[22]

Calle and colleagues[23] investigated the relationship between postmenopausal estrogen use and fatal colorectal cancer in a large prospective study of adults in the United States. Eight hundred and seventy-nine colon cancer case patients were compared to 421,476 noncase subjects. Ever use of ERT was associated with a significantly decreased risk of fatal colon cancer (RR = 0.71; 95% CI = 0.61 to 0.83). Reduction in risk was strongest among current users (RR = 0.55; 95% CI = 0.40 to 0.76) compared to former estrogen users. There was a significant trend of decreasing risk with increasing years of estrogen use among all users (p = .0001). Those women who used estrogen for ≤ 1 year had a RR = 0.81, whereas users of ≥ 11 years had a RR of 0.54 (95 percent CI = 0.39 to 0.76). These associations were not altered in multivariate analyses controlling for age, race, parental history of colon cancer, body mass index, exercise, parity, type of menopause, age of menopause, oral contraceptive pill use, aspirin use, and smoking.

Vasomotor Instability

The menopausal state most commonly produces vasomotor instability and genital organ atrophy. Vasomotor symptoms affect 70 percent of postmenopausal women but only about 30 percent seek medical assistance. For 25 percent of menopausal women, these symptoms may persist for > 5 years and may be lifelong in others. Vasomotor instability is more commonly termed "hot flushes" or "hot flashes." The frequency, severity, or diurnal variation with which hot flushes occur can result in significant disruptions of sleep and daytime function. Menopausal symptoms are the most common side effect associated with the use of adjuvant chemotherapy for breast cancer, with approximately two-thirds of women experiencing symptoms classified as moderate to severe.[24] This effect may be compounded by tamoxifen therapy, which also leads to vasomotor instability.

Urogenital Atrophy

Because the vagina and urethra share a common embryologic origin, it is believed that estrogen deficiency causes atrophy of both structures. Atrophy of the vaginal epithelium may cause vaginal itching, dryness, and dyspareunia, with resulting inflammation. One effect of estrogen deficiency is to cause changes in the vaginal pH, which predispose women to urinary tract infections that cause urgency, incontinence, frequency, nocturia, and dysuria. The loss of estrogen on periurethral tissues will contribute to pelvic laxity and stress incontinence. Recurrent urinary tract infections can be prevented with systemic estrogen therapy, and low-dose topical estrogen is effective in managing atrophic vaginitis. Estrogen provides relief of these symptoms and may protect against recurrent urinary tract infections.

EXPOSURE TO EXOGENOUS OR ENDOGENOUS ESTROGEN DURING BREAST CANCER DEVELOPMENT

The decision whether or not to take hormone replacement remains difficult for the postmenopausal woman because of conflicting risks and benefits and is even more difficult for the breast cancer survivor for whom there is even less data. One can therefore analyze situations in which women are inadvertently exposed to exogenous or endogenous estrogen at a time when they may have been harboring subclinical breast cancer. Does such exposure adversely affect survival outcome for these patients?

Such situations include those in which the diagnosis of breast cancer is made in postmenopausal women receiving ERT at the time of diagnosis or in whom the diagnosis is made in pregnancy or during lactation, or in those women with a history of oral contraceptive pill use around the time of diagnosis of breast cancer.

Breast Cancer in Women on Estrogen Replacement Therapy

Bergkvist and co-workers[25] compared 261 women who developed breast cancer while on ERT to 6,617 breast cancer patients who had no recorded treatment with estrogen. The relative survival rate over an 8-year period was higher in the breast cancer patients who had previously received ERT. This corresponded to a 32 percent reduction in excess mortality. Gambrell,[26] in a prospective study, also evaluated the effect on survival in breast cancer patients diagnosed while on ERT. Mortality was 22 percent among those diagnosed with breast cancer while on ERT compared to 46 percent among those who had never received hormone replacement. Henderson and colleagues[27] observed a 19 percent reduction in breast cancer mortality among 4,988 previous ERT users, compared to 3,865 nonusers who subsequently developed this disease.

Breast Cancer Associated with Pregnancy

Pregnancy coincident with, or subsequent to, the detection of breast cancer provides another excellent opportunity to evaluate the outcome of breast cancer patients inadvertently exposed to high levels of estrogen at times when they were harboring occult disease. During pregnancy, the serum levels of estriol increase 50-fold. Only 0.5 to 4 percent of all breast cancers are diagnosed during pregnancy. Because the average breast cancer remains occult in the breast some 5 to 8 years prior to diagnosis, some authors include in this category women in whom a diagnosis of breast cancer has been made within 12 months of delivery. The outcome in women with subclinical breast cancers exposed to elevated levels of progesterone and estrogen under these circumstances could provide insight into the influence of these hormones on the malignant disease process.

The physiologic changes and engorgement that occur in the breast during pregnancy often hinder early detection of breast cancer. This results in a diagnosis at more advanced stages in pregnant and lactating women. Comparisons to nonpregnant women matched for similar age stage of breast cancer and reproductive capacity do not suggest a worse prognosis for the pregnant patients with breast cancer.[28,29] von Schoultz[30] performed a comparison of women diagnosed with breast cancer 5 years before pregnancy to women without a pregnancy during the same time period. There was no survival disadvantage to the women who were pregnant 5 years prior to the diagnosis of breast cancer. These and other studies have discouraged the practice of prohibiting breast cancer survivors from becoming pregnant on clinical grounds. Subsequent pregnancies do not negatively affect survival outcomes.

Anderson and colleagues[31] reported their experience at the Memorial Sloan Kettering Cancer Center with breast cancer in women < 30 years of age. Two hundred and twenty-seven cases were identified, of whom 22 had pregnancy-associated breast cancer. The authors confirmed that pregnancy-associated breast cancers were usually larger and present in more advanced stages at the time of diagnosis, compared to a similar group who were not pregnant. However, the survival probability for women with early stage disease was independent of pregnancy status.

The experience of women who have completed term pregnancies after treatment of antecedent breast cancer is another situation that deserves analysis. There are inherent biases associated with evaluation of this particular group of subjects. This cohort is representative of the young women who did well after primary breast cancer therapy; since pregnancy data is not uniformly coded in cancer registry databases, the true denominator of postbreast cancer pregnancies is unknown. Clark[32] reported a 71 percent 5-year survival in a series of 136 women with pregnancies after breast cancer (stages I to III). Equivalent survival outcomes were reported by von Schoultz[30] for breast cancer patients with no subsequent pregnancy, compared to those who became pregnant within 5 years of their diagnosis.

Breast Cancer in Oral Contraceptive Pill Users

Given the long natural history of this neoplasm, it is certain that a large number of patients subsequently diagnosed with breast cancer have used oral contraceptive pills (OCP) during the genesis and progression of their malignant disease process; they are another group that deserves examination.

Rosner[33] evaluated 347 women < 50 diagnosed with breast cancer, of whom 112 were OCP users. The distribution of tumor size, estrogen-receptor status, and family and reproductive history was the same between the two cohorts. There was no difference in disease-free survival or survival between the two groups. Women who used OCP within a year of diagnosis of their breast cancer had a similar survival to those who had discontinued use > 1 year before. There was no difference in survival among those who used OCP ≥ 10 years prior to their diagnosis of breast cancer.

Schonborn and colleagues[34] evaluated the influence of a positive history of OCP use on survival. Four hundred and seventy-one breast cancer patients were investigated. Two hundred and ninety-seven patients (63 percent) had used OCP during any period of their life, and 92 (20 percent) still used them at the time of diagnosis. Sixty months after diagnosis, the OCP users had a significantly increased overall survival ($p = .037$). Survival rates amounted to 79.5 percent and 70.3 percent for OCP users and nonusers, respectively.

Sauerbrei[35] investigated the relationship between OCP use and standard prognostic factors, and the effect of OCP use on disease-free survival and overall survival, in 422 premenopausal node-positive patients from two trials of the German Breast Cancer Study Group. One hundred and thirty-seven OCP users (32.5 percent) were younger than those who did not use OCP (mean age 41.5 years versus 45 years). Noteworthy was the fact that the percentage of patients with smaller tumors was higher in the group of OCP users. No significant effect of OCP use on either disease-free or overall survival could be demonstrated in univariate and multivariate analyses after adjustment for tumor size and other prognostic factors.

STUDIES ON ESTROGEN-REPLACEMENT THERAPY IN BREAST CANCER SURVIVORS

DiSaia[36] reported on 71 breast cancer survivors who received ERT. There was no exclusion based on time interval from diagnosis, stage, age, receptor status, or lymph node status. Women received combination therapy with progestin only if they had not previously undergone hysterectomy. Later, the author reported a comparison of 41 of these ERT survivors to 82 non-ERT breast cancer subjects, matched for both age and stage of disease.[37] Survival analysis did not indicate a significant difference between the two groups. An updated series of 145 patients who received ERT for at least 3 months after diagnosis has identified 13 recurrences. The duration of estrogen use prior to the diagnosis of recurrent breast cancer ranged from 4 months to 11.5 years (Figures 15–1 and 15–2).

Other authors have reported their experience of ERT in breast cancer survivors. Eden[38] reported six recurrences among 90 women receiving ERT. These ERT users were matched two to one with control subjects with no history of hormone use after diagnosis of breast cancer. The recurrence rate was 7 percent in the ERT users and 30 percent in the non-ERT users. Bluming[39] reported on 155 breast cancer patients who received ERT for between 1 and 56 months, among whom 7 recurrences were identified. The only published prospective randomized trial is being undertaken by Vas-

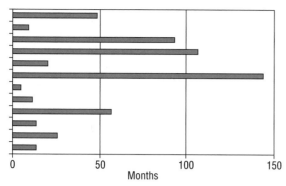

Figure 15–1. Subjects with recurrent breast cancer. The interval between initiation of use of estrogen replacement therapy and diagnosis of recurrent breast cancer.

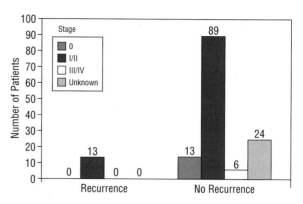

Figure 15–2. Comparison by known stage of subjects who received estrogen replacement therapy.

silopoulou-Sellin.[40] Subjects are randomized to either a placebo or ERT without a progestational agent. Ninety women have been randomized and 49 have received ERT for a minimum of 2 years. No breast cancer recurrences have been observed in the ERT arm. The single recurrence was in the placebo arm.

The series discussed above are representative of the reported experience of ERT in 499 female breast cancer survivors (Table 15–2). This group of women is very heterogeneous with respect to breast cancer stage, the interval between diagnosis of breast cancer and initiation of ERT, the hormonal combinations prescribed, estrogen-receptor status, and finally in the duration of use of estrogen. Despite these limitations, it remains obvious that the use of estrogen is not associated with a rash of occurrences. Overall, the data do not suggest that ERT has an adverse effect on breast cancer outcome.

CONCLUSION

The fear that administration of estrogen to women with a history of breast cancer will result in the activation of quiescent metastatic foci, as well as the climate of medical litigation, are the basis of much of the reluctance of physicians to prescribe this agent. The standard of care no longer supports prophylactic oophorectomy in young women who do not become amenorrheic after cytotoxic therapy. In addition, many women continue to menstruate regularly after treatment and may even complete pregnancies. If castration and pregnancy termination are not routinely recommended, why then should the replacement of estrogen at a much lower dose than is physiologic be prohibited?

Fifty-year-old women have a 13 percent lifetime probability of developing breast cancer and a 3 percent probability of dying from it; they have a 46 percent chance of developing coronary

Table 15–2. ESTROGEN-REPLACEMENT THERAPY IN BREAST CANCER SURVIVORS

Study	No. of Patients	Stage of Disease	Duration of ERT	Recurrences
Stoll[43]	Unknown	Early stage	3–6 mo	None
Wile et al[44]	25	All stages	24–82 mo	3
Powles et al[45]	35	All stages	1–44 mo	8
Eden et al[38]	90	Local	4–144 mo	6
Vassilopoulou-Sellin et al[40]	49	0–III (ER negative only)	24–142 mo (oral or vaginal estrogen only)	0
Bluming et al[39]	155	Local	1–56 mo	7
Brewster et al*	145	All stages	3–144 mo	13

*In press.
ERT=estrogen-replacement therapy; ER=estrogen replacement.

heart disease and a 31 percent probability of dying from it. While breast cancer claims 43,000 lives per year in the United States, coronary heart disease will kill approximately 233,000 women annually. Nearly 65,000 women die each year from the complications of hip fracture.

No guarantee can be made that ERT will be accompanied with freedom from recurrent breast cancer, because some women will have recurrent disease coincident with renewed hormonal exposure. However, should one discuss the risks and benefits of estrogen replacement therapy with patients to help them make an informed decision?

REFERENCES

1. Early Breast Cancer Trialists' Collaborative Group. Systemic treatment of early breast cancer by hormonal, cytotoxic, or immune therapy: 133 randomized trials involving 31,000 recurrences and 24,000 deaths among 75,000 women. Lancet 1992;339:1–15, 71–85.

2. Mehta RR, Beattie CW, Das Gupta T. Endocrine profile in breast cancer patients receiving chemotherapy. Breast Cancer Res Treat 1991; 20:125–32

3. Colditz GA, Hankinson SE, Hunter DJ, et al. The use of estrogens and progestins and the risk of breast cancer in postmenopausal women. N Engl J Med 1995;332:1589–93.

4. Stanford JL, Weiss NS, Voigt LF, et al. Combined estrogen and progestin hormone replacement therapy in relation to risk of breast cancer in middle age women. JAMA 1995;274:137–41.

5. Dhodapkar MV, Ingle JN, Ahmann DL. Estrogen replacement therapy withdrawal and regression of metastatic breast cancer. Cancer 1995;75: 43–6.

6. Sacks FM, Walsh BW. The effects of reproductive hormones on serum lipoproteins: unresolved issues in biology and clinical practice. Ann NY Acad Sci 1990;592:272–85.

7. Gebera OC, Mittleman MA, Walsh BW, et al. Fibrinolytic potential is significantly increased by oestrogen treatment in postmenopausal women with mild dyslipidemia. Heart 1998;80:235–9.

8. Koh KK, Mincemoyer R, Bui MN, et al. Effects of hormone-replacement therapy of fibrinolysis in postmenopausal women. N Engl J Med 1997;336:683–90.

9. Grady D, Rubin SM, Petitti DB, et al. Hormone therapy to prevent disease and prolong life in postmenopausal women. Ann Intern Med 1992;117:1016–37.

10. Hunt K, Vessey M, McPherson K, Coleman M. Long-term surveillance of mortality and cancer incidence in women receiving hormone replacement therapy. Br J Obstet Gynaecol. 1987;94:620–35.

11. Bush TL, Barrett-Connor E, Cowan LD, et al. Cardiovascular mortality and noncontraceptive use of estrogen in women. Circulation 1987;75: 1102–9.

12. Stampfer MJ, Colditz GA, Willet WC, et al. Postmenopausal estrogen therapy and cardiovascular disease. Ten-year follow-up from the Nurses' Health Study. N Engl J Med 1991;325:756–62.

13. The Writing Group for the PEPI Trial. Effects of estrogen or estrogen/progestin regimens on heart disease risk factors in postmenopausal women. The Postmenopausal Estrogen/Progestin Interventions (PEPI) Trial. JAMA 1995; 274:199–208.

14. Grodstein F, Stampfer MJ, Colditz GA, et al. Postmenopausal hormone therapy and mortality. N Engl J Med 1997;336:1769–75.

15. Paganini-Hill A, Henderson VW. Estrogen replacement therapy and risk of Alzheimer's disease. Arch Intern Med 1996;156:2213–17.

16. Tang MX, Jacobs D, Stern Y, et al. Effect of oestrogen during menopause on risk and age at onset of Alzheimer's disease. Lancet 1996;348: 429–32.

17. Jacobs DM, Tang MX, Stern Y, et al. Cognitive function in nondemented women who took estrogen after menopause. Neurology 1998;50: 368–73.

18. Kampen DL, Sherwin BB. Estrogen use and verbal memory in healthy postmenopausal women. Obstet Gynecol 1994;83:979–83.

19. Rice MM, Graves AB, McCurry SM, Larson EB. Estrogen replacement therapy and cognitive function in postmenopausal women without dementia. Am J Med 1997;103:26S–35S.

20. Ernst RL, Hay JW. The US economic and social costs of Alzheimer's disease revisited. Am J Public Health 1994;84:1261–4.

21. Davis RA, Fern F Jr. Effects of ethinyl estradiol and phenobarbital on bile acid synthesis and biliary bile acid and cholesterol excretion. Gastroenterology 1976;70:1130–5.

22. Lointier P, Wildrick DM, Bowman BM. The effects of steroid hormones on a human cancer cell line in vitro. Anticancer Res 1992;12: 1327–34.

23. Calle EE, Miracle-McMahill HL, Thun MJ, Heath CW Jr. Estrogen replacement therapy and the risk of fatal colorectal cancer in a prospective cohort of postmenopausal women. J Natl Cancer Inst 1995;87:517–23.

24. Canney PA, Hatton MQF. The prevalence of menopausal symptoms in patients treated for breast cancer. Clin Oncol 1994;6:297–9.

25. Bergkvist L, Adami HO, Persson I, et al. Prognosis after breast cancer diagnosis in women exposed to estrogen and estrogen progesterone replacement therapy. Am J Epidemiol 1992; 130:221–8.

26. Gambrell DR. Proposal to decrease the risk and improve the prognosis in breast cancer. Am J Obstet Gynecol 1984;150:119–28.

27. Henderson BE, Paganini-Hill A, Ross RK. Decreased mortality in users of estrogen replacement therapy. Arch Intern Med 1991;151:75–8.

28. Holleb AI, Farrow JH. The relation of carcinoma of the breast and pregnancy in 283 patients. Surg Gynecol Obstet 1962;115:65.

29. Nugent P, O'Connell TX. Breast cancer and pregnancy. Arch Surg 1985;120:1221–4.

30. von Schoultz E, Johansson H, Wilking N, Rutqvist LE. Influence of prior and subsequent pregnancy on breast cancer prognosis. J Clin Oncol 1995;13:430–4.

31. Anderson BO, Petrek JZ, Byrd DR, et al. Pregnancy influences breast cancer stage at diagnosis in women 30 years of age and younger. Ann Surg Oncol 1996;3:204.

32. Clark RM, Chua T. Breast cancer and pregnancy: the ultimate challenge. Clin Oncol (R Coll Radiol) 1989;1:11–8.

33. Rosner D, Lane W. Oral contraceptive use has no adverse effect on the prognosis of breast cancer. Cancer 1986;57:591–6.

34. Schonborn I, Nischan P, Ebeling K. Oral contraceptive use and the prognosis of breast cancer. Breast Cancer Res Treat 1994;30:283–92.

35. Sauerbrei W, Blettner M, Schmoor C, et al. The effect of oral contraceptive use on the prognosis of node positive breast cancer patients. German Breast Cancer Study Group. Eur J Cancer 1998 Aug;34(9):1348–51.

36. DiSaia PJ, Odicino F, Grosen EA, et al. Hormone replacement therapy in breast cancer [letter]. Lancet 1993;342:1232.

37. DiSaia PJ, Grosen EA, Kurosaki T, et al. Hormone replacement therapy in breast cancer survivors. A cohort study. Am J Obstet Gynecol 1996; 174:1494–8.

38. Eden JA, Bush T, Nand S, Wren BG. A case control study of combined continuous estrogen-progestin replacement therapy among women with a personal history of breast cancer. Menopause 1995;2:67–72.

39. Bluming AZ, Waisman JR, Dosik GM. Hormone replacement therapy (HRT) in women with previously treated primary breast cancer. Update III. Proc Am Soc Clin Oncol 1997;16A:463,131a.

40. Vassilopoulou-Sellin R, Therriault R, Klein MY. Estrogen replacement therapy in women with prior diagnosis and treatment for breast cancer. Gynecol Oncol 1997;65:89.

41. Falkeborn M, Persson I, Adami HO, et al. The risk of acute myocardial infarction after oestrogen and oestrogen-progestogen replacement. Br J Ob Gyn 1992;99:821–8.

42. Psaty BM, Heckbert SR, Atkins D, et al. The risk of myocardial infarction associated with the combined use of estrogens and progestins in postmenopausal women. Arch Intern Med 1994;154:1333–9.

43. Stoll BA. Hormone replacement therapy in women treated for breast cancer. Eur J Cancer Clin Oncol 1989;25:1909–13.

44. Wile AG, Opfell RW, Margileth DA. Hormone replacement therapy in previously treated breast cancer patients. Am J Surg 1993;165:372–5.

45. Powles TP, Casey S, O'Brien M, Hickish T. Hormone replacement after breast cancer. Lancet 1993;342:60.

16

Surveillance of the Breast Cancer Patient

JANARDAN D. KHANDEKAR, MD

In recent years, extensive clinical trials have established the roles for conservative surgery, radiation, and adjuvant chemo/hormonal therapy in the primary therapy of breast cancer. It may seem self-evident that repeated postoperative contact between cancer patients and their physicians, that is, follow-up, is a good thing. Follow-up practice patterns vary greatly, with some oncologists frequently following their breast cancer patients with various intensive investigation and others only doing sporadic follow-up. The possible beneficial effects of follow-up include:

1. Management of postsurgical complications. This is essential and need not be elaborated upon here.
2. Early detection of recurrence or of new primaries.
3. Reassuring patients. This can be a double-edged sword, as some patients are reassured by the process while others are made anxious by an impending visit to the physician.
4. Measurement of quality control of outcomes. Participation in clinical trials or American College of Surgeons-sponsored audits can be helpful.

This chapter evaluated criteria for follow-up and provides background on the principal of screening and economic analysis.

DEFINITIONS

It will be useful to review some of the terms used in analyzing the surveillance data. The *decision matrix* is a term most commonly applied to the simple decision of whether the disease is present (D+) or absent (D-) when the test is abnormal, that is, positive (T+) or normal, that is negative (T-). When these two binary results are plotted on a 2 × 2 table, four possible combinations form the ratios shown below.[1–3]

The true positive (TP) ratio represents the proportion of positive tests in all patients who have the disease. The ratio therefore expresses the sensitivity of the test and can be expressed as:

$$\text{sensitivity} = \frac{\text{diseased subjects with positive test}}{\text{all diseased subjects tested}} \times 100$$

More simply stated, sensitivity is determined by the false-negative (FN) ratio, which is the proportion of negative tests in all patients with the disease. The TP and the FN ratio then represent the sensitivity of the test.

The false-positive (FP) ratio is the proportion of positive tests in all patients who do not have the disease. The true-negative (TN) ratio is the proportion of negative tests in all patients who do not have the disease. The FP and TN ratios then express specificity, defined as:

$$\text{sensitivity} = \frac{\text{nondiseased subjects with negative test}}{\text{all nondiseased subjects tested}} \times 100$$

The sensitivity of a test under consideration is usually determined by evaluating its efficacy against a known standard. Depending on the sensitivity of that standard, the sensitivity can be spuriously high or low. For example, the sensitivity of a bone scan is usually evaluated in relation to radiography, a technique which itself is not very sensitive. Therefore, the sensitivity of the bone scan is very high, in the vicinity of about 99 percent. However, if in the future even more sensitive tests for detecting bone metastasis become available, such as use of either better imaging techniques and/or polymerase chain reaction-based molecular assays, the sensitivity of the bone scan will decrease. The specificity of the test is also dependent upon the FP ratio. Generally, the FP rate increases with more data, and the initial specificity of a given diagnostic test decreases with time. These factors then govern the sensitivity and specificity of various diagnostic tests. When sensitivity and specificity of a test are determined, it is possible to calculate the predictive value (PV).

The positive PV is defined as the likelihood that a subject yielding a positive test actually has the disease. Conversely, a negative PV indicates the likelihood that a subject with a negative test does not have the disease. This likelihood is related to the actual prevalence of disease in the total population. More simply stated, PV for positive tests can be defined as the percentage of time that a positive test will detect the diseased individual. The PV of a positive test can be calculated as follows:[4]

$$PV = \frac{\text{number of diseased subjects (or proportion) with positive test}}{\text{total number (or proportion) of subjects with positive test}} \times 100$$

The PV of a negative test can be calculated as follows:

$$PV = \frac{\text{number (or proportion) of nondiseased persons with positive test}}{\text{total number (or proportion) of persons with positive test}} \times 100$$

The usefulness of a diagnostic test is therefore directly proportional to the prevalence of the target disease in the population. The FP rate of a test is usually constant and is often related to the test and not the disease itself. Therefore, when the prevalence of the target disease is low, the PV of the positive test is also low since FP is constant. On the other hand, if there is a higher prevalence of the disease, the PV of a positive test will also be high.

The evaluation of various diagnostic tests are also affected by various biases that significantly affect the interpretation of the data. These are outlined below.

Lead-Time Bias

The apparent increased duration of survival simply reflects a longer time that the recurrence was clinically known but there is no true gain in longevity. In other words, there is an illusion of an increased survival because of the longer duration of observation but there is no impact on mortality rate. It is because of this consideration that reduction of mortality rate has become the "gold standard" in evaluating the impact of a diagnostic or therapeutic intervention.

Length-Time Bias

An event such as cancer detected in an asymptomatic phase often has an indolent course and is therefore detected at the time of evaluation rather than between the visits. Cancers that are aggressive will often present with symptoms in the intervening visits, creating the illusion that more intensive surveillance would have resulted in detecting of the disease earlier and a better outcome.

EVALUATION OF VARIOUS TESTS USED IN BREAST CANCER

The American Society of Clinical Oncology (ASCO) established an expert panel to evaluate the use of various tests in breast cancer.[5] The panel modified the scale developed by the Canadian Taskforce on Periodic Health Examination to evaluate various tests (Table 16–1).[6] There are only two prospective randomized trials that have evaluated the impact of a multitude of surveillance tests on the overall survival and quality of life in breast cancer patients. They fulfill the criteria of providing Level 1, that is, highest level of evidence. However, beginning with studies published in 1979 by Winchester and colleagues,[7] a large database has been developed that has retrospectively analyzed the value of various diagnostic tests in the follow-up of breast cancer patients. These studies have tried to answer some of the following questions:

1. Do the available tests diagnose early asymptomatic recurrence in breast cancer? If so, which tests are useful?
2. Does early detection and recurrence result in better therapy and thus improve quality and quantity of survival? (This is the most important question).
3. What is the cost-benefit analysis for the possible improved quality or quantity of life?

Winchester and colleagues analyzed 87 patients with recurrent breast cancer for patterns of recurrence and methods of detection.[7] In 79 of 87 patients, recurrence was detected by symptoms such as pain or shortness of breath, while physical examination detected an additional 5 patients with recurrence. Review of the literature indicates that only 12 to 22 percent of recurrences occur in truly asymptomatic women.[8–14] In the prospective intergroup for cancer care evaluation trial (GIVIO), 31 percent of the recurrences were detected in asymptomatic patients in the intensely investigated group compared to 21 percent of recurrences in the control group.[11] However, there was no effect on survival in patients detected in the asymptomatic phase. It has been argued that patients with local recurrence only those who undergo aggressive therapy have a 50 percent 5-year survival, and may therefore have an improved outcome. However, it can be argued that patients with local recurrence may have more biologically inert disease, as these were retrospective studies. Dewar and Kerr in an English study reported that of 546 breast cancer patients followed with 6,863 clinic visits, only 1 percent of the visits were associated with recurrences that were curable.[14] These authors have therefore questioned even routine physical examination. In their studies, recurrences were found five times more often during spontaneous visits than during routine visits, illustrating the lead-time bias. Dewar and Kerr suggest that negative physical examinations may give false assurance to patients, leading to an even further delay in diagnosis of a recurrence.

Table 16–1. MODIFIED CANADIAN CRITERIA FOR EVALUATING DIAGNOSTIC TEST EVIDENCE

Level of Evidence	Type of Evidence for Recommendation
Level 1 (highest level)	Meta-analysis or large high-powered concurrently controlled studies with a primary objective to evaluate the utility of a given test
Level 2	Prospective clinical trials designed to test given hypothesis
Level 3	Large size retrospective trials
Level 4	Similar to Level 3, but even less reliable. Comparative and correlative descriptive and case studies can be included.
Level 5	Case reports and clinical examples

Adapted from Khandekar JD. Preoperative and postoperative follow up of cancer. In: Winchester DJ, Scott Jones R, Murphy GP, editors. Surgical oncology for the general surgeon. Philadelphia, PA: Lippincott, Williams and Wilkins; 1999.p. 43–54.

Scanlon and colleagues carefully analyzed the information from the last examination to recurrence in 93 patients.[8] They reported that 43 percent of recurrences were detected within 3 months of the last examination, 64 percent within 6 months, and 94 percent within 1 year. They therefore recommended that examinations be conducted every 3 months for the first 2 to 3 years after primary therapy for breast cancer, and then at a reduced interval.

The vast majority of recurrences are detected by history and physical examination. Although the impact of such detection on overall survival is unknown, it may have the psychological benefit of reassuring the patient of having had a contact with their physician. Since the cost of such surveillance is approximately $150 per annum per patient and allows evaluation of other parameters such as the effects of primary therapy, physical and psychosocial rehabilitation, and detection of contralateral primary, the current author agrees with ASCO's recommendation that the patients should be seen at 3-month intervals for the first 2 years then every 6 months for the next 3 years.[5]

Chemistry

An abnormal chemical evaluation has been the first evidence of recurrent breast cancer in approximately 1 to 12 percent of patients.[7,14] An abnormal blood count is rarely seen as a first indicator of recurrent breast cancer. Hannisdal and colleagues reviewed their experience with 430 patients.[15] In 8 of 430 patients, an elevated erythrocyte sedimentation rate, gamma glutamyl transferase, and alkaline phosphatase values heralded recurrences. The sensitivity and specificity of these tests for relapse was 55 and 91 percent, respectively.[15] The ASCO panel recommends no laboratory tests in the follow-up.[5] However, the chemotherapeutic drugs used as adjuvant therapy can be leukemogenic, and periodic blood tests may have to be undertaken to detect these changes. Further, many patients with breast cancer have other concurrent dis-

eases and/or can develop new problems. Therefore, an occasional blood test may be warranted.

Tumor Markers: CA-15-3 and CEA

Hayes and colleagues defined the marker that represents qualitative or quantitative alteration or deviation from normal of a molecule, substance, or process that can be detected by some type of assay.[16] This includes measurement of a gene, RNA, a product such as protein, carbohydrate, a lipid, or a process such as vascular density. Markers used in follow-up are considered below.

CA-15-3

The CA-15-3[16] marker measures the serum level of a mucin-like membrane glycoprotein that is shed from the tumor cells into the blood stream. Recently, the Food and Drug Administration approved the Truquant assay which uses a monoclonal antibody, CA-27-29, to measure CA-15-3-like antigen. This marker is elevated only in patients with advanced disease.[16] The level of CA-15-3 is highest in patients with liver or bone metastasis. The ASCO panel evaluated 12 studies reporting on the value of CA-15-3 in detecting asymptomatic recurrent breast cancer. Of these studies, only seven could be properly analyzed.[5] Of 1,672 patients followed in these trials, 352 developed recurrence. About two-thirds of these were detected by an elevated CA-15-3 before other parameters revealed recurrence. The mean lead-time from marker elevation to clinical diagnosis was 5 to 7 months. However, the sensitivity of the test was only 57 to 79 percent. It is also not known whether such early detection leads to improved survival. If and when new therapies for the treatment of metastatic breast cancer are developed, the role of CA-15-3 may need re-evaluation.

CEA

The value of CEA[5] in detecting recurrent breast cancer is even less than that of CA-15-3. At present, there are no indications for using CEA in routine surveillance of breast cancer patients.

Mammography

Patients with breast cancer are at higher risk for developing contralateral breast cancer. Further, patients with breast cancer who have undergone conservative therapy with lumpectomy or radiation are at risk for ipsilateral recurrence. Currently, it is recommended that patients who have undergone unilateral mastectomy should undergo contralateral mammography on a yearly basis. Patients who have been treated with conservative techniques and develop local recurrence can be salvaged by appropriate treatment such as mastectomy. In the GIVIO trial,[11] patients randomized to intensive follow-up had an 11.4 percent incidence of contralateral breast cancer, versus 6.6 percent in the group with only routine follow-up. Local therapy for ipsilateral breast cancer recurrence or detection of a new primary in the contralateral breast will improve quality and quantity of life.

Routine Chest Radiography

Several investigators have studied the value of annual chest radiography in patients with breast cancer. In general, only 0.2 to 4 percent of radiographs were abnormal in truly asymptomatic patients. As pointed out by Loprinzi,[17] the only value of routine annual chest radiography is to detect lymphangitic pulmonary metastasis before it causes significant pulmonary symptoms and thus impairs quality of life. Although the ASCO panel does not recommend annual chest radiography,[6] the current author agrees with Loprinzi[17] that it may be beneficial up to 3 years following primary therapy. It is unlikely that this will improve survival, but it can be helpful in preserving quality of life. Patients with aggressive breast cancer tend to recur in the first 2 years following primary therapy, meaning that the annual radiograph can be ceased after 3 years of follow-up.[3]

Bone Scans

In 1979, it was proposed on the basis of Bayes decision analysis that since there is no evidence that early detection and therapy for metastatic breast cancer alters the clinical course of the patient, bone scans should be performed only in symptomatic patients. Since then, several studies have confirmed this recommendation. The Eastern Cooperative Group confirmed the finding in the mid-1980s.[18] The National Surgical Adjuvant Breast and Bowel Project (NSABP) followed 1,989 patients on the B-09 arm of their study.[19] Of these patients, 779 had treatment failure, of whom roughly one-fifth had recurrences limited to bone. Only 52 (0.6%) patients had screening scans that were useful in detecting lesions in asymptomatic patients. The NSABP changed their recommendation about surveillance of breast cancer patients in 1994 based on this study.

In the GIVIO trial, in which patients were randomized between intensive follow-up versus observation only, compliance was > 80 percent in both groups.[11] At a median follow-up of 71 months, there was no difference in overall survival in the two groups. The study also showed no impact on the quality of life because of intensive intervention. Another Italian trial, that of Del Turco and colleagues,[12] evaluated 1,243 consecutive patients with intensive intervention versus minimum follow-up. In this study, there was increased detection of isolated intrathoracic and bone metastasis in the intensive follow-up group compared to clinical follow-up group. No difference was observed, however, for other sites, and 5-year overall mortality was 18.6 versus 19.5 percent (statistically insignificant difference) between the two groups.

The bone scan has a false-positive rate of approximately 15 percent.[2] If the prevalence of metastasis is low, the predictive value of a positive test will be low and the patient may be subjected to additional unnecessary interventions. On the basis of Baye decision analysis, it was pointed out that routine bone scans in surveillance of a breast cancer patient will lead to a low predictive value of a positive test and unnecessary and expensive interventions.[2] It is therefore recommended that bone scans be performed only in breast cancer patients who are symptomatic with bone pain or with significant elevations in their alkaline phosphatase.

Imaging Studies of the Liver

There have been no prospective studies comparing sensitivity and specificity of CT and MRI evaluations in the postoperative surveillance of breast cancer patients. However, on the basis of evaluation in preoperative breast and lung cancers, it is safe to conclude that in the absence of symptoms and abnormal liver function tests, these imaging techniques will be of little or no value. The Italian GIVIO investigators performed liver echography in their intervention group. In that study, 6.5 percent of patients had their first recurrence diagnosed by liver echography, versus 6.1 percent in the control group, who had echography because of abnormal examination and/or hepatic function tests.[11] Based on these studies, it can be concluded that routine imaging techniques for detecting liver metastasis are not warranted.

Table 16–2 summarizes recommendations for follow-up of breast cancer patients who have completed their primary therapy, and, when appropriate, adjuvant chemotherapy.

IMPLICATIONS FOR HEALTH-CARE COSTS

In response to spiraling health-care costs, managed care was aggressively introduced.[20] Managed care is under intense pressure these days, and its future is uncertain. However, the silver lining of managed care has been that it has forced clinicians to critically evaluate their practices. This has resulted in developing pathways and guidelines for various illnesses. Cohen and colleagues argue that physicians have a responsibility to assure the delivery of appropriate health care without sacrificing the quality of care.[21] The upper limit for an acceptable cost-effectiveness ratio remains controversial. Moreover, it is important to bear in mind that not only quantity of life but the impact of an intervention on the quality of life should be measured.[22] Measurement of quality of life is still somewhat subjective, but as new tools are developed, it must be incorporated into cost analyses.

In two prospective clinical trials conducted in Italy,[11,12] no cost-effective analysis was available. Schapira attributed savings of $636 million in 1990 costs and projected a $1 billion saving in the year 2,000[23] when a minimal follow-up schema, as described here, is employed. However, it is unclear whether his analysis includes additional expenses incurred as the result of FP tests, which can lead to additional interventions. The negative psychological impact of an FP test cannot be quanti-

Table 16–2. PROPOSED FOLLOW-UP SCHEDULE

Procedure	Low-Risk*	High-Risk†
History and physical examination	3 mo × 2 yr and then 6 mo × 3 yr then yearly	3 mo × 2 yr 6 mo × 3 yr then yearly
Complete blood count and chemistry	Every 6 mo × 2 yr and then yearly	3 mo × 2 yr 6 mo × 3 yr then yearly
Markers: CEA, CA-15-3	—	—
Mammogram	Yearly	Yearly
Chest radiograph	Yearly	Yearly
Scans (bone, liver)	—	—

*Patients with negative nodes and/or positive receptors.
†Patients with positive nodes and/or received chemotherapy.
Adapted from Khandekar JD. Preoperative and postoperative follow up of cancer. In: Winchester DP, Scott Jones R, Murphy GP, editors. Surgical oncology for the general surgeon. Lippincott Williams and Wilkins; 1999. p.

fied at this time, but needs to be evaluated in future analyses.

In summary, the minimal surveillance schema proposed has considerable implications for health-care costs. Reallocation of health-care resources to areas that will lead to improved survival and quality of life is an important aspiration for health-care policy.

LEGAL IMPLICATIONS

In our litiginous society, there is apprehension about the legal consequences of a delayed diagnosis, even for the metastatic disease. It is important to educate the public as well as the legal profession on the differentiation between diagnosis of a primary breast cancer and that of a metastatic disease. If in the future better and more effective treatments become available that change the natural history of the disease, detection at an earlier time may become important. The guidelines developed by associations such as ASCO[5] and the Society of Surgical Oncology[21] are helpful for physicians protecting against these legal threats.

CONCLUSION

It is only in recent years, primarily because of economic pressure, that guidelines for surveillance have been developed and adapted. In 1999, about $1.3 trillion will be spent on health care.[24] Several studies as well as the analysis presented here indicate that a minimal surveillance approach is clearly warranted.[17,25] One can argue that there need not be any follow-up for breast cancer patients after primary intervention. Although routine history and physical examinations may not have a direct benefit in terms of survival, they have an immense psychological effect. Most patients need reassurance, which leads to self-confidence. Visits also provide time to educate patients and discuss psychosocial and physical rehabilitation—it is imperative that patients do not feel abandoned by their physicians. These visits also allow diagnosis of local and regional recurrences as well as new contralateral breast cancers, which can be cured. Although controversial, the current author continues to believe that an annual radiograph for the first 3 years after primary treatment and occasional blood tests are indicated. On the other hand, more expensive tests such as bone scans, ultrasound, and CT scans of the chest, brain, and liver, and measurement of tumor markers, are not indicated.

At this time, there is no evidence that metastatic disease, when detected early, can be cured by present techniques. However, the recommendation of minimal follow-up may need to be altered if early intervention in recurrent breast cancer will lead to improved survival. Patients who are in clinical trials should have a more intensive follow-up to differentiate the disease-free interval and overall survival in the control and experimental groups. However, the clinical trial should keep these diagnostic tests to a minimum so that managed care and other healthcare providers do not object to extra expenses. To improve therapy, it is important that an increasing number of patients be enrolled in clinical trials. Therefore, true collaboration needs to be developed between various cooperative groups and healthcare providers. It is important to improve the health-care of patients while giving appropriate consideration to the problem of escalating health-care costs.

REFERENCES

1. McNeil BJ, Keller E, Adelstein SJ. Primer on certain elements of medical decision-making. N Engl J Med 1975;293:211.
2. Khandekar JD. Role of routine bone scans in operable breast cancer: an opposing viewpoint. Cancer Treat Rep 1979;63:1241.
3. Khandekar JD. Preoperative and postoperative follow-up of cancer. In: Winchester DP, Scott Jones R, Murphy GP, editors. Surgical oncology for the general surgeon. Philadelphia, PA: Lippincott, Williams & Wilkins; 1999. p. 43–54.
4. Vecchio TJ. Predictive value of a single diagnostic test in unselected populations. N Engl J Med 1966;274:1171.

5. ASCO Special Article. Recommended breast cancer surveillance guidelines. J Clin Oncol 1997; 15:2149.

6. Canadian Medical Association. The Canadian task force on the periodic health examination. Can Med Assoc J 1979;121:1193.

7. Winchester DP, Sener SF, Khandekar JD, et al. Symptomatology as an indicator of recurrent or metastatic breast cancer. Cancer 1979;43:956.

8. Scanlon EF, Oviedo MA, Cunnigham MP, et al. Preoperative and follow-up procedures on patients with breast cancer. Cancer 1980;46:977.

9. Gerber FH, Goodreau JJ, Kirchner PT, Fouty WF. Efficacy of preoperative and postoperative bone scanning in the management of breast carcinoma. N Engl J Med 1977;297:300.

10. Burke W, Daly M, Garber J, et al. Recommendations for follow-up care of individuals with an inherited predisposition to cancer. II. BRCA1 and BRCA2. JAMA 1997;277:997.

11. The GIVIO Investigators. Impact of follow-up testing on survival and health-related quality of life in breast cancer patients. A multicenter randomized controlled trial. JAMA 1994;271:1587.

12. Del Turco MR, Palli D, Cariddi A, et al. Intensive diagnostic follow-up after treatment of primary breast cancer. A randomized trial. JAMA 1994; 271:1593.

13. Tomin R, Donegan WL. Screening for recurrent breast cancer: its effectiveness and prognostic value. J Clin Oncol 1987;5:62.

14. Dewar JA, Kerr GR. Value of routine follow-up of women treated for early carcinoma of the breast. BMJ 1985;291:1464.

15. Hannisdal E, Gundersen S, Kvaloy S, et al. Follow-up of breast cancer patients stage I-II: a baseline strategy. Eur J Cancer 1993;29A:992–7.

16. Eskelinen M, Hippelainen M, Carlsson L, et al. A decision support system for predicting a recurrence of breast cancer; a prospective study of serum tumor markers TAG 12, CA 15-3 and MCA. Anticancer Res 1992;12:1439–42.

17. Loprinzi CL. It is now the age to define the appropriate follow-up of primary breast cancer patients. J Clin Oncol 1994;12:881.

18. Pandya KJ, McFadden ET, Kalish LA, et al. A retrospective study of earliest indicators of recurrence in patients on Eastern Cooperative Oncology Group adjuvant chemotherapy trials for breast cancer. A preliminary report. Cancer 1985;55:202.

19. Wickerham L, Fisher B, Cronin W. The efficacy of bone scanning in the follow-up of patients with operable breast cancer. Breast Cancer Res Treat 1984;4:303.

20. Bodenheimer T. The American health care system: physicians and the changing medical marketplace. N Engl J Med 1999;340:584–8.

21. Cohen AM, Bland KI, Gardner B, Winchester DP. Society of Surgical Oncology and Practice Guidelines. Oncology 1997;11:869.

22. Cella D, Fairclough DL, Bonomi PB, et al. Quality of life (QOL) in advanced non-small cell lung cancer (NSCLC) results from Eastern Cooperative Oncology Group (ECOG) study E5592. Proc ASCO 1997;16(4):2a.

23. Schapira DV, Urbrn N. A minimalist policy for breast cancer surveillance. JAMA 1991;265:380.

24. Modern Healthcare. Economic data: some things never change. Modern Healthcare 1999;29:16.

25. Schapira DV. Breast cancer surveillance: a cost-effective strategy. Breast Cancer Res Treat 1993;25:107.

17

Treatment of Metastatic Breast Cancer

DOUGLAS E. MERKEL, MD

Despite the improvements in prognosis achieved for many patients with breast cancer, approximately 46,000 women die of this disease each year. The increase in incidence of breast cancer seen through the early 1990s has been successfully offset by two factors: widespread application of screening mammography, permitting more frequent early diagnosis and, more recently, the decrease in recurrence and mortality rates achieved through the now standard application of effective systemic adjuvant therapy.[1] Unfortunately, similar gains have not been achieved for women who present with metastatic breast cancer or for those with distant disease relapse after initial treatment. For these women, palliation of symptoms and some prolongation of survival is possible but there is no known curative treatment. In fact, the death rate for this disease has remained stubbornly constant over decades.[2] Metastatic breast cancer is the second most common cause of cancer death among women.

While only 6 percent of patients present initially with metastatic breast cancer,[2] metastases will eventually develop in at least 30 percent of patients with node-negative primary breast cancer and 50 percent of those with positive nodes at diagnosis. The event rate for recurrence is relatively constant over the first 10 years for women who receive adjuvant therapy, that is, each year healthy survivors face the same risk for recurrence as they did in the preceding year.[1]

The most common sites of metastatic involvement are bone, lungs, and liver.[3] While both infiltrating ductal carcinoma and infiltrating lobular carcinoma will relapse at the same rate over time based on their size and degree of nodal involvement, a predilection for certain sites of involvement can be related to histology. Infiltrating lobular carcinomas are more likely to recur in bone marrow, peritoneum, pelvic organs, and meninges than are infiltrating ductal carcinomas. On the other hand, lung metastases are more common with infiltrating ductal cancers.[4–6]

When metastatic breast carcinoma is first diagnosed, a brief staging workup is indicated to determine the extent of disease and thus treatment priorities. In the absence of symptoms, chest radiography, abdominal CT scan, and bone scan are needed. Any abnormalities on bone scan should be further pursued with bone radiographs, to confirm metastatic disease and determine whether it is lytic or blastic in nature. The finding of lytic disease, particularly in weight-bearing bones, has specific palliative implications. In addition to the above studies, any symptoms should be fully investigated.

Prior to beginning treatment for metastatic disease, biopsy to confirm clinical suspicions should be considered mandatory in all but the most unusual of circumstances. The diagnosis of incurable metastatic disease has obvious and profound prognostic implications, and often commits a patient to lifelong systemic treatment. The possibility of a benign lesion must therefore be excluded. In a disease such as breast cancer, which may recur many years after initial treatment, the possibility of a second primary carcinoma must also be considered and excluded. In addition to confirming the diagnosis of metastatic cancer, the tumor should be analyzed for estrogen receptor, progesterone receptor, and *HER2/c-erb*B2 protein,[7] as these results will largely determine the options for systemic therapy.

The prognosis for metastatic breast cancer is related to a number of variables, perhaps most importantly to the disease-free interval, or the duration of time between initial diagnosis and recurrence. This duration provides some measure of the growth rate of the cancer; longer survivals are reported when the disease-free interval exceeds several years.[8] The extent of metastatic involvement, or the number of involved sites, also has an impact on survival, as does location.[9] There is a particularly good prognosis observed for patients with a single metastatic focus amenable to surgery or radiotherapy.[10] Survival in excess of 2 years is also common when the disease is limited to bone but is not expected when there is visceral involvement.[11] Finally, improved survival is reported for estrogen receptor-positive metastatic breast cancer,[12] although other markers such as ploidy, S-phase fraction, and *HER2* status are not informative.[13] The relationship of estrogen receptor status and prognosis may not be independent of other factors, however, as these metastases are also more likely to be found in bone and soft tissue, and to occur at a longer disease-free interval, than those lacking estrogen receptors.[14]

As many patients will present initially with only a single site of metastasis, or a dominant lesion, treatment considerations for specific sites of metastases will be surveyed below. Systemic measures designed to palliate symptoms and offer some hope of delaying the progression of metastatic disease will then be discussed.

BRAIN METASTASES

Brain metastases are diagnosed in 16 to 25 percent of all women with breast cancer, but the brain is seldom the first site of relapse.[15] Thus, while brain imaging with gadolinium-enhanced MRI is not part of the routine initial workup for newly diagnosed metastatic breast cancer, any patient with new neurologic complaints should be promptly evaluated. Most commonly, a progressively worsening headache develops over days to weeks. Other common clinical features of brain metastases include behavioral or cognitive changes, focal weakness, ataxia, speech disorders, and seizures.[16]

Papilledema is present in only 15 percent of patients, and the screening neurologic exam may be negative. Any of the above symptoms are thus indications for scheduling a gadolinium-enhanced MRI. Computed tomography (CT) scan is less sensitive and more likely to result in equivocal or false-positive findings. These scans cannot detect meningeal involvement and should only be obtained where MRI is unavailable.[17]

Corticosteroids, usually dexamethasone at a dosage of 4 mg every 6 hours, can produce immediate but shortlived improvement in neurologic symptoms and are indicated as initial treatment in all patients with strongly suspected or newly diagnosed brain metastases.[18] Anticonvulsants, however, should be reserved for the 20 to 30 percent of patients who suffer focal or generalized seizures.[19]

Treatment of brain metastases may consist of either surgical extirpation, whole brain radiotherapy, or stereotactic "gamma-knife" radiosurgery. As retrospective analyses and a single randomized trial have demonstrated improved neurologic control and survival for patients undergoing surgery for brain metastases, resection must be the first consideration for all appropriate patients.[20] The most appropriate candidates for resection have single, accessible lesions, particularly those that are relatively bulky and thus unlikely to respond completely to radiotherapy. The surgical candidate should also be one whose other sites of metastatic disease are responding, or are likely to respond to systemic therapy; for those whose expected survival is limited, surgical intervention has little or no advantage over radiotherapy.

Radiation therapy is indicated as initial palliative treatment for all other patients, for example, those with multiple lesions or poorly controlled systemic disease. Median survival for patients treated in this fashion is 3 to 6 months but a majority receive symptomatic benefit.[21] Those who survive for ≥ 1 year or longer after whole brain radiotherapy are at risk for a variety of complications ranging from subtle cognitive deficits to leukoencephalopathy manifesting as progressive dementia with ataxia. This is primarily a concern in good-risk patients and has made the use of adjuvant whole brain radiotherapy following surgical removal of a solitary brain metastasis controversial.

Stereotactic radiosurgery is a new technique that delivers a single, large, tightly focused dose of radiation to a metastatic site, using multiple beams. This technique is highly effective for tumors < 3 cm, can be performed on an outpatient basis, and appears to result in far less risk of long-term damage to surrounding normal tissue.[22] While the current treatment of choice for recurrent disease after whole brain radiotherapy, and for patients with surgically inaccessible lesions, this technique may in time replace primary surgery for some patients.

Perhaps surprisingly, brain metastases from breast cancer have been reported to respond favorably to systemically administered chemotherapy[23] or tamoxifen.[24] While currently no trials have established this as frontline therapy for brain metastases, this approach can certainly be tried in patients who relapse following whole-brain radiotherapy, or those who decline to undergo it.

LEPTOMENINGEAL CARCINOMATOSIS

Involvement of the leptomeninges occurs in up to 5 percent of patients with breast cancer, usu-

ally in the setting of disseminated, progressive disease.[25] As mentioned above, this complication is more commonly observed in patients with infiltrating lobular cancer. The majority of patients will present with neurologic signs referable to some combination of cerebrum, cranial nerves, and spinal cord, although the patient may complain only of a single symptom.[26] The single-most common complaint is weakness of the legs, perhaps accompanied by pain or paresthesias. Cranial nerve involvement can produce diplopia, facial numbness or weakness, and hearing loss. Involvement of the cerebral cortex is heralded by headache, impaired memory, lethargy, and nausea.

Definitive diagnosis of leptomeningeal carcinomatosis is difficult, as initial cytologic examination of the cerebrospinal fluid (CSF) is falsely negative in up to 46 percent of patients.[27] Elevated CSF protein levels and monocytosis may be observed, and repeated sampling may yield positive cytology. Gadolinium-enhanced MRI of any areas of clinical involvement should be obtained, both to rule out parenchymal brain metastases or epidural cord compression and to detect enhancing, nodular meningeal enhancement—this may be seen along the convexity of the cerebrum, along the brain stem, or involving spinal nerve roots in up to 70 percent of patients.[28]

Treatment of leptomeningeal carcinomatosis is difficult, as it often arises in the midst of progressive systemic breast cancer and there has been no optimal approach established. Radiation therapy is usually administered to areas of bulky or symptomatic disease, although studies to establish this practice are lacking. Radiation therapy to the entire neuraxis is to be avoided as it can result in severe and prolonged myelosuppression, thus preventing the subsequent administration of systemic chemotherapy.

As the entire neuraxis is potentially at risk for leptomeningeal spread, direct CSF installation of chemotherapy is also indicated. Because of improved distribution of drug throughout the CSF, intraventricular administration via an

Ommaya reservoir is preferred over lumbar puncture. Methotrexate 12 mg two or three times weekly has been used most often, with improvement reported in 60 to 80 percent of patients.[26,29] The most common complication is transient aseptic meningitis, manifesting as headache, fever, and stiff neck. Particularly with simultaneous cranial radiotherapy, a necrotizing leukoencephalopathy with impaired mentation and focal defects may develop.[29] Leakage of methotrexate outside of the CSF may result in mucositis or myelosuppression but may be counteracted by concurrent administration of oral or intravenous folinic acid. The median survival for patients who develop carcinomatosis meningitis is 3 to 6 months, although responders may live in excess of 1 year.

MALIGNANT EFFUSIONS

Breast cancer is the most common cause of malignant pleural effusions in women. They are more commonly seen ipsilateral to the primary tumor, suggesting that the effusion sometimes arises via direct extension through the chest wall or through involvement of internal mammary lymph nodes. While 80 percent of malignant pleural effusions arise in the presence of other sites of metastatic involvement,[30] they are usually symptomatic and require specific treatment.

In a previously untreated patient with newly metastatic breast cancer, an attempt may be made to relieve the malignant pleural effusion with therapeutic thoracentesis and initiation of systemic chemotherapy or hormonal therapy. In this setting, a positive response to systemic therapy is likely and may be sufficiently rapid to prevent reaccumulation of fluid. In patients with previously treated metastatic disease, however, the likelihood of objective response to any systemic therapy is certainly < 50 percent; definitive treatment with chest tube drainage and sclerosis is recommended. Failure to adequately manage a malignant pleural effusion can result in a trapped lung, with permanent dyspnea, cough, and pain.

The purpose of chest tube placement and suction drainage is to empty the pleural space to permit approximation of the visceral and parietal pleura. When chest tube output is minimal, any of a variety of topical irritants is instilled and the patient repositioned every 15 minutes for 2 hours to distribute the irritant throughout the pleural space. The goal is to create adhesions between the irritated visceral and parietal pleura to prevent subsequent massive reaccumulation of fluid with atelectasis. There have been a variety of agents employed, including talc slurry, tetracycline, bleomycin, and other chemotherapeutic agents. In a randomized trial comparing the first three agents, an insufficient number of patients was accrued; in the absence of a direct comparison, talc appears to have the highest success rate.[31]

Pericardial effusions are not uncommon and may eventually occur in up to 25 percent of all women with metastatic breast cancer.[32] The presenting complaint is typically exertional dyspnea. Chest radiography and resting arterial oxygen saturation may both be normal, requiring this diagnosis to be specifically considered in the dyspneic patient.[33] As pericardial effusions occur not infrequently in conjunction with malignant pleural effusions but go unrecognized on chest radiography, pericardial effusions should also be considered whenever pleural effusions are diagnosed. Physical exam may show tachycardia, an absent precordial cardiac impulse, a pericardial friction rub, atrial fibrillation, and pulsus paradoxus. Electrocardiogram will show decreased voltages in the precordial leads. Definitive diagnosis of pericardial effusion requires echocardiography, which may also demonstrate cardiac tamponade with diastolic collapse of the right atrium and ventricle.[34]

Patients with symptomatic or hemodynamically significant pericardial effusions should undergo immediate drainage. Immediate catheter drainage can prevent cardiovascular collapse in patients with tamponade but does not provide definitive treatment. The creation of a subxiphoid pericardial window is a relatively simple surgical solution with a high success rate.[35] Open thoracotomy with pericardial stripping has a much higher morbidity and is required only for rare patients with constrictive pericarditis.

Malignant ascites can develop as a manifestation of peritoneal metastases, occurring more frequently in patients with infiltrating lobular carcinoma. Symptoms include bloating, distension, early satiety, and shortness of breath. Both ultrasound and CT scan can demonstrate ascites, with the latter also revealing peritoneal studding or omental thickening in some patients. While the most satisfactory control of malignant ascites is achieved with effective systemic therapy, this is often not possible where ascites occurs as a late complication of advanced disease. Therapeutic paracentesis may provide transient relief of symptoms. Repeated drainage of several liters of ascitic fluid may result in hypotension or hypoalbu-

minemia, however. Diuretics are seldom helpful in managing malignant ascites.

BONE METASTASES

Bone is the most frequent site of metastatic spread, with autopsy series revealing skeletal involvement in 85 percent of all breast cancer patients. The axial skeleton is most commonly affected, for example, the pelvis, spine, ribs, skull, and proximal long bones (Figure 17–1).[36] Constant, dull, progressive pain is the usual presentation, and any such complaint should be investigated radiographically, particularly if the pain is unrelieved by rest. Plain radiographs most often show lytic lesions, although 15 percent of breast carcinomas are associated with blastic lesions and both patterns may be evident.[37] Technetium bone scans are more sensitive but less specific than plain films, as bone

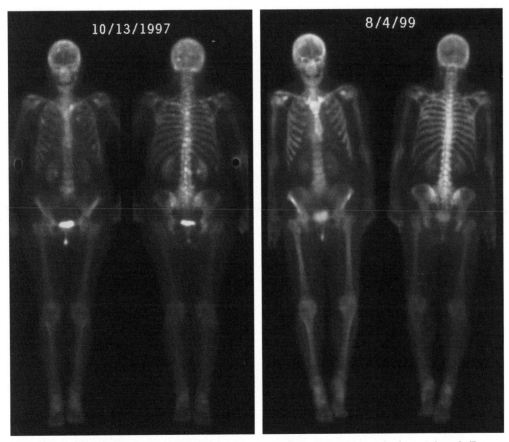

Figure 17–1. A bone scan with multiple focal areas of increase radionuclide uptake (e.g., spine, skull) responding over time to hormonal therapy.

loss of up to one-third may occur before becoming visible. The first discovery of a bone metastasis in a patient should prompt a bone scan to determine the extent of disease. Unfortunately, available serum markers of osteoblastic activity such as alkaline phosphatase or tumor markers such as CA15-3 antigen are insufficiently sensitive to rule out bone metastases in a patient with bony pain.[37]

External beam radiation therapy is the mainstay of palliating the pain of bone metastases and will provide at least some relief in 90 percent of patients.[38] Relief may be experienced early on as a result of decreasing periosteous inflammation, with maximal palliation within 3 weeks. The main side effect of radiation therapy to the axial skeleton is myelosuppression, which may be cumulative and prolonged when large fields or multiple sites are treated. As this may preclude effective dosing of chemotherapy, radiation should be reserved for sites of severe or dominant symptoms, to prevent fracture of long bones, or in patients unsuitable for, or unlikely to respond to, chemotherapy.

Surgical stabilization is required in patients with impending fractures of the femur or for occasional patients with extensive and painful humeral lesions. The proximal femur is at particular risk of pathologic fracture due to the high mechanical stresses of ambulation; an aggressive approach to prevention is appropriate due to the catastrophic effects of this complication. Prediction of an impending fracture is not entirely accurate, but the usual criteria for prophylactic stabilization are cortical destruction of > 50 percent or proximal lesions > 1 inch.[39] Lytic lesions are more prone to fracture than is blastic disease. Depending on location, a variety of orthopedic approaches may be required; the use of methylmethacrylate cement permits early reambulation.[40] Following fixation, adjuvant radiotherapy to the involved bone is usually indicated to prevent progressive destruction of bone, with resulting destabilization.

Recently, medical therapy has been able to more directly address the pathophysiology of bone metastases. Bisphosphonates are a class of drugs related to pyrophosphate that bind to hydroxyapatite crystals, stabilizing bone and inhibiting reabsorption. The bisphosphonate pamidronate, administered intravenously, has been shown to produce sclerosis or stabilization of lytic metastases in 50 percent of breast cancer patients.[41] This results in a decrease in the rate of pathologic fractures, in the need for radiotherapy, and in the use of analgesics,[42] suggesting an important palliative role for pamidronate. Similar trials using orally absorbed bisphosphonates such as alendronate have also been completed.

Strontium 89 is an emitter of β-radiation that is taken up by sites of active bone destruction, and can be administered intravenously. Improvement in bone pain is reported by 80 percent of patients,[43] and toxicity is largely limited to myelosuppression. Indications include widespread, painful bony metastases in patients who will not be candidates for chemotherapy and recurrent pain in sites already treated by external beam radiotherapy.

LOCAL RECURRENCE

Recurrence of cancer within a breast after lumpectomy and radiation therapy has different implications from a recurrence involving the skin or chest wall following mastectomy.[44] Treatment involves mastectomy and often a course of systemic "pseudoadjuvant" chemotherapy or change in hormonal adjuvant therapy. No randomized trials have addressed this issue, however.

Initial recurrence in the skin overlying a mastectomy site is associated with synchronous presentation of distant metastatic disease in one-third of patients. Discovery of local recurrence should therefore prompt restaging with a bone scan and CT scan of chest and liver.[45] If distant metastasis are not discovered, the skin recurrence, usually in the form of one or several dermal or subdermal nodules, should receive local treatment. Complete excision of isolated, small nodules should be attempted. Wide excision with partial or full-thickness chest wall resection are seldom indicated, however, due to morbidity and a 50 percent failure rate.[46] Rather, radiation therapy delivered to the entire chest wall at a dose of 45 to 50 cGy, with a boost to the site of recurrence, should be considered standard therapy. This will yield 5-year local control rates of 85 percent if the tumor is first excised or 63 percent if radiation is given without excision.[47]

Nearly all patients with isolated local recurrence will subsequently develop distant metastases. Only 30 percent remain free from distant metastases after 5 years, with the disease-free interval between mastectomy and skin recurrence the most important predictive factor. Only 20 percent of those suffering local recurrence within 2 years will be free of distant disease 3 years later, compared to 36 percent of those who first recurred > 2 years after mastectomy.[48] This suggests that most patients could potentially benefit from systemic therapy following local recurrence. The benefits of postrecurrence hormonal therapy with tamoxifen have been established in a randomized trial for patients with estrogen receptor-positive tumors.[49] Unfortunately, similar benefits have not been established for chemotherapy in receptor-negative patients.

SYSTEMIC THERAPY

When metastatic breast cancer presents clinically as an isolated, symptomatic site, specific palliative measures, discussed above, are indicated. Many patients, however, present with visceral or multi-site disease, or will be found to have additional metastases upon restaging. While widely metastatic breast cancer is incurable, lessening of the symptomatic burden and prolongation of survival are possible for most women through judicious use of systemic hormone therapy and chemotherapy. It is important to understand that the goal of systemic therapy is ultimately palliation, so that every decision must involve weighing the potential improvement in quality of life against the expected toxicities of treatment.

HORMONAL THERAPY

In this context, hormonal therapy is almost always preferred as initial therapy for women with estrogen receptor-positive metastatic breast cancer. Whenever possible, and particularly for women who relapse after adjuvant hormonal therapy, this decision should be based on receptor assays performed on a biopsy of the metastatic disease. While in the absence of intervening therapy the receptor status of metastatic disease is predicted by that of the primary tumor, estrogen receptor becomes negative in one-third of patients and progesterone receptor becomes negative in one-half of patients who receive tamoxifen in the interval before relapse.[50]

There will be a complete or partial response obtained by initial hormonal therapy in over three-quarters of women with estrogen receptor and progesterone receptor-positive metastatic disease and no prior therapy.[51] If the estrogen receptor assay is negative, the response rate drops to less than half, and to one-third if the progesterone receptor assay is negative. If neither receptor is detected, response is seen in < 10 percent of patients; in this circumstance, chemotherapy is often a preferable option. Hormonal therapy is also contraindicated in women with lymphangitic carcinomatosis or extensive metastases to the liver, due to the need for a rapid response. Finally, if biopsy of a metastatic site is not possible, the decision to employ hormone therapy can be based on those clinical criteria (eg, a long disease-free interval, disease limited to bone or soft tissue, and elderly patients) associated with the receptor-positive phenotype.

Estrogen Antagonists

The likelihood of response to initial hormonal therapy is similar for several classes of drugs, and so initial treatment can often be selected based on their side-effect profiles. In previously untreated patients, or for those several years removed from adjuvant hormonal therapy, competitive inhibitors of estrogen binding are usually the first choice.

The oldest and most widely prescribed estrogen antagonist is tamoxifen,[52] but toremifene has also been approved for this indication. Raloxifene is currently marketed for prevention of osteoporosis and may also have some efficacy against metastatic breast cancer, although further study is clearly required.[53] Tamoxifen appears to be effective for both pre- and post-menopausal women with advanced, receptor-positive disease.[54] Common side effects of tamoxifen include hot flashes (particularly in perimenopausal women), disruption of menstrual cycles, and vaginal dryness or discharge.[55] In addition, weight gain and mild fluid retention are frequent, with nocturnal leg cramps not uncommonly reported. Patients with bone metastasis may suffer a syndrome of "tumor flare," typically 7 to 10 days after initiation of tamoxifen. This is seen in 1 to 3 percent of patients and consists of increased pain at sites of metastases; it may lead to hypercalcemia. As this is predictive of subsequent response to tamoxifen, therapy should be continued, with supportive measures as needed. Approximately 1 percent of healthy patients on tamoxifen will develop deep-vein thrombosis, although women with metastatic breast cancer also have an increased incidence of thromboembolic disease.[56] Other, rare complications such as cataract formation or an increased incidence of endometrial cancer are seldom of concern to women with metastatic disease.

The average duration of response to initial hormone therapy is approximately 1 year. Women whose disease stabilizes on tamoxifen appear to do as well as those achieving objective remissions. While responses lasting for years are not uncommon (particularly if there has been a long disease-free interval), eventually most tumors will develop resistance to tamoxifen, leading to clinical progression. This may occur due to outgrowth of receptor-negative clones within a heterogenous population or to acquired, specific resistance to estrogen antagonists. Once a responding tumor progresses on tamoxifen, other agents in this class have little activity. Indeed, a fraction of such patients will briefly improve when tamoxifen is withdrawn, suggesting that changes in the receptor or the cellular estrogen-response machinery has led to the drug behaving as an estrogen agonist.[57]

Aromatase Inhibitors

About half of women who initially respond to tamoxifen will also respond to second-line hormonal therapy. Randomized trials have suggested somewhat greater efficacy, lesser side effects, and perhaps slight improvement in survival when specific aromatase inhibitors are compared to oral progestins in this setting.[58,59] The new generation of aromatase inhibitors—anastrozole, letrozole, and others not yet approved for use—have replaced the older drug aminoglutethimide due to much improved safety profiles. Anastrozole and letrazole work by binding competitively to the porphyrin nucleus of the aromatase enzyme, which is responsible for estrogen production from androstenedione. This extraovarian pathway is important only in postmenopausal women, therefore anastrozole and letrazole should be used only after menopause. The most common side effects seen with these drugs are headache and mild nausea. Prior to the development of these agents, aminoglutethimide had been employed as an aromatase inhibitor, but has now fallen into disuse because of its high frequency of unacceptable side effects, including rash, lethargy, and ataxia.

Progestins

Before the development of the newer aromatase inhibitors, second-line hormonal therapy for most women consisted of progestins, usually oral megestrol acetate or parenteral medroxyprogesterone acetate.[60,61] Up to half of women receiving these drugs will respond with improvement or stabilization of their disease. Unlike other hormonal agents, there is evidence of a dose-response effect with progestins, although their mechanism of action is unknown. These drugs also produce an increased sense of well-being, improved appetite, and suppress hot flashes. Unfortunately, the side effects of chronic weight gain, fluid retention, and dyspnea make them unacceptable to many.

Ovarian Ablation

For premenopausal women with receptor-positive disease, medical or surgical castration is also an effective approach to hormonal therapy. The endocrinologic effect of castration is achieved by two analogs of gonadotropin-releasing hormone, goserelin and leuprolide, which suppress follicle-stimulating hormone and luteinizing hormone, and thus estrogen production by the ovary.[62,63] Either agent will achieve the same benefit as oophorectomy, that is, a 45 percent likelihood of disease regression or stabilization, but require parenteral administration on a monthly or trimonthly basis. Side effects are limited to pain at the injection site and menopausal symptoms such as hot flashes, mood swings, and dry skin. Once disease progresses after either medical or surgical castration, the alternate approach has little chance of benefit. Obviously, castration by either technique can only be of benefit to premenopausal patients, where the ovary is the primary site of estrogen production.

There have been a number of studies that have attempted to combine hormonal agents for more effective control of metastatic disease.[64] In general, a small increase in response rate is seen with combinations, but time-to-progression is not improved over the use of the same agents employed sequentially and there is clearly no survival advantage. Additional toxicity is often reported when hormonal agents are used in combination; since the goal of all such therapy is palliative, this approach is not recommended.

CHEMOTHERAPY

Systemic chemotherapy is often indicated to control disseminated breast cancer and relieve symptoms. While prolonged remissions may be achieved, there is no evidence that metastatic breast cancer can be cured by chemotherapy. Thus, the ultimate goals are again palliative, and the toxicity of chemotherapy must be carefully weighed against a realistic appraisal of benefits. With this caveat, chemotherapy is commonly indicated as frontline therapy for metastases to liver or lung, those arising from estrogen receptor-negative tumors, and those that fail to respond to initial or subsequent hormonal treatments.

There are a wide variety of chemotherapeutic agents that show some activity against metastatic breast cancer. Response rates are affected by site of disease, with soft tissue metastases typically most responsive, and liver metastases least responsive, to many agents. Prior treatment history has a major effect on the likelihood of response, due to the phenomenum of pleiotropic drug resistance, which occurs when cancer cells undergoing treatment become resistant not only to that particular agent but also to unrelated classes of cytotoxic drugs. Attempts to overcome drug resistance have included the use of chemotherapeutic agents in combination and at increased dose intensity. These approaches have resulted in higher response rates, but the average duration of response to initial chemotherapy remains < 1 year. High dose chemotherapy with bone marrow or stem cell rescue has not demonstrated any survival advantage when compared to conventional regimens in strictly randomized prospective trials and should remain investigational. The use of alternative agents after progression of disease is marked by lower response rates and shorter durations of response, so much so that patients rarely benefit from more than three sequential chemotherapy regimens. The major classes of useful cytotoxic agents are reviewed below.

Anthracyclines

Doxorubicin has long been considered the benchmark drug for treatment of metastatic breast cancer, with a single-agent response rate of 40 to 50 percent.[65] Increases in the dose of doxorubicin, sometimes given with granulocyte colony-stimulating factor support, can yield response rates as high as 80 percent, but at the price of increasing toxicity.[66] As this higher response rate does not result in any noticeable improvement in survival, dose-intense schedules cannot be recommended at present. Common toxicities include moderate nausea, mucositis, neutropenia, and a cumulative dose-related risk of congestive cardiomyopathy. Despite these toxicities, doxorubicin, often given in combination, has become the standard frontline chemotherapy for metastatic breast cancer. Several randomized trials have established that doxorubicin-containing combinations are superior to similar regimens lacking an anthracycline.

Mitoxantrone is a potentially less toxic derivative of doxorubicin that is also widely used for palliative treatment of metastatic disease. It is clearly less emetogenic and appears to have less cardiotoxicity than the parent compound, although cardiotoxicity is cumulative and additive to that induced by prior doxorubicin exposure.[67] In direct comparison to doxorubicin, either alone or in combination, response rates were lower for mitoxantrone, although overall survival was not compromised.[68] The most effective use of mitoxantrone may be in combination with 5-fluorouracil and folinic acid, which is associated with a response rate of up to 65 percent and quite manageable toxicity.[69] Another approach to lessening the toxicity of doxorubicin is to encapsulate the drug in lipid liposomes.[70] This strategy permits more selective tissue uptake, resulting in less nausea, neutropenia, and cardiotoxicity, although various cutaneous reactions are seen with the currently available formulation. Studies using liposomal doxorubicin are still in progress and the drug is not currently approved for treatment of breast cancer.

Taxanes

The complex, semisynthetic paclitaxel and the synthetic docetaxol have recently established themselves to be of equal or greater single-agent efficacy than doxorubicin and maintain significant activity in patients previously treated with doxorubicin.[71,72] Paclitaxel administered by 24-hour infusion has achieved response rates as high as 60 percent, but the optimum dose and schedule for this drug have not been established. Toxicities include neutropenia, a delayed arthralgias/myalgia syndrome occurring 48 hours after administration, and a peripheral neuropathy with higher cumulative doses. Bradycardia is observed but is seldom clinically significant. Frequent type I hypersensitivity reactions require premedication with steroids and antihistamines. These toxicities are lessened by administration on a weekly rather than triweekly schedule.

Docetaxol has recently been introduced for treatment of metastatic breast cancer, where it has demonstrated a higher response rate and more durable remissions than doxorubicin.[72] Toxicity consists of neutropenia and a capillary leak syndrome, resulting in peripheral edema and pleural or pericardial effusions, which are preventable with a 3-day course of corticosteroids.[73] These taxanes have been combined by a number of investigators, but thus far both activity and toxicity appears to be additive rather than synergistic. An exception is the combination of doxorubicin and paclitaxel, which appears to produce a very high response rate but results in cardiotoxicity at lower than expected cumulative doxorubicin doses.[74]

Alkylating Agents

Cyclophosphamide has reasonable single-agent activity but is usually used in combination with other agents such as doxorubicin or methotrexate and fluorouracil. Toxicity is limited at conventional doses to neutropenia, moderate nausea, mucositis, and occasional hemorrhagic cystitis. Ifosfamide, an analog of cyclophosphamide, appears to have similar efficacy, and is not entirely cross-resistant to cyclophosphamide. In addition to neutropenia, toxicity includes frequent hemorrhagic cystitis (requiring the use of a urothelial protective agent), interstitial nephritis, and temporary encephalopathy. These toxicities have limited the use of ifosfamide.

Antimetabolites

Five-fluorouracil, a pyrimidine analog that binds to thymidylate synthase, is widely employed in the treatment of breast cancer. Intermittent bolus administration, as is found in many classic cytotoxic combinations, is probably the least effective schedule for this cell-cycle active agent, given its short half-life. Continuous infusion of 5-fluorouracil will yield responses in even heavily pretreated patients, with manageable toxicity consisting largely of palmar/planter dermatitis.[75] Alternatively, the intracellular binding of fluorouracil to thymidylate synthase can be stabilized by coadministration of folinic acid. Again, higher response rates are seen, although neutropenia, mucositis, and diarrhea become significant.[76] Methotrexate, a folic acid analog, has a low single-agent response rate in metastatic breast cancer but is occasionally useful, primarily to provide biochemical synergy with fluorouracil.

Vinca Alkaloids

Whereas vincristine has little activity against breast cancer, vinblastine yields response rates as high as 37 percent when given by 120-hour infusion.[77] Toxicity is limited to myelosuppression but the schedule is inconvenient. Vinblastine was given as a bolus in many earlier combinations but probably added little. Vinorelbine, a newer vinea derivative, yields a single-agent response rate of 35 to 40 percent when given as a weekly bolus.[78] Toxicity consists of neutropenia, peripheral neuropathy, myalgias, and short-lived pain at sites of metastatic disease.

Other Agents

Cisplatin is an active single agent in previously untreated metastatic breast cancer, but dosage is inconvenient due to the need for prolonged hydration to prevent nephrotoxicity; also, the drug has a poor response rate in previously treated patients. Gemcitabine may be non-crossresistant with anthracyclines and taxanes, with toxicity limited to fatigue and mild myelosuppression, suggesting that this drug may find a role in previously treated patients.[79] Further study is required, however, and neither this drug nor cisplatin has been approved for treatment of breast cancer. Finally, capecitabine, an oral drug, has recently been approved for use in previously treated patients with metastatic breast cancer. Once absorbed, this drug is converted to fluorouracil, explaining its similar toxicity spectrum.

The higher response rates seen with combination chemotherapies often justify their initial use over single agents. After progression on frontline treatment, however, the toxicity of multiagent therapy may make adequate dosing impossible and obviate any advantage seen with this approach. Thus, the sequential use of single agents, especially after initial treatment, may provide a higher quality of life, equal palliative benefit, and no compromise of overall survival.

In patients who achieve a complete response or whose disease stabilizes after a partial response, the question of duration of chemotherapy arises. Several small studies have suggested that the time-to-treatment failure is extended by several months and that quality of life is improved by continuing with maintenance therapy once a response is achieved, rather than withholding further therapy until relapse.[80]

IMMUNOTHERAPY

Earlier studies in which the nonspecific immunostimulants bacille Calmette-Guerin or levamisole were added to chemotherapy showed no advantage to this procedure. In the last 2 years, however, studies using specific immunotherapy with the humanized murine monoclonal antibody trastuzumab have yielded promising results. This antibody recognizes and binds to a transmembrane tyrosine kinase coded for by the *c-erb*B2 or *HER2* gene, which is amplified and/or overexpressed in up to one-third of all breast cancer specimens (Figure 17–2). When given to a heavily pretreated group of patients whose tumors overexpressed this gene product, trastuzumab produced a 16 percent objective response rate.[81] Toxicity was minimal, consisting of fever and chills after the first weekly infusion, and mild pain, asthenia, nausea, diarrhea, and dyspnea. In addition, 5 percent of patients had evidence of cardiac dysfunction.

Trastuzumab was also studied in a placebo-controlled study involving women simultaneously receiving chemotherapy with either doxorubicin-cyclophosphamide or paclitaxel.[82] When added to doxorubicin-cyclophosphamide, the response rate increased from 43 to 52 percent, with a 3.6-month prolongation of responses. When trastuzumab was added to paclitaxel in patients who had prior exposure to doxorubicin, response rate increased from 16 to 42 percent, and duration of response from 4.4 to 11 months. Unfortunately, cardiotoxicity was seen in 27 percent of women receiving the doxorubicin combi-

nation plus antibody treatment and in 12 percent receiving paclitaxel plus antibody. The mechanism of this synergy, manifest both in increased response rates and cardiotoxicity, is not yet understood, and a wide variety of trials have begun to define the role of trastuzumab in the treatment of metastatic breast cancer.

CONCLUSION

Metastatic breast cancer is responsible for over 40,000 deaths of American women each year, with most of these women having lived with metastatic disease for 2 or more years prior to their death. During this time, many symptoms can be palliated or avoided by addressing both local problematic sites with surgery or radiation therapy and the overall course of the disease with hormonal therapy or chemotherapy. At all times, the impact of a therapeutic intervention on quality of life must be weighed, as many options, particularly second- or third-line therapies, offer little chance of prolonging life.

Improvements in breast cancer prevention, early detection, and postsurgical adjuvant therapy are likely to reduce the overall mortality of breast cancer by reducing the number of women who suffer metastatic recurrence. Those women who nonetheless are forced to contend with metastases will have an increasing number of options in coming years. Newer chemotherapeutic drugs, hormonal agents, and immunologic approaches offer the hope of more selective, less toxic, and ultimately more effective treatments for metastatic breast cancer.

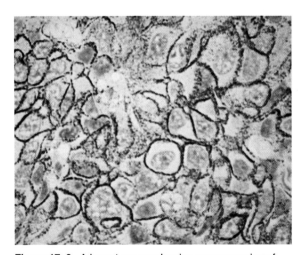

Figure 17–2. A breast cancer showing overexpression of membrane associated *HER-2* protein. Metastatic breast cancer with this phenotype demonstrates a 16% response rate to trastuzumab when employed as a single agent.

REFERENCES

1. Early Breast Cancer Trialists' Collaborative Group. Tamoxifen for early breast cancer: an overview of the randomised trials. Lancet 1998;351:1451–67.
2. Landis S, Murray T, Bolden S, et al. Cancer statistics, 1999. CA Cancer J Clin 1999;49:8–31.
3. Valagussa P, Bonadonna G, Veronesi U. Patterns of relapse and survival following radical mastectomy. Cancer 1978;41:1170.
4. Borst MJ, Ingold JA. Metastatic patterns of inva-

sive lobular versus invasive ductal carcinoma of the breast. Surgery 1993;114:637.

5. Harris M, Howell A, Chrissohou M, et al. A comparison of the metastatic pattern of infiltrating lobular carcinoma and infiltrating duct carcinoma of the breast. Br J Cancer 1984;50:23.

6. Lamovec J. Metastatic pattern of infiltrating lobular carcinoma of the breast: an autopsy study. J Surg Oncol 1991;48:28.

7. Van De Vijver M, Mooi W, Wisman P, et al. Immunohistochemical detection of the neu protein in tissue sections of human breast tumors with amplified neu DNA. Oncogene 1988;2:175-8.

8. Rouesse J, Friedman S, Guash-Jordan I, et al. Survival effect of systemic therapy on patients developing metastatic breast carcinoma. Breast Cancer Res Treat 1990;15:13.

9. Perez JE, Machiavelli M, Leone BA, et al. Bone-only versus visceral-only metastatic pattern in breast cancer: analysis of 150 patients. Am J Clin Oncol 1990;13:294.

10. Blumenschein GR, Pinnamaneni K, Buzdar AU. Combined regional and systemic therapy in breast cancer patients with an isolated metastasis with or without prior chemotherapy. In: Jones SE, Salmon SE, editors. Adjuvant therapy of cancer. IV. Orlando: Grune and Stratton; 1984. p. 311.

11. Vogel C, Azevedo S, Hilsenbeck S, et al. Survival after first recurrence of breast cancer. Cancer 1992;70:129-35.

12. Clark G, Sledge G, Osborne C, et al. Survival from first recurrence: relative importance of prognostic factors in 1,015 breast cancer patients. J Clin Oncol 1987;5:55-61.

13. Blanco G, Holli K, Heikkinen O, et al. Prognostic factors in recurrent breast cancer: relationships to site of recurrence, disease-free interval, female sex steroid receptors, ploidy and histological malignancy grading. Br J Cancer 1990;62:142-6.

14. Qazi R, Chuang JL, Drobyski W. Estrogen receptors and the pattern of relapse in breast cancer. Arch Intern Med 1984;144:2365-7.

15. DiStefano A, Yap HY, Hortobagyi GN, et al. The natural history of breast cancer patients with brain metastases. Cancer 1979;44:1913.

16. Posner JB. Neurologic complications of systemic cancer. Med Clin North Am 1979;63:783.

17. Davis PC, Hudgins PA, Peterman SB, et al. Diagnosis of cerebral metastases: double-dose delayed CT vs contrast-enhanced MR imaging. AJNR Am J Neuroradiol 1991;12:293.

18. Galicich JH, French LA, Melby J. Use of dexamethasone in treatment of cerebral edema associated with brain tumors. Lancet 1961;1:46.

19. Cohen N, Strauss G, Lew R, et al. Should prophylactic anticonvulsants be administered to patients with newly diagnosed cerebral metastases? a retrospective analysis. J Clin Oncol 1988;6:1621.

20. Patchell R, Tibbs P, Walsh J, et al. A randomized trial of surgery in the treatment of single metastases to the brain. N Engl J Med 1990;322:494-500.

21. Borgelt B, Gelber R, Kramer S, et al. The palliation of brain metastases: final results of the first of two studies by the Radiation Therapy Oncology Group. Int J Radiat Oncol Biol Phys 1980;6:1.

22. Flickinger JC, Kondziolka D, Lansford LD, et al. A multi-institutional experience with stereotactic radiosurgery for solitary brain metastases. Int J Radiat Oncol Biol Phys 1994;28:979.

23. Rosner D, Taukuma N, Lane W. Chemotherapy induces regression of brain metastases in breast carcinoma. Cancer 1986;58:832.

24. Colomer R, Cosos D, Del Campo JM, et al. Brain metastases from breast cancer may respond to endocrine therapy. Breast Cancer Res Treat 1988;12:83.

25. Tsukada Y, Fouad A, Pickren JW, et al. Central nervous system metastasis from breast carcinoma: autopsy study. Cancer 1983;52:2349.

26. Ongerboer de Visser BW, Somers R, Nooyen WH, et al. Intraventricular methotrexate therapy of leptomeningeal metastasis from breast carcinoma. Neurology 1983;33:1565.

27. Wasserstrom WR, Glass JP, Posner JB. Diagnosis and treatment of leptomeningeal metastases from solid tumors: experience with 90 patients. Cancer 1982;49:759.

28. Sze G, Soletsky S, Bronen R, et al. MR imaging of the cranial meninges with emphasis on contrast enhancement and meningeal carcinomatosis. AJNR Am J Neuroradiol 1989;10:965.

29. Yap HY, Yap BS, Rasmussen S, et al. Treatment for meningeal carcinomatosis in breast cancer. Cancer 1982;49:219.

30. Raju RN, Kardinal CG. Pleural effusion in breast carcinoma: analysis of 122 cases. Cancer 1981;48:2524.

31. Hausheer FH, Yarbro JW. Diagnosis and treatment of malignant pleural effusion. Semin Oncol 1985;12:54.

32. Hagemeister FB, Buzdar AU, Luna MA, et al. Causes of death in breast cancer. Cancer 1980;46:162.

33. Cham WC, Freiman AH, Carstens PHB, et al. Radiation therapy of cardiac and pericardial metastases. Ther Radiol 1975;114:701.

34. Gillam LD, Guyer DE, Gibson TC, et al. Hydrodynamic compression of the right atrium: a new echocardiographic sign of cardiac tamponade. Circulation 1983;68:294.

35. Vaitkus PT, Herrmann HC, LeWinter MM. Treatment of malignant pericardial effusion. JAMA 1994;272:59.

36. Tubiana-Hulin M. Incidence, prevalence and distribution of bone metastases. Bone 1991;12 Suppl 1:S9

37. O'Brien DP, Horgan PG, Gough DB, et al. CA 15-3: a reliable indicator of metastatic bone disease in breast cancer patients. Ann R Coll Surg 1992;74:9.

38. Poulsen HS, Nielsen OS, Klee M, et al. Palliative irradiation of bone metastases. Cancer Treat Rev 1989;16:41.

39. Harrington KD. Orthopaedic management of metastatic bone disease. St Louis: CV Mosby; 1988. p. 7.

40. Yazawa Y, Frassica FJ, Chao EYS, et al. Metastatic bone disease: a study of the surgical treatment of 166 pathologic humeral and femoral fractures. Clin Orthop 1990;251:213.

41. Morton AR, Cantrill JA, Pillai GV, et al. Sclerosis of lytic bone metastases after disodium aminohydroxypropylidene bisphosphonate (APD) in patients with breast carcinoma. BMJ 1988; 297:772.

42. van Holten-Verzantvoort ATM, Kroon HM, Bijvoet OLM, et al. Palliative pamidronate treatment in patients with bone metastases from breast cancer. J Clin Oncol 1993;11:491.

43. Robinson RG, Blake GM, Preston DF, et al. Strontrium-89: treatment results and kinetics in patients with painful metastatic prostate and breast cancer in bone. Radiographic 1989;9:271.

44. Recht A, Schnitt SJ, Connolly JL, et al. Prognosis following local or regional recurrence after conservative surgery and radiotherapy for early stage breast carcinoma. Int J Radiat Oncol Biol Phys 1989;16:3.

45. Andry G, Suciu S, Vico P, et al. Locoregional recurrences after 649 modified radical mastectomies: incidence and significance. Eur J Surg Oncol 1989;15:476.

46. Dahlstrom KK, Andersson AP, Andersen M, et al. Wide local excision of recurrent breast cancer in the thoracic wall. Cancer 1993;72:774.

47. Kenda R, Lozza L, Zucali R. Results of irradiation in the treatment of chest wall recurrent breast cancer [abstract]. Radiother Oncol 1992;24 Suppl:S41.

48. Aberizk WJ, Silver B, Henderson IC, et al. The use of radiotherapy for treatment of isolated locoregional recurrence of breast carcinoma after mastectomy. Cancer 1986;58:1214.

49. Borner M, Bacchi M, Goldhirsch, et al. First isolated locoregional recurrence following mastectomy for breast cancer: results of a phase III multicenter trial comparing systemic treatment with observation after excision and radiation. J Clin Oncol 1994;12:2071.

50. Hull D, Clark G, Osborne K, et al. Multiple estrogen receptor assays in human breast cancer. Cancer Res 1983;43:413–6.

51. Wittliff JL. Steroid-hormone receptors in breast cancer. Cancer 1984;53:630.

52. Jaiyesimi IA, Buzdar AU, Decker DA, Hortobagyi GN. Use of tamoxifen for breast cancer: twenty eight years later. J Clin Oncol 1995;13:513–29.

53. Gradishar WJ, Jordan VC. Clinical potential of new antiestrogens. J Clin Oncol 1997;15:840–52.

54. Sunderland MC, Osborne CK. Tamoxifen in premenopausal patients with metastatic breast cancer: a review. J Clin Oncol 1986;9:1283–97.

55. Fisher B, Costantino J, Wickerham D, et al. Tamoxifen for prevention of breast cancer: report of the national surgical adjuvant breast and bowel project p-1 study. J Natl Cancer Inst 1998;90:1371–88.

56. McDonald CC, Alexander FE, Whyte BW, et al. Cardiac and vascular morbidity in women receiving adjuvant tamoxifen for breast cancer in a randomized trial. The Scottish Cancer Trials Breast Group. BMJ 1995;311:977–80.

57. Howell A, Dodwell DJ, Anderson H, Redford J. Response after withdrawal of tamoxifen and progestins in advanced breast cancer. Ann Oncol 1992;3:611–7.

58. Dombernowsky P, Smith I, Falkson G, et al. Letrozole, a new oral aromatase inhibitor for advanced breast cancer: double-blind randomized trial showing a dose effect and improved efficacy and tolerability compared with megestrol acetate. J Clin Oncol 1998;16:453–61.

59. Buzdar A, Jonat W, Howell A, et al. Anastrozole versus megestrol acetate in the treatment of postmenopausal women with advanced breast carcinoma. Cancer 1998;83:1142–52.

60. Muss H, Case D, Cappizzi RL, et al. High versus standard dose megesterol acetate in women with advanced breast cancer: a phase III trial of the Piedmont Oncology Association. J Clin Oncol 1990;8:1797–1805.

61. Cavalli F, Goldhirsch A, Jungi F, et al. Randomized trial of low versus high dose medroxyprogesterone acetate in the induction treatment of postmenopausal patients with advanced breast cancer. J Clin Oncol 1984;2:414–9.

62. Taylor CW, Green S, Dalton WS, et al. Multicenter randomized clinical trial of goserelin versus surgical ovariectomy in premenopausal patients with receptor-positive metastatic breast cancer: an intergroup study. J Clin Oncol 1998;16:994–9.

63. Harvey HA, Lipton A, Max DT, et al. Medical castration produced by the GnRH analogue leuprolide to treat metastatic breast cancer. J Clin Oncol 1985;3:1068–72.

64. Ingle JN, Green SJ, Ahmann DL, et al. Randomized trial of tamoxifen alone or combined with aminoglutethimide and hydrocortisone in women with metastatic breast cancer. J Clin Oncol 1986;4:958–64.

65. Taylor SG, Gelber RD. Experience of the Eastern Cooperative Oncology Group with doxorubicin as a single agent in patients with previously untreated breast cancer. Cancer Treat Rep 1982;66:1594.

66. Bronchud MH, Howell A, Crowther D, et al. The use of granulocyte colony-stimulating factor to increase the intensity of treatment with doxorubicin in patients with advanced breast and ovarian cancer. Br J Cancer 1989;60:121.

67. Myers CE, Chabner BA. Anthracyclines. In: Chabner B, Collins JM, editors. Cancer chemotherapy: principles and practice. Philadelphia: JB Lippincott; 1990. p. 356.

68. Cowan JD, Neidhart J, McClure S, et al. Randomized trial of doxorubicin, bisantrene, and mitoxantrone in advanced breast cancer: a Southwest Oncology Group study. J Natl Cancer Inst 1991;83:1077.

69. Hainsworth JD, Andrews MG, Johnson DH, et al. Mitoxantrone, fluorouracil, and high-dose leucovorin: an effective, well-tolerated regimen for metastatic breast cancer. J Clin Oncol 1991; 9:1731.

70. Lyass O, Uziely B, Heching NI, et al. Doxil in metastatic breast cancer (MBC) after prior chemotherapy: therapeutic results in two consecutive studies. Proc Am Soc Clin Oncol 1998.

71. Reichman BS, Seidman AD, Crown JPA, et al. Paclitaxel and recombinant human granulocyte colony-stimulating factor as initial chemotherapy for metastatic breast cancer. J Clin Oncol 1993;11:1943–51.

72. Chan S, Friedrichs K, Noel D, et al. A randomized phase III study of taxotere (T) versus doxorubicin (D) in patients (pts) with metastatic breast cancer (MBC) who have failed an alkylating containing regimen: preliminary results. ASCO 1997;540.

73. Riva A, Fumoleau P, Roche H, et al. Efficacy and safety of different corticosteroid (C) premedications (P) in breast cancer (BC) patients (PTS) treated with taxotere (T). Proc Am Soc Clin Oncol 1997;16:188a.

74. Gianni L, Munzone E, Capri G, et al. Paclitaxel by 3-hour infusion in combination with bolus doxorubicin in women with untreated metastatic breast cancer: high antitumor efficacy and cardiac effects in a dose-finding and sequence-finding study. J Clin Oncol 1995;13:2688–99.

75. Huan S, Pazdur R, Singhakowinta A, et al. Low-dose continuous infusion 5-fluorouracil. Cancer 1989;63:419–22.

76. Swain SM, Lippman ME, Egan EF, et al. Fluorouracil and high-dose leucovorin in previously treated patients with metastatic breast cancer. J Clin Oncol 1989;7:890–9.

77. Fraschini G, Yap HY, Hortobagyi N, et al. Five-day continuous-infusion vinblastine in the treatment of breast cancer. Cancer 1985;56:225–9.

78. Romero A, Rabinovich MG, Vallejo CT, et al. Vinorelbine as first-line chemotherapy for metastatic breast carcinoma. J Clin Oncol 1994;12(2):336–41.

79. Carmichael J, Possinger K, Phillip P, et al. Advanced breast cancer: a phase II trial with gemcitabine. J Clin Oncol 1995;13:2731–6.

80. Muss HB, Case LD, Richards F. Interrupted versus continuous chemotherapy in patients with metastatic breast cancer. N Engl J Med 1991; 325:1342.

81. Cobleigh MA, Vogel CL, Tripathy D, et al. Efficacy and safety of herceptin (humanized anti-HER2 antibody) as a single agent in 222 women with HER2 overexpression who relapsed following chemotherapy for metastatic breast cancer. Proc Am Soc Clin Oncol 1998;17:97a.

82. Slamon D, Leyland-Jones B, Shak S, et al. Addition of herceptin (humanized anti-HER2 antibody) to first line chemotherapy for HER2 overexpressing metastatic breast cancer (HER2+/ MBC) markedly increases anticancer activity: a randomized, multinational controlled phase III trial. Proc Am Soc Clin Oncol 1998b;17:98a.

Index